The Little Black Book of International Medicine

Series Editor: Daniel K. Onion

William A. Alto, MD, MPH, FABFM
Professor of Community and Family Medicine
Dartmouth Medical School and
Maine Dartmouth Family Medicine Residency Program
Fairfield, ME

JONES AND BARTLETT PUBLISHERS

Sudbury, Massachusetts

BOSTON   TORONTO   LONDON   SINGAPORE

World Headquarters

Jones and Bartlett Publishers
40 Tall Pine Drive
Sudbury, MA 01776
978-443-5000
info@jbpub.com
www.jbpub.com

Jones and Bartlett Publishers
Canada
6339 Ormindale Way
Mississauga, Ontario L5V 1J2
Canada

Jones and Bartlett Publishers
International
Barb House, Barb Mews
London W6 7PA
United Kingdom

Jones and Bartlett's books and products are available through most bookstores and online booksellers. To contact Jones and Bartlett Publishers directly, call 800-832-0034, fax 978-443-8000, or visit our website, www.jbpub.com.

The authors, editor, and publisher have made every effort to provide accurate information. However, they are not responsible for errors, omissions, or for any outcomes related to the use of the contents of this book and take no responsibility for the use of the products and procedures described. Treatments and side effects described in this book may not be applicable to all people; likewise, some people may require a dose or experience a side effect that is not described herein. Drugs and medical devices are discussed that may have limited availability controlled by the Food and Drug Administration (FDA) for use only in a research study or clinical trial. Research, clinical practice, and government regulations often change the accepted standard in this field. When consideration is being given to use of any drug in the clinical setting, the healthcare provider or reader is responsible for determining FDA status of the drug, reading the package insert, and reviewing prescribing information for the most up-to-date recommendations on dose, precautions, and contraindications, and determining the appropriate usage for the product. This is especially important in the case of drugs that are new or seldom used.

Production Credits

Executive Publisher: Christopher Davis
Associate Editor: Kathy Richardson
Senior Editorial Assistant: Jessica Acox
Production Director: Amy Rose
Production Editor: Mike Boblitt/Daniel Stone
Marketing Manager: Ilana Goddess

V.P., Manufacturing and Inventory Control:
   Therese Connell
Composition: Auburn Associates
Cover Design: Kristin E. Parker
Printing and Binding: Malloy, Inc.
Cover Printing: Malloy, Inc.

Library of Congress Cataloging-in-Publication Data
Alto, William A.
   The little black book of international medicine / William A. Alto.
      p. ; cm. — (Little black book)
Includes bibliographical references and index.
   ISBN-13: 978-0-7637-5451-8
   ISBN-10: 0-7637-5451-X
   1. Medical assistance—Developing countries—Handbooks, manuals, etc.   2. Missions, Medical—Developing countries—Handbooks, manuals, etc.   I. Title. II. Series: Little black book series.
      [DNLM: 1. Medical Missions, Official.   2. Cultural Competency.   3. Developing Countries.   4.   Health Promotion. W 323 A4688t 2009]
   RA390.A2A48 2009
   610.73'7—dc22

                                                                                          2008026536

6048

Printed in the United States of America
12   11   10   09   08   10   9   8   7   6   5   4   3   2   1

Dedication

This book is dedicated to Sam Pickens, MD, who promoted my interest in international health and told me to go to Papua New Guinea; Mary Lois Jung, MD, who helped me select a location there and served as my mentor; and my wife, Sue, whose continuing support made possible all these adventures.

Contents

Preface

Do something for someone every day for which you do not get paid.

Albert Schweitzer

Every year thousands of medical, nursing, dental, and public health students and experienced practitioners travel abroad to spend a medical elective, or to begin a lifetime of helping others, working in and experiencing the culture and medical system of a foreign country. This book is to help these people prepare for the experience and to serve as a guide once they begin their daunting tasks. It is based on the authors' experiences in remote areas of developing countries. and is dedicated to the principle that health promotion and disease prevention are the best approaches to improving the well being of the people you will serve. The chapters offer practical management using World Health Organization protocols and formulary. Local practices will vary, and readers are strongly encouraged to follow standard management and treatment, soliciting expert advice as necessary.

Please contact the author with suggestions, corrections, or stories of your experiences. Best of luck in your adventures.

William A. Alto

Acknowledgments

Several physicians graciously allowed me to excerpt parts of their *Little Black Books* for incorporation into this text.

Stephen D. Sears, MD, MPH and **Robert P. Smith, MD, MPH**
Immunizations

Daniel K. Onion, MD, MPH, FACP
Professor of Community and Family Medicine, Dartmouth
Medical School and Director (Emeritus)
Maine-Dartmouth Family Practice Residency Program

Other physicians helped in reviewing chapters of this book.

Samuel Pickens, MD: Surgery, Orthopedics,
Obstetrics and Gynecology

Peter Selley, MBBS: Editing

Steven Witkin, MD: Opthalmology

Jim Schmidt, DDS: Dental

Contributor List

Acculturation (Chapter 3)
Letizia Alto, MD, MA (Anthropology),
Resident in Family Medicine
Swedish Medical Center, Cherry Hill
Seattle, Washington

Health Promotion in Developing Countries (Chapter 4)
Bryan Cooke, PhD, MPH, CHES
Professor (Retired)
Department of Community Health and Nutrition
College of Health and Human Services
University of Northern Colorado
Greeley, Colorado

HIV/AIDS (Chapter 14)
Donn Colby, MD, MPH
In-Country Medical Director
Vietnam-CDC-Harvard Medical School AIDS Partnership
Ho Chi Minh City, Vietnam
  and
Dimitri Prybylski, PhD (Epidemiology)
Senior Technical Officer, Evaluation, Surveillance and Research
Family Health International
Bangkok, Thailand

Pediatrics (Chapter 34)
Chi Jokonya, MD, DTM&H
Faculty
Maine Dartmouth Family Medicine Residency
Augusta, Maine

Medical Abbreviations

AB	abortion	BCG	Bacille Calmette-Guerin
Abx	antibiotics		
ACEI	angiotensin-converting enzyme inhibitor	BL	borderline lepromatous (leprosy)
ADH	antidiuretic hormone	BMI	body mass index
AFB	acid fast bacilli	BP	blood pressure
AGN	acute glomerulonephritis	BT	borderline tuberculoid (leprosy)
AIDS	acquired immune deficiency syndrome	BUN	blood urea nitrogen
		BV	bacterial vaginosis
ALT	SGPT; alanine transferase	BW	birth weight
AMS	acute mountain sickness	Ca	calcium
		CAD	coronary artery disease
AP	anterior-posterior X-ray	CBC	complete blood count
ARDS	adult respiratory distress syndrome	CDC	Centers for Disease Control and Prevention
ARF	acute rheumatic fever		
ARI	acute respiratory infection	CDD	control diarrheal disease
ART	antiretroviral therapy	CHF	congestive heart failure
ASA	aspirin	Cl	chloride
AST	SGOT; aspartate transferase	CMV	cytomegalovirus
		CMS	chronic mountain sickness
ATN	acute tubular necrosis		
AV	atrial-ventricular	CNS	central nervous system
AZT	azido-thymidine	CNVS	Catholic Network of Volunteer Services
BAL	British anti-Lewisite	CO	corneal opacity
BB	borderline (leprosy)		

CPD	cephalopelvic disproportion	DTP	diphtheria, tetanus, pertussis
CPK	creatine phosphokinase	dx	diagnosis or diagnostic
CPYLS	cost per year life saved		
Cr	creatinine	E	ethambutol
C-Section	cesarean section	EBV	Epstein-Barr virus
CSF	cerebralspinal fluid	EDC	estimated date of confinement (delivery)
CT	computerized tomography		
CTX	Co-trimoxazole	EIA	enzyme immunoassays
Cu	copper	EKG	electrocardiogram
CXR	chest X-ray	ELISA	enzyme-linked immunosorbent assay
D	day(s)	ENL	erythema nodosum leprosum
D&C	dilatation and curettage	EPI	WHO Expanded Program on Immunisation
DDT	dichloro-diphenyl-trichloroethane		
DEC	diethylcarbamazine	ERCP	endoscopic retrograde cholangiopancreatography
DEET	diethyltoluamide		
DHF	dengue hemorrhagic fever	ESR	erythrocyte sedimentation rate
DHFR	dihydrofolate reductase-thymidylate synthase		
		FCTC	Framework Convention on Tobacco Control
DIC	disseminated intravascular coagulation		
DIP	distal intraphalangeal joint	FDC	fixed drug combinations
DM	diabetes mellitus	FSME	formaldehyde inactivated purified whole virus
DOT	directly observed therapy		
DPG	diphosphoglycerate	FTA	fluorescent treponemal antigen
DSS	dengue shock syndrome		
DTaP	diphtheria, tetanus, acellular pertussis	G6PD	glucose 6 phosphate dehydrogenase

GAVI	Global Alliance for Vaccines and Immunizations	HEM	high energy milk
		HF	hemorrhagic fever
		HFRS	hemorrhagic fever with renal syndrome
GC	*Neisseria gonorrhea*		
GERD	gastroesophageal reflux disease	HgbA$_1$C	hemoglobin A$_1$C level
		HIV	human immunodeficiency virus
GI	gastrointestinal		
GLN	glomerulonephritis	HIV+	human immunodeficiency virus positive
gm	gram		
GU	genitourinary	HPF	high power field
		HPV	human papillomavirus
H	isoniazid	HR	heart rate
H&H	hemoglobin and hematocrit	hr	hour(s)
		HT	hypertension
H$_2$ blocker	histamine 2 receptor blocker	HTC	HIV testing and counseling
HAART	highly active antiretro viral therapy	HTIG	human tetanus immune globulin
HACE	high altitude cerebral edema	HTLV	human T-cell lymphotropic virus
HAPE	high altitude pulmonary edema	I&D	incision and drainage
HAPH	high altitude pulmonary hypertension	I&O	intake and output
		IARC	International Agency for Research on Cancer
Hb	hemoglobin		
HBM	Health Belief Model		
HCG	human chorionic gonadotropin	IBD	inflammatory bowel disease
HCO$_3$	bicarbonate	ICVP	International Certificate of Vaccination or Prophylaxis
HCS	hemoglobin color scale		
HCV	hepatitis C virus		
HCW	healthcare worker	id	intradermal
HDCV	human diploid cell rabies vaccine	IDU	injection drug use
		IFA	immunofluorescence assay
HELLP	hemolysis, elevated liver tests, low platelets	IM	intramuscular

IMCI	Integrated Management of Childhood Illnesses	LMP	last menstrual period
		LP	lumbar puncture
		LPF	low power field
IO	intraosseous	LR	lactated Ringer's solution
IP	intraocular pressure		
IRIS	immune reconstitution inflammatory syndrome	LV	left ventricle
		LVH	left ventricular hypertrophy
IRRB	Institutional Research Review Board		
		MAC	mycobacterium avium complex
ITN	insecticide-treated bed nets		
		MB	multibacillary
IU	international units	MCH	maternal-child health
IV	intravenous	MCP	metacarpophalangeal joint
IVP	intravenous pyelogram		
		MCV	mean cell volume
JBE	Japanese B encephalitis	MDR	multidrug resistant (TB)
K	potassium	MDT	multidrug therapy
KCl	potassium chloride	Mgm	milligram
Kg	kilogram	$MgSO_4$	magnesium sulfate
KOH	potassium hydroxide	MI	myocardial infarction
		min	minute(s)
LBBB	left bundle branch block	MMR	measles, mumps, rubella vaccine
LBW	low birth weight	MP	metacarpal phalangeal joint
LDH	lactate dehydrogenase		
LDL	low density lipoprotein	MRI	magnetic resonance imaging
LEEP	loop electrosurgical excision procedure		
		MSF	Medecins Sans Frontieres
LFT	liver function test		
LGV	lymphogranuloma venereum	MVA	motor vehicle accident
LIP	lymphocytic interstitial pneumonitis	Na	sodium
		NaCl	sodium chloride
LL	lepromatous (leprosy)	NG	nasogastric
LLQ	lower left quadrant		

NGO	nongovernment organization	PEM	protein energy malnutrition
NGT	nasogastric tube	PEP	postexposure prophylaxis
NNRTI	nonnucleoside reverse transcriptase inhibitor	PHC	primary health care
		PHO	provincial health office (officer)
NNT	number needed to treat		
nPEP	nonoccupational postexposure prophylaxis	PID	pelvic inflammatory disease
		PIP	proximal interphalangeal joint
NPO	nothing by mouth (fasting)	PMI	point of maximum impulse
NRTI	nucleoside/nucleotide reverse transcriptase inhibitor	PML	progressive multifocal leukoencephalopathy
NS	normal saline		
NSAIDS	nonsteroidal anti-inflammatory drugs	PMTCT	prevention of mother-to-child transmission
		PO	per os, orally
O&P	ova and parasites	PPD	purified protein derivative (Mantoux)
OCP	oral contraceptive pill		
OI	opportunistic infection	PPH	postpartum hemorrhage
OPV	oral polio virus vaccine		
ORS	oral rehydration solution	PPI	proton pump inhibitor
		PPV	positive predictive value
ORT	oral rehydration therapy	PrEP	pre-exposure prophylaxis
OTC	over-the-counter		
		PROM	premature rupture of membranes
PB	paucibacillary		
PCP	pneumocystis carinii (jiroveci) pneumonia	PT	protime
		PTB	pulmonary tuberculosis
PCR	polymerase chain reaction	PTSD	posttraumatic stress disorder
PCEC	purified chick embryo cell vaccine	PUD	peptic ulcer disease
		PV	vaginal insertion

PVC	premature ventricular contraction	SQ	subcutaneously
		SS	sickle cell
q	every	SSPE	subacute sclerosing panencephalitis
R	rifampicin	SSRI	selective serotonin reuptake inhibitor
RAM	rapid assessment and management	STI	sexually transmitted infection
RBBB	right bundle branch block	susp	suspension
RBC	red blood cell	sx	symptoms
RHD	rheumatic heart disease	T	thioacetazone
RLQ	right lower quadrant	TB	tuberculosis
r/o	rule out	TBA	traditional birth attendants
ROM	range of motion	TF	trachomatous inflammation-follicular
RPR	rapid protein reagin		
RSV	respiratory syncytial virus		
RUQ	right upper quadrant	TI	trachomatous inflammation-intense
RV	right ventricle		
RVA	rabies vaccine adsorbed		
		TL	tubal ligation
S	streptomycin	TLC	total lymphocyte count
SBE	subacute bacterial endocarditis		
SBET	standby emergency self-treatment	TMP	trimethoprin
		TS	trachomatous scarring
SBP	spontaneous bacterial peritonitis	TSH	thyroid stimulating hormone
sc	subcutaneous	tsp	teaspoon
SMX (also CTX)	sulfamethoxazole	TT	tetanus toxoid
		TT	tuberculoid (leprosy)
SOB	short of breath	UA	urinalysis
SP	severe pneumonia	UGI	upper gastrointestinal
SP	sulfadoxine-pyrimethamine	UNICEF	United Nations Children's Fund

URI	upper respiratory tract infection	WBC	white blood cell
		WHO	World Health Organization
USD	United States dollars		
UTI	urinary tract infection	WHR	waist-hip ratio
		wk	week(s)
VDRL	venereal disease research lab	WPW	Wolff-Parkinson-White syndrome (short PR interval)
VIP	ventilation improved performance	x	times
		XDR	extensively drug resistant (TB)
VL	viral load		
VSP	very severe pneumonia	yr	year(s)
Vtach	ventricular tachycardia	Z	Pyrazinamide

Journal Abbreviations

Acad Emerg Med	Academic Emergency Medicine
AIDS	Acquired Immune Deficiency Syndrome
Am Fam Physician	American Family Physician
Am J Clin Nutr	American Journal of Clinical Nutrition
Am J Hum Genet	American Journal of Human Genetics
Am J Public Health	American Journal of Public Health
Am J Respir Crit Care Med	American Journal of Respiratory and Critical Care Medicine
Am J Surg	American Journal of Surgery
Am J Trop Med Hyg	American Journal of Tropical Medicine and Hygiene
Ann Emerg Med	Annals of Emergency Medicine
Ann Intern Med	Annals of Internal Medicine
Ann Pharmacother	Annals of Pharmacotherapy
Ann Trop Med Parasitol	Annals of Tropical Medicine and Parasitology
Arch Dermatol	Archives of Dermatology
Arch Dis Child	Archives of Diseases in Childhood
BMC Nephrol	BMC Nephrology
Br J Psychol	British Journal of Psychology
Breast J	The Breast Journal
Bull WHO	Bulletin of World Health Organization
Clin Infect Dis/CID	Clinical Infectious Diseases
Clin Orthop	Clinical Orthopedics
Clin Orthop Relat Res	Clinical Orthopaedics and Related Research
Cochrane Database Syst Rev	Cochrane Database of Systematic Reviews
Com Eye Health	Community Eye Health Journal
Crit Care Med	Critical Care Medicine

Emerg Infect Dis/EID	Emerging Infectious Diseases
Emerg Med Clin North AM	Emergency Medicine Clinics of North America
Emerg Med J	Emergency Medicine Journal
Fam Pract Manag	Family Practice Management
J Gen Intern Med	Journal of Internal Medicine
Health Aff	Health Affairs
Health Policy Plan	Health Policy and Planning
Health Promo Intern	Health Promotions International
High Alt Med Biol	High Altitude Medicine & Biology
Inf(ect) Dis Clin North Am	Infectious Disease Clinics of North America
Inj Prev	Injury Prevention
Int J Cardiol	International Journal of Cardiology
Int J Epidemiol	International Journal of Epidemiology
J Am Acad Dermatol	Journal of the American Academy of Dermatology
JAMA	Journal of the American Medical Association
J Chemother	Journal of Chemotherapy
J Clin Path	Journal of Clinical Pathology
J Gen Intern Med	Journal of General Internal Medicine
J Infect Chemother	Journal of Infection and Chemotherapy
J Infect Developing Countries	Journal of Infection in Developing Countries
J Infect Dis	Journal of Infectious Diseases
J Pediatr Gastroenterol Nutr	Journal of Pediatric Gastroenterology and Nutrition
J Travel Med	Journal of Travel Medicine
J Urol	Journal of Urology
Lancet	The Lancet
Lancet Infect Dis	The Lancet Infectious Diseases

Matern Child Nutr	Maternal & Child Nutrition
Mayo Clin Proc	Mayo Clinic Proceedings
Med J Aust	The Medical Journal of Australia
Med Lett Drugs Ther	The Medical Letter on Drugs and Therapeutics
MMWR	Morbidity and Mortality Weekly Report
N Engl J Med	New England Journal of Medicine
Obstet Gynecol	Obstetrics and Gynecology
Pacific Health Dialog	Pacific Health Dialog
Parasitologia	Parasitología Latinoamericana
Pediatr Clin North Am	Pediatric Clinics of North America
Pediatr Infect Dis J	Pediatric Infectious Disease Journal
PNG Med J	Papua New Guinea Medical Journal
Postgrad Med J	Postgraduate Medical Journal
Primary Care	Journal of Primary Care
Redox Rep	Redox Report: Communications in Free Radical Research
S Afr Med Journal	South African Medical Journal
Soc Sci Med	Social Science & Medicine
Trans R Soc Trop Med Hyg	Transactions of the Royal Society of Tropical Medicine and Hygiene
Trop Med Int(ern) Health	Tropical Medicine & International Health
UNAIDS	The Joint United Nations Programme on HIV/AIDS
UNAIDS/WHO	United Nations AIDS/World Health Organization
UNODC/UNAIDS	United Nations Office on Drugs and Crime/United Nations AIDS
Vaccine	Vaccine
WHO/UNODC/UNAIDS	World Health Organization/United Nations Office on Drugs and Crime/United Nations AIDS

Notice

We have made every attempt to summarize accurately and concisely a multitude of references. However, the reader is reminded that times and medical knowledge change, transcription or understanding error is always possible, and crucial details are omitted whenever such a comprehensive distillation as this is attempted in limited space. And the primary purpose of this compilation is to cite literature on various sides of controversial issues; knowing where "truth" lies is usually difficult. We cannot, therefore, guarantee that every bit of information is absolutely accurate or complete. The reader should affirm that cited recommendations are reasonable still, by reading the original articles and checking other sources, including local consultants as well as recent literature, before applying them.

Drugs and medical devices are discussed that may have limited availability controlled by the Food and Drug Administration (FDA) for use only in research study or clinical trial. The drug information presented has been derived from reference sources, recently published data, and pharmaceutical tests. Research, clinical practice, and government regulations often change the accepted standard in this field. When consideration is being given to use of any drug in the clinical setting, the clinician or reader is responsible for determining FDA status of the drug, reading the package insert, and prescribing information for the most up-to-date recommendations on dose, precautions, and contraindications and determining the appropriate usage for the product. This is especially important in the case of drugs that are new or seldom used.

Chapter 1
Getting Started

1.1   Locating a Position

Before embarking on an overseas medical assignment, be it a 2-week stint at a medical mission or a life-long commitment, it is critical to take the time to consider your goals, expectations, adaptability, and the skill sets you can offer. Your success and value to the people you will serve depends on careful preparation and an appropriate match with a supportive organizational environment.

It has been said that there are 3 kinds of expatriates to be found in developing countries: missionaries, mercenaries, and misfits. Although an oversimplification of caregivers, these polarities offer a starting point in contemplating one's own motivations and in finding an organization or position that matches and supports your interests and skills.

There is a critical shortage of healthcare workers for several reasons (N Engl J Med 2007;356:2564; see Figure 1.1). The "brain drain" of skilled medical providers from developing countries is driven by more than economic incentives. Stop and consider these issues as you prepare:

- How much time can I commit? Contracts of one year and longer are worth a site visit before signing up.
- Will this be a single volunteer commitment, or is there the possibility of repeat visits?
- Can I use my language and cultural skills?

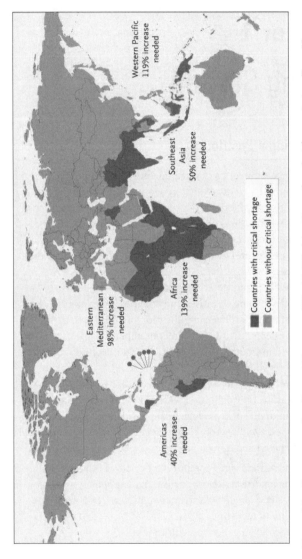

Figure 1.1 Countries with a Critical Shortage of Health Workers. Reproduced with permission. From Kumar. Providing the Providers—Remedying Africa's Shortage of Health Care Workers. *N Engl J Med* 2007;356:2565. Copyright 2007 Mass. Medical Society. All Rights reserved.

- Will special equipment, facilities, and staff be required and available to effectively use my medical skills?
- Am I willing and prepared to work outside my specialty? Can I deal with diagnostic uncertainty, work beyond my experience, and care for critically ill patients?
- What about my significant other (security, employment, interests, boredom)?
- What are the educational possibilities for children (local, home school/correspondence)?
- Is local healthcare adequate and acceptable for me and my family?
- Do I have income requirements and loan payments and require health and malpractice insurance?
- Who will be my colleagues, and will they be professionally and personally supportive?
- Am I interested in training others, especially local health workers?
- What are the licensing requirements, if any?
- Contact someone who has worked there and read about the area.

Religious organizations often sponsor overseas medical missions. The advantages of volunteering or contracting through them is an extensive support service and usually a smoothly functioning infrastructure of clinics and hospitals. Disadvantages are that you usually must be a member of that particular church, be willing to integrate into a tightly-knit mission community, and follow their tenets and customs. Some churches accept nonmembers, such as the Catholics for example. Some helpful sites you can search include the following:

- Catholic Network of Volunteer Services (CNVS) links
- Mission Finder: links to numerous missions[*]
- Nonreligious sites:

---

[*]Medical student electives

- Global Health Education Consortium (GHEC): a good place to start, especially for medical students but useful for all. (http://www.globalhealth-ec.org)
- Yale/J & J Physician Scholars in International Health Program: 1- to 2-month volunteer postings (Am J Trop Med Hyg 1999;61:1019)
- International Medical Volunteers Association: numerous links, some out-of-date
- Remote Area Medical (RAM)*
- International Center for Equal Healthcare Access (ICEHA)
- Doctors of the World
- Doctors for Global Health (http://www.dghonline.org)*
- INMED
- Health Volunteers Overseas
- AAFP International Health Care Opportunities in Family Medicine
- Project Hope
- Operation Smile
- International Rescue Committee (IRC)
- Medics Travel
- American Medical Students' Association (AMSA)
- Student BMJ: student elective reports*
- Children's Surgery International
- Canadian Society for International Health: paid and volunteer positions

Organizations that provide package experiences:
- Himalayan Health Exchange*
- Child Family Health International (CFHI)*
- Elwin International Tours*
- Project Abroad*
- Red R Recruitment Services
- Long-term clinical employment:

---

*Medical student electives

- CUSO: Canadians
- Voluntary Services Overseas (VSO): 2 years experience and commitment
- Volunteer Service Abroad (VSA): New Zealand residents only
- Australian Volunteers International (ACI): Australian citizens only except PACTAM (short-term consultants)
- International Committee of the Red Cross (ICRC)
- Various governments: contact the Ministry of Health
- Doctors without Borders: experienced providers, long term
- International SOS: minimum 5 years GP/emergency experience
- Development Executive Group: long-term positions for experienced providers (http://www.DevelopmentEx.com)

Numerous other possibilities and Web sites are out there; simply search International Medical Volunteer. Medical, nursing, and physicial assistant students can check with their dean's office, and residents with their program directors. Local medical societies are another source, or you can contact a hospital directly and offer your services. St. Jude's Hospital, Vieux Fort, St. Lucia, is one example of a Catholic hospital that welcomes volunteers.

Start your planning a year in advance and good luck!

- *Developing Global Health Curricula: A Guidebook for US Medical Students*. Available from AMSA.
- *Staying Alive: Safety and Security Guidelines for Humanitarian Volunteers in Conflict Areas*. ICRC 2006.
- Finding Work in Global Health and Global Health Directory. http://www.globalhealth.org.

1.2 Prepare for Overseas Work

Courses

International Health in the Developing World: Clinical and Community Care. University of Arizona. Dr. Ron Pust. Syllabus online. http://www.globalhealth.arizona.edu. Highly recommended.

Annual Tropical Medicine Course for Medical Students. Universidad Peruana Cayetano Hospital. April in Lima, Peru. Morning lectures and afternoon clinics, laboratories, and ward rounds. http://www.upch.edu.pe/tropicales. Highly recommended (in English).

The Gorgas Expert Course in Tropical Medicine. Lima, Peru. Two week bedside course in August. info@gorgas.org or 1-800-UAB-MIST.

The Gorgas Diploma Course in Tropical Medicine for Physicians. Lima, Peru. February-March. E-mail above.

The Gorgas Memorial Institute offers live cases online at http://www.gorgas.org.

GHEC: course modules, series of PowerPoint presentations on international health.

Topics in International Health on CD ROM. http://www.wellcome.ac.uk/node5810.html.

Tropical medicine courses approved by ASTMH:

Bernhard Nocht Institute and Humboldt University, both in Germany.

Liverpool School of Tropical Medicine and London School of Hygiene and Tropical Medicine, Johns Hopkins, Tulane, Marshall, and Uniformed Services Universities. http://www.astmh.org/certification/certificate.

Useful Books and Resources

World Health Organization (WHO) publishes a number of excellent books, which are listed throughout the chapters. Check out their online library with many books free to download.

WHO *Good Clinical Diagnostic Practice*: very useful in arriving at a diagnosis.

WHO *Model Formulary*: Pharmacology of common drugs and disease treatment.

International Workbook Guide for Students and Residents, University of Ottawa.

Oxford Handbook of Tropical Medicine.

Online Resources

Medline Plus: Herbal Medicine, http://www.nlm.nih.gov/medlineplus/herbalmedicine.html.

Surgery in Africa, http://www.ptolemy.ca/members.

MSF (Doctor's without Borders), http://www.doctorswithout borders.org/publications.

1.3 Research

If you are planning to undertake a research project overseas, the requirements are daunting. Apart from the usual preparation of a research proposal, you should obtain clearance from the Institutional Research Review Board (IRRB) at your local institution. Any project that involves human subjects, be it a drug trial or a health behavior survey, should have IRRB consideration and board approval if necessary. Speak with the chairperson of your IRRB for approval procedures.

Also consider how you can obtain approval locally for your research. Community participatory research (section 4.7) is to be encouraged, but it takes time and flexibility, often not available to a medical student or resident. You always require local approval prior to collecting data.

Most Ministries of Health have a research council that authorizes medical and sometimes anthropological research. Contact them if appropriate. Your IRRB should be able to advise you.

To avoid all these hassles, plan a simple observational study; do not collect any person's name or identifying data and check with your IRRB before you leave. Remember your research will be considered unethical and unable to be published without appropriate clearance and approval.

Chapter 2

Preparations

2.1 Overview

(Disease-a-Month 2006;52:259-338; two issues devoted to volunteering and travel medicine)

Preparing for overseas medical work, be it a short elective at a rural clinic to a long-term posting with one's family, requires some planning. Your sponsoring agency, non-government organization (NGO), or training institution may have suggestions, but ultimately it is your responsibility. A visit to a travel medicine specialist is highly recommended if your plans are complicated by extensive travel, involve time in remote locations, are for long periods, involve your family and children, or you have any illness that might complicate matters, such as previous splenectomy or immunosuppression.

Deaths in American travelers are largely due to the following:

- motor vehicle accidents, 27.7%
- other causes, 28.5%
- airplane crashes, 7.2%
- drowning, 16.4%
- homicide, 9.2%
- poisoning, 7.2%
- burns, 3.6%

Wear a seat belt and avoid riding motorcycles, traveling at night, and riding open-back trucks. Look to the left and right when crossing streets. If you can, pick your pilot carefully. Forget sex unless you bring your partner.

Common problems in travelers:

- fever 2%
- diarrhea 30%–80%, 1%–3% lasting > 2 weeks duration
- skin rashes and sunburn
- sexually transmitted diseases
- URIs

2.2 Visas

If you are going to be employed (and earn wages) to deliver healthcare, you will almost always require a work permit and an "employment permitted" visa stamped on your passport. Work permits and the appropriate visa should be obtained prior to your departure, and this can take months. Your sponsoring agency or government ministry will arrange all this for you. A common mistake is to arrive on a tourist visa, find a job, and then try to obtain the appropriate papers while in-country. You will usually have to leave and apply outside the country—a costly and time-consuming (and occasionally impossible) task.

If you are a volunteer, the situation may still be complex. Your sponsoring agency should be able to advise you. Often a tourist visa is used, but then you should apply as a tourist and not add details about the medical work you will be carrying out. Be certain to allow time for the volunteering and some sightseeing.

2.3 Medical License

Strictly speaking a medical license is necessary to practice medicine in any country. Applications are time consuming and frustrating and may take up to one year in some cases.

Alternately, the agency you are working with may have an agreement with the government, which will allow you to work under their umbrella. Be sure to find out early in the application process.

Bring along notarized copies of all your certificates, licenses, and anything else that seems pertinent. The author has been required to produce a letter from his residency director detailing training and successful completion of residency, and a letter from the local chief of police attesting to moral character.

2.4   Personal Medical Kit and Checklist

Unless you are certain that adequate supplies will be available, it is essential and perhaps lifesaving that you bring your own medical kit. Make certain that all medications are in a properly labeled bottle, are adequate for your time away, and are not out of date. Over-the-counter (OTC) narcotics, such as low dose codeine combinations, may be illegal in other countries and may result in arrest. Remember, if appropriate, the following:

- necessary immunizations, start early (chapters 5 and 43)
- traveler's diarrhea medications (chapter 5)
- something for monilia vaginitis
- topical antibiotics and antifungals
- contraceptives/condoms
- HIV/AIDs antiretroviral prophylaxis (chapter 14; MMWR 2005;54(RR09):1–17)
- malaria prophylaxis and presumptive therapy (chapter 10)
- mountain sickness prophylaxis (chapter 32)
- antibiotic for skin infection
- surgical masks for TB protection; safety glasses for surgery
- surgical gloves; examination gloves
- medical superglue
- water filter

- chemical treatment for water purification
- hand sanitation lotion
- sun block, hat, sunglasses (high altitude?)
- Are you taking any sun-sensitizing medications?
- medical tools, extra batteries, voltage converters, and electrical plugs
- motion sickness medications
- analgesics
- extra supply of any prescription medicines you take
- insect repellent; buy a bed net at your destination
- travel insurance
- medical evacuation insurance
- visas, licenses, etc.
- reference books or programs on palm pilot or computer
- journal

Chapter 3

Acculturation

Letizia Alto

3.1 Introducing Cultural and Medical System Bias

> Clinicians need to acknowledge that the Western medical
> model of ill health is not the only valid one available.
> They have to recognize that there are many other ways,
> world-wide, of interpreting human suffering, and many dif-
> ferent ways of relieving it.
>
> *Helman 2000:107*

The biomedical system of healthcare, which is practiced in
hospitals, clinics, and outpatient facilities across the globe, is
deeply ingrained within the European and North American
cultures. The tenets of the medical system of the United States,
for example, reflect and truly embrace the values of scientific
thought, individuality, professional healthcare provider training and licensing, separation from religion, and monetary fee for
services, seen within American culture as a whole. As children,
future physicians are trained to value scientific thought and, as
medical students, overtly counseled to rely on physiological over
subjective reasoning. They view the world, including the realm of
medicine, in terms of their own experience within their culture.
In fact, working outside of the boundaries of so-called western
thought (by this I mean Euro-American centered beliefs) within

the confines of the biomedical model of healthcare proves to be extremely difficult. The biomedical system of healthcare leaves little room for explanations based on the supernatural and not on physiology.

Understanding the interconnection between western culture and the biomedical model of medicine is particularly important for the healthcare provider traveling abroad, leaving both his/her native society and familiar medical facilities. The knowledge that the western model of medicine, biomedicine, is indoctrinated by western cultural beliefs allows the traveling provider to come to terms with his or her own inherent bias and to ultimately open his or her mind to the fact that patients and even other healthcare personnel have different and yet legitimate ways of viewing medicine, illness, and health. Learning a patient's explanation for what has happened in a particular situation can often prove more helpful toward fully understanding causation than a traditional history filled with subjective facts alone.

Finally, it is important to remember that there is variability not only among the beliefs and practices of patients in other locales but also of practitioners themselves. While the biomedical model of healthcare may go by the same name in other areas of the world, the type of medicine practiced and the manner of thinking about health and illness both within the confines of healthcare institutions and outside in the community may well be very different than what is found at home. A biomedical trained doctor in Mexico, for example, may blend traditional beliefs of what constitutes a hot vs cold illness and appropriate medications according to this theory along with biomedical explanations of physiology to create an understanding for himself and his patients that is congruent with their cultural framework for viewing the world. People's cultural background, whether physician or patient, influences the way that they view society, their life, their state of health and illness, and their ideas about what medicine and medical care does and should do.

3.2   Culturally Competent Care: At Home and Abroad

Over the last several years considerable interest and dialogue
among medical practitioners has centered on the issue of culturally competent healthcare. Health fairs and advanced education courses are rarely without a speaker devoted to advocating
cultural competence, knowledge of patient population, cultural
practices and beliefs, and similar issues. Cultural-based care has
become in vogue. Despite the healthcare community's recent
expanding interest in all things cultural, the concept and,
therefore, the practice of cultural competence frequently remains
vague and ill-defined. Conference speakers champion the concept without delving into the concrete reality of what it means
to practice cultural competence in the real world. Since cultural
competence is undoubtedly required in the successful practice
of medicine among patients whose culture is different from that
of the healthcare provider, this section of the chapter will begin
by exploring the concepts of culture, individuality, and cultural
competence and sensitivity in an attempt to tease out the reality
of what it means in practice to be culturally competent and how
each medical practitioner can go about preparing for and interacting with patients from a culture different from their own.

If culture is defined as the sum total of the customs, beliefs,
attitudes, values, goals, laws, traditions, and moral codes of a people (King 1966:4:1), the practice of cultural competency involves
possessing knowledge, awareness, and respect for other cultures
(Am Fam Phys 2005;72:2267). A healthcare provider must be
aware of a patient's background and community in order to give
context to that patient's medical complaint and, ultimately, to
provide the best treatment. In order to become culturally competent, the medical practitioner is obliged to have a basic understanding of the dominant cultural beliefs and practices of the
groups to whom his or her patients belong. Within the United
States, for example, healthcare professionals working in areas

ACCULTURATION

with large Hispanic populations prioritize learning about the hot/cold theory of disease, while other healthcare providers devote time to learning about common ancient Chinese medicine in order to better communicate with their Asian patients. In addition to being aware of cultural diversity, however, the medical practitioner must respect the differences between his or her own culture and theory of medicine and allow for flexibility in dealing with his or her patients from other cultures. This means both acknowledging to the patient that other explanations of causation and varieties of treatments exist for a particular condition and that this particular healthcare provider's explanation and treatment is based on his or her training under the biomedical model combined with what has been presented in the history and gathered in the physical exam. For example, if a patient believes that his facial paralysis (Bell's palsy) is related to seeing a ghost, rather than disparaging the patient's belief, a culturally competent physician might note that while many of his other patients have expressed similar opinions regarding the causation of facial paralysis, studies done by the biomedical community have shown a relationship between the onset of Bell's palsy and other conditions such as Lyme disease. For this reason, he would suggest gathering more laboratory tests in order to better identify a possible cause of this kind of facial paralysis. In this way, the physician recognizes this common cultural belief, does not dismiss it as incorrect, informs the patient of the biomedical approach to this medical problem, and gives a suggestion of what he thinks should be done. Obviously, practicing cultural competency in this manner requires a certain amount of knowledge, awareness, and respect for another culture, as well as the recognition that the healthcare provider is representing the culture of biomedicine and is, by definition, biased.

Though the examples above serve to teach about how to practice cultural competency in the real world, they also clearly present an underlying ambiguity between the theory and practice of cultural competency, which has not yet been addressed. Namely, the theory of cultural competency, in embracing the model of culture as a set of ideas and practices held by a group, misses the complexity of the individual as part of the culture. Just as cultures are not static and immune from outside influences, neither are individuals within a culture unchanging and homogenous in their beliefs. As Juckett expounds in an essay on approaching cross-cultural medicine: "Generalizations [about patient cultural beliefs and practices] can serve as a starting point and do not preclude factoring in individual characteristics such as education, nationality, faith, and acculturation. Every patient is unique" (Am Fam Phys 2005;72:2267). Just because a particular patient may appear to be of Asian descent to a physician does not mean that the patient identifies himself as Asian and believes in traditionally held Asian medical beliefs. This patient may think of himself as Thai first, not Asian, and specifically as northern Thai. Even more confusing, the patient may have spent a majority of his life living in a predominately white middle-class community in Nebraska and consider himself American first. What medical beliefs he shares with a Chinese immigrant who recently moved from a rural farm near Mongolia and lives in Chinatown in New York City may not be readily apparent. In fact, some immigrants transitioning between belief systems may hold several viewpoints simultaneously (Am Fam Phys 2005;72:2267). Therefore, while attempting to gain cultural competence by learning about cultural practices of a particular group, the healthcare provider must always be aware that not all members follow cultural norms and that some members may hold several beliefs at once. Moreover, as Helman cautions, "generalizations [of group behavior] can also be dangerous, for they often lead to the development of stereotypes and then to cultural misunderstandings, prejudices, and discrimination (Helman 2000:3). A patient, then, should be approached as part of a culture, not as a product of that culture.

ACCULTURATION

Given the risks of generalizing about cultural beliefs and the wide range of heterogeneity in seemingly similar patient populations, what is the healthcare provider striving for cultural competency to do? Certainly cultural competency, in all of its complexity, is a worthy (and when traveling abroad, very necessary) practice. Balancing the generalizations of a culture and the specificity of the individual over the course of a several minute visit, often in another language, poses a challenge. Fortunately, much work has been done on practicing cultural competence through the patient interview. The patient interview presents the opportunity for the culturally competent medical provider to successfully communicate with a patient, ultimately delivering superior healthcare across the cultural chasm. For this reason, the following section will delve into the specifics of how a culturally competent provider can conduct a culturally sensitive patient interview.

3.3   Interviewing the Patient

> The diversity of responses within cultural groups means that generalization about any given ethnic group will not be useful in the care of individual patients.
>
> *Candib 2002:218*

Much of the advice presented in this section can be found in more detail in the numerous works of Arthur Kleinman, a preeminent medical anthropologist and psychiatrist, as well as texts by other researchers interested in exploring the intersection between culture and healthcare.

Conducting a successful cross-cultural interview of the patient begins before the medical provider even leaves home. The first, and most obvious, step is to recognize that a cultural difference exists. Going into another country expecting that everyone has the same familiar set of values and thinks about medicine and illness in the same way is bound to result in a failure of communication. Moreover, as noted in previous sections, realizing that the biomedical professional brings his or her own biases into the healthcare encounter can ultimately aid in furthering communication and understanding.

Speaking a patient's native language aids in improving the patient-provider relationship and in building trust and is the best case scenario of delivering medical care across cultures. Realistically, however, expecting a medical provider traveling abroad to learn a new language is not realistic. Nevertheless, the visiting provider should attempt to learn at least the most frequently used 5 to 10 words, such as greetings, to further create solidarity and rapport both when working abroad or working with a culturally different group within the United States or Canada.

Both prior to traveling to a country and while staying in a specific locale, an effort should be made to learn as much as possible about its culture. Important topics to cover include family structure, politics, values, economics, status, health and disease, traditional healers, and medicines. A healthcare provider may seek out such information in more obvious texts, such as up-to-date historical and anthropological nonfiction works, but he or she should also examine works done by local artists including novelists and playwrights (King 1966:4:3). Reading a novel written by an author of a specific cultural group, for example, can teach a foreign medical staff person not only about local beliefs but also about areas of cultural conflict and change. Outside of the written text, the healthcare provider also may consider meeting with an anthropologist working in the area or becoming friends with educated members of the society, such as hospital staff, who are familiar with local customs as well as the culture of the visiting provider. Finally, it is vital that the healthcare practitioner continue to make observations and ask questions. Noting local customs, clothing, food products, and common practices while visiting a village may prove invaluable at a later time when a patient presents with medical complications resulting from a common daily practice such as weaving or working in the fields. Healthcare providers also should consider questioning their patients about customs and practices, even when those questions are not obviously related to immediate medical illnesses. Inquiring about local customs shows interest in the patient and ultimately builds trust.

Though the power of observation continues to be useful in cross-cultural encounters, providers cannot always assume that they are correctly identifying the significance of body language and spoken language. Body language, including the acceptable distance between 2 communicating individuals, differs between cultural groups and even within a specific culture based on the relationship between individuals. Among some Apache communities, for example, "the Whiteman" is viewed as impolite in his insistence to make eye contact, to have unnecessary physical contact, and to ask about people's emotional or physical states and because he talks "too loud, too fast, and too tense" (Basso 1979:45). The healthcare provider, as a member of his or her own culture, must make a special effort to learn about foreign customs governing body language and personal space and to abide by them.

With whom to speak regarding a patient's illness and diagnosis is an important part of the medical provider-patient interview process. The current dominant culture of the United States values the individual over the family as the unit of healthcare. Healthcare providers meet with their patients individually beginning in the teens and have a code of confidentiality with the patient to the exclusion of the family. Medical information and diagnoses are shared exclusively between the patient and the provider. Although as recently as 1961 a majority of US-based physicians did not reveal the diagnosis or prognosis of cancer to their patients (more likely involving the patient's family instead), currently 98% of US-based physicians report that they disclose such diagnoses directly to the patient involved (Candib 2002:213). Even within the borders of the United States, the biomedical individual patient-provider model described above cannot be assumed to always be the desirable form of interaction with patients and their families. Researchers working with patients from a wide variety of ethnic backgrounds in Los Angeles found that 47% of Korean Americans, 65% of Mexican Americans, 87% of European Americans, and 89% of African Americans believed that a physician should share a diagnosis of cancer with a patient. The remainder of patients believed that the family should be told and, in many cases, that the family and not the patient should make decisions about end-of-life care (JAMA 1995;247:820). The medical provider is likely to face dilemmas regarding patient vs family involvement in healthcare when attempting to export the biomedical medical model into different societies abroad. In many developing countries (and among ethnically diverse populations in the United States, as noted above), the family may be considered the main unit. A patient may arrive at the hospital with all his or her relatives and anticipate that these family members will make the major care decisions. Patients may not want to be given choices regarding care (the American model of shared clinical decision making) but instead want to be directed to a choice by the healthcare provider (Chelminski, Annuals IntMed 2007:67). Again, it is important to remember that there is diversity within cultural groups, and what you may expect to be a patient preference based upon cultural background may be very different from the reality of what that patient expects for care. The healthcare professional should be willing to ask patients who they would like to involve in their medical care and to what extent they would like to make healthcare decisions for themselves.

When conducting a medical interview across cultures, the biomedical practitioner may find it useful to ask several specific questions in each encounter to help shed light on cultural beliefs

ACCULTURATION

relating to illness. In their text, Kleinman et al. suggest the following questions based upon an "Explanatory Model" to understand how a patient is approaching his/her medical illness (Ann Int Med 1978;88:251):

• What do you think has caused your problem?
• Why do you think it started when it did?
• What do you think your sickness does to you?
• How does it work?
• Will it have a short or long course?
• What kind of treatment do you think you need? What treatment have you sought prior to visiting the physician/hospital?
• What are the most important results you hope to receive from this treatment?
• What are the chief problems your sickness has caused for you? What do you fear most about your sickness?

These questions should be added to the normal history of present illness questions. Finally, after inquiring about the specifics of the illness and treatment, do not forget to reflect upon your own personal experiences, social background, and cultural beliefs and consider how they might be altering the way that you are viewing the situation. After all "one cannot really understand other people's inner motivations and beliefs without, to some extent, understanding one's own" (Helman 2000:107).

3.4 Using Translators

Communication between a clinician and a patient is always a delicate transaction. Even in the best of circumstances, with both being native English speakers and with a well-educated, well-informed patient, the opportunities for miscommunication are plentiful—and the consequences potentially profound.

Health Aff 2006;25:811

Frequently healthcare providers travel abroad to work in developing countries with rudimentary language skills. They may be eager to try out the French that they learned in high school or the Spanish they picked up in college 15 years ago. Unfortunately, basic language skills and restaurant and shopping-related vocabulary are not enough to allow for facile communication between physicians and patients. In fact, attempting to stumble through a patient-physician interview with such limited language ability can result in medical error and misunderstandings between the 2 parties involved (Fam Pract Manag 2004:38). Using a translational service could make the difference between diagnosing a patient with gastroenteritis based upon a history of chronic abdominal pain versus recognizing that this specific type of symptomatology is a common presentation of depression and stress in that particular culture. Therefore, it is not surprising that healthcare practitioners who are not fluent in a particular language or culture are generally discouraged from acting as translators. The "gold standard" when interacting with a patient from a different culture who speaks a language in which you are not fluent is to use a language interpreter who has experience and training in medical terminology and the healthcare system (Am Fam Phys 2005;72:2269). An additional reason to use interpreter services besides reducing medical error is that, in a study of interpreter services and healthcare quality, researchers found that patients perceived the quality of the interpreter to be strongly associated with the quality of care received overall (J Gen Intern Med 2005;20:1050). To the patient, the medical provider's advice seems only as good as the translating service that is provided. Optimal use of language translation services results in actual and perceived improved medical care for the patient.

In a patient-provider interaction, a wide variety of people can and do serve as interpreters. In a study of residents completed in 157 academic health center hospitals across the United States, researchers found that, when facing language barriers, 77% of

ACCULTURATION

residents said that they sometimes or often used professional interpreters, 84% used ad hoc interpretation by adult family members and friends, 77% used other hospital employees, and 22% used children (JAMA 2006;296:1052). Among members of the healthcare community, using lay people such as patients' husbands and friends, clinic secretaries, and staff members mentioned above, however, is considered "reliably unreliable" (Health Aff 2006;25:812). This is both because patient family members are often untrained in medical terminology and may misinterpret information to either party and because interpreters who have an active relationship with the patient may purpose-fully misinterpret information if they have reason to hide it from the healthcare provider. The patient also may be less likely to share potentially important information with a physician when his or her family members or neighbors are in the room. Imagine a mother attempting to consult a doctor regarding her heavy menses and being faced with having her 6-year-old son acting as the translator. Although these examples undoubtedly are the extreme of the possibilities that a medical practitioner and patient may face when using a family member or close friend as an ad hoc translating service, they serve as an important lesson to remind the healthcare provider of the pitfalls of using untrained translators.

In the United States, medically trained translators have a formal education in interpreting and abide by a professional code of ethics (Fam Pract Manag 2004:38). They are familiar with medical terminology, have experience in healthcare, and some-times have attended accredited training programs for medical interpreters. In developing countries, interpreters will very likely not have any formal education in translation. Often other physi-cians and nurses who have cultural insight as well as experience working in the medical field serve as useful translators.

The finest interpreters translate both cultural and bio-medically related information; they should have a "good understanding of common health problems and diseases experienced by patients in a given culture and should have a solid grasp of their folk traditions and healthcare beliefs" (Lecca et al. 1998:71). An interpreter should be a linguistic and cultural tool to the medical provider. A good interpreter "can save time and resources in the long run by decreasing the number of callbacks, misdiagnoses and unnecessary tests, and increasing patient comprehension, compliance and satisfaction" (Fam Pract Manag 2004:39).

In the text *Cultural Competency in Health*, the authors present 3 distinct models for using an interpreter (Lecca et al. 1998:71). A translator can be used as an interviewer, as a tool, or as a partner to the healthcare provider.

In the translator-as-an-interviewer model, the translator gains some control in the direction of a meeting and can ask the patient questions not originating from the healthcare provider. In this model, the interpreter can gain the trust of the patient and can elicit cooperation. This may work particularly well if the translator senses that the patient is presenting with a common folk illness.

In the second model, the interpreter acts as a tool of the medical provider, translating literally, adding no cultural nuances or meaning to the physician's questions. The provider is in complete control in this situation and may not gain access to cultural meanings or information.

Finally, in the Lecca et al. model, the interpreter and interviewer are partners. This allows them to communicate among themselves and also with the patient. In this situation, the interpreter acts both as the voice of the healthcare practitioner and as a cultural broker, translating any cultural health beliefs that the patient may have expressed. Although translators in the United States are often encouraged to follow more of the interpreter-as-a-tool model (Fam Pract Manag 2004:37), there is much to be gained by allowing the interpreter some freedom in informing the

ACCULTURATION

provider about unfamiliar practices and cultural beliefs. Medical professionals abroad will likely find a particular model that appeals to them through experimentation with different interpreters in a variety of situations.

The following guidelines are from a useful overview titled "Getting the Most from Language Interpreters" available on the Web site of the American Academy of Family Physicians (http://www.aafp.org/fpm). I have also added some details that I find to be useful. An in-house interaction between healthcare provider, translator, and patient can benefit from adhering to some of the following suggestions.

- Confidentiality: Make sure to remind the patient (and the family when applicable) and interpreter that all information exchanged during the interview will be kept in confidentiality.
- Addressing the patient: Maintain eye contact with the patient (if culturally appropriate), keep appropriate distance between yourself and the patient; and speak to the patient directly, not to the translator. Speak in the first person to the patient.
- Timing: Keep sentences brief and pause to allow extra time for interpreting. Use diagrams and pictures when available. Listen without interrupting and frequently ask the patient to repeat information back to you to check for understanding.

At the end or anytime during the interview, it may be useful to ask the translator what he or she thinks about the patient's presentation. The translator may have inside cultural information that may be of use to the physician unfamiliar with cultural customs, beliefs, or even the politics or common practices of the community.

3.5   Working with Local Healers and Folk Practitioners

When working abroad, biomedical practitioners sometimes disregard local healers, village midwives, and folk practitioners as possessing little medical knowledge and training, as practicing unproven methods, and even as being dangerous. Biomedically trained providers may shun local healers and discourage patients from seeking their advice. The consequence of such insular practice is that patients will not disclose past and current medical experiences when seeking medical care. A hostile relationship between healthcare provider and the local healer, often a powerful figure of the local community, also will result. Local healers and folk practitioners often have years of knowledge in their subject area, familiarity with the politics of the area, and a vital role in the community. They can educate the visiting provider and aid in improving the healthcare of their area. Local healers should not be dismissed as "false" practitioners with little to add to the biomedical healthcare system; rather the biomedical professional should make an effort to reach out to practicing local healers and folk practitioners to build mutual understanding and to improve the ability to refer patients across medical system borders depending on patient condition and need.

Much literature exists relating to successful interactions between the biomedical and folk medical systems. Perhaps one of the most common examples referenced is the model of traditional healer as purveyor of oral rehydration therapy (ORT) to patients outside of the hospital (http://rehydrate.org/dd/dd48.htm; Bastien 1992). In this particular example, which has been applied in numerous countries in South America and Africa, traditional medical practitioners working in the community are recruited to increase the usage of ORT among mothers in rural locations. As seen in Bolivia, oftentimes traditional healers are already using plant-based teas to treat children with diarrhea, and the biomedical community needs only to convince these practitioners to add particular electrolytes to the solution and to provide ORT packets (Bastien, 1992). For further reading on culturally acceptable and integrating traditional healers into preventive medicine programs, find Somma and Bodiang's 2003 text on HIV/

ACCULTURATION

AIDs prevention campaigns in Africa using theater groups and traditional healers http://www.sdc-health.ch/priorities_in_health/communicable_diseases/hiv_aids/cultural_approach_to_hvi_aids_prevention or read one of Joseph Bastien's books on integrating biomedicine and ethnomedicine in Bolivia.

In addition to acting as rural representatives in health-care campaigns, traditional healers, as integrated members of a culture, can teach biomedical practitioners about local customs and beliefs. Most societies have several examples of *cultural-bound syndromes*, a set of somatic and psychiatric symptoms that is recognizable only within a specific cultural context. Among members of the dominant cultures of the West, some cultural-bound syndromes include anorexia nervosa, abduction phenomenon (ie, being kidnapped by aliens), and Gulf War syndrome. For other examples of culture-bound syndromes, refer to DSM-IV Appendix I or Juckett's review article on cross-cultural medicine (Am Fam Phys 2005; 72:2267). Culture-bound syndromes are generally treated by folk healers and often not well understood by biomedical personnel. For this reason, the biomedical provider who identifies a patient suffering from a culture-bound syndrome may find it useful to refer that patient to a local traditional healer for successful treatment of this psychosocial based illness.

While existing practices of traditional healers can often be modified slightly from their original form to increase their benefit to the patient (according to biomedical standards), sometimes practices that are deemed to be of negative value by the biomedical community can be found in particular locations. *Negative value practices* are those considered to be dangerous to the patient according to the tenets of biomedicine (King 1966:4:4), such as female circumcision. In cases of negative value practices, biomedical practitioners must delicately navigate between cultural sensitivity, their cultural beliefs, and the doctrine of human rights. How best to address specific cases is dependent on numerous variables including the people involved, the risk of the practice, and the politics of the situation.

3.6   Returning Home

For some people returning home from a developing country poses a challenge. Transitioning from a healthcare system burdened beyond its capacity by financial hardship to a Western hospital replete with technology and frequently a relative disregard for healthcare economics may prove frustrating. Having witnessed deaths that could have been avoided by simple interventions unavailable in the developing world, healthcare resource waste on unnecessary procedures can try a provider's patience.

Even outside of the medical domain, healthcare workers can experience difficulty reintegrating into a society filled with so many options. Someone having spent numerous years abroad once mentioned to me that they felt overwhelmed by all of the food choices in grocery stores in the United States. Other people have difficulty empathizing with the fears and concerns of their friends in the developed world after experiencing the level of adversity abroad.

Finally, there is often a disinterest of other physicians and lay people regarding your experiences overseas. Having had a life changing encounter in a developing country, physicians and medical staff are eager to speak with others about the experience. They may be disappointed that others, whether jealous of their opportunity, disinterested, or too busy in their own lives, do not care to learn about their trip. Fortunately, many physicians and medical staff have some friends or colleagues who share their passion for working with underserved communities throughout the world.

So, what can be done to decrease this experience of culture shock? Speaking with like-minded individuals who have had a similar experience abroad often aids in reintegration. Also, physicians and healthcare workers can draw strength from knowing that what they have done in the developing world and what they continue to do daily in the west has improved and saved the lives of many individuals.

3.7 Bibliography

Basso KH. *Portraits of "The Whiteman": Linguistic play and cultural symbols among the Western Apache*. New York: Cambridge University Press; 1979.

Bastien JW. *Drum and Stethoscope: Integrating Ethnomedicine and Biomedicine in Bolivia*. Salt Lake City: University of Utah Press; 1992.

Bastien JW. *Healers of the Andes: Kallawaaya Herbalists and Their Medicinal Plants*. Salt Lake City: University of Utah Press; 1987.

Candib LM. Truth telling and advance planning at the end of life: problems with autonomy in a multicultural world. *Families, Systems, & Health*. 2002:20(3).

Cross T, Bazron B, Dennis, Isaacs M. *Towards a Culturally Competent System of Care*. Vol. 1. Washington DC: Georgetown University Child Development Center; 1989.

Cultural Competence. http://www.faqs.org/nutrition/Ca-De/Cultural-Competence.html.

Getting the most from Language Interpreters. http://www.aafp.org/fpm.

Helman CG. *Culture, Health, and Illness*. Boston: Butterworth and Heinemann; 2000.

King M. *Medical Care in Developing Countries: A Symposium from Makerere*. London: Oxford University Press; 1966.

Kleinman A. *Patients and Healers in the Context of Culture: An Exploration of the Borderland Between Anthropology, Medicine, and Psychiatry*. Los Angeles: University of California Press; 1980.

Lecca PJ, Quervalu I, Nunes JV, Gonzales HF. *Cultural Competency in Health, Social, and Human Services: Directions for the Twenty-First Century*. New York: Garland Publishing, Inc.; 1998.

Oral Rehydration Therapy. http://rehydrate.org/dd/dd48.htm.

Chapter 4

Health Promotion in Developing Countries

Bryan Cooke

4.1 Introduction

It would be too presumptuous of me to begin to enumerate
the dos and don'ts of health promotion strategies that work in
developing countries, as much advice has been provided on this
subject by many experts like John Bryant, Kenneth Newell, and
Kreuter et al. Other helpful sources may include WHO, Pan
American Health Organization, the Rockefeller Foundation,
Centers for Disease Control and Prevention, Agency for Interna-
tional Development, Rotary International, the US Peace Corps,
Partners of the Americas, the World Bank, and Doctors Without
Borders Web site (http://www.doctorswithoutborders.org).

The concepts shared in this chapter are based not only on
the literature but also on my limited experiences while working
as the US Peace Corps' first medical and health specialist coor-
dinator in Malaysia, a Fulbright Fellow in Australia and India,
a partner for Partners of the Americas in Brazil, and as a rotary
professor in a Developing Country-India.

Probably the first thing to realize about addressing international health problems is that it can be a very satisfying
and rewarding experience; so have fun and enjoy the journey.

However, it can be so daunting a task, as Dr Carroll Behrhorst explained that curing the ailing from clinics and hospitals in jungles, savannas, and mountains was like trying to empty the Atlantic Ocean with a teaspoon. It made the toiler feel active and useful and caused everyone to exclaim: "My, what a beautiful teaspoon!"

Before health can supplant disease among the 2 billion rural poor of the world, Behrhorst believes that the following problems must be tackled aggressively:

- social and economic injustice
- land tenure
- agricultural production and marketing
- population control
- malnutrition
- health training
- curative medicine

One of the first lessons to be learned when working on health problems in an international setting is to build positive relationships and develop trust with your target population. This takes time and could be a challenge for the medical student or team, who is on a tight schedule and must complete their research project in a few weeks.

Much can be done ahead of time by studying the culture, their history, belief systems, attitudes, and behaviors. When in-country, be sensitive to cross-cultural differences and involve the local people to identify and prioritize their perceived health needs and encourage them to come up with possible solutions. This builds their confidence and empowers them to take owner-ship of the project. Meanwhile, you become accepted as part of a bottom-up team as opposed to a top-down foreign expert possess-ing all the answers.

So, if you go into a developing country with the attitude that you have all the answers and will single-handedly rescue them by fixing their health problems, you may, as the story goes, be "giving them a fish and feeding them for a day." While you may feel good addressing their health problem as seen through your eyes, it may not be their top health problem as perceived through their eyes. But, if you approach the village council members and leaders and key informants and ask for their help, you could identify their perceived health needs and the available community assets and resources. By identifying the enlightened and influential community leaders, you could develop a team, and through teamwork, you could "teach them to fish," thereby feeding them for a lifetime and creating a self-sustaining society. Remember TEAM stands for Together Everyone Achieves More.

4.2 Identifying Community Needs, Assets, and Resources

It is true that for a community to be sustainable, it values a hand-up much more than a hand-out.

Perhaps the best example of identifying community needs, assets, and resources is illustrated in community medicine doctors Mabelle and Rajanikant Arole's comprehensive rural health project in Jamkhed, India.

This Johns Hopkins trained couple conceived a plan to provide a viable and effective healthcare system for a population of 40,000 in several villages. They explained to the community leaders that they were interested in meeting the basic health needs of the people through curative, preventive, and promotional methods, provided they participated actively in making a building available for health activities in each village, provided they participated in active health promotional and preventive activities such as the mass immunization of infants and children, and provided volunteers would help the health personnel in their work.

They used the following 4 criteria:

- Local communities should be motivated and involved in decision making and must participate in the health promotion program so that ultimately they owned the program in their respective villages.
- The program should be planned at the grass roots and develop a referral system to suit the local conditions.
- Local resources, such as buildings, manpower, and agriculture, should be used to solve local health problems.
- The community needs total healthcare and not fragmented care.

The community responded by providing 7 acres of land on which to put up permanent buildings. Volunteers were provided to plan and supervise the building work. Some communities repaired access roads so that the health team could reach them, and youth groups donated blood.

When the project began, the area was facing drought, and the Aroles discovered that the priorities were not health but food and water. They focused on the most vulnerable groups—under 5 years old and mothers. They organized a community kitchen, finding firewood, large cooking pots, and volunteers to cook and keep records. By using local resources, wells were dug and the farmers who benefited from the water donated land to grow food. Tractors were donated to cultivate the fields, and the crop was shared by the owner and communities for community kitchens. The project now has a small poultry farm and dairy to meet the nutritional needs of patients in the center.

The 2 mobile health teams consist of a physician, nurse supervisor, social worker, auxiliary nurse midwife, driver, paramedical worker, and a village health worker. The teams are trained and each member has a role in the delivery of health services.

By finding resources within the community and activating people to identify and help solve their own problems, the Arole's Jamkhed Project is self sustaining with the help of Village Health Workers. By empowering them and building their confidence, it became easier for the local participants to take ownership of the project, and the power passed from the Aroles to them much like a relay runner passes the baton.

4.3   Building Relationships

How do we develop relationships? I use a mnemonic called *FORM*. I connect with people by asking about the following:

F is for Family; people love to talk about themselves and their families.

O is for Occupation, or what they do for work.

R is for Recreation, or what they like to do for fun.

M is for Message, or what health benefits they expect to get out of our interaction.

This helps us to find their perceived health wants, needs, desires, dreams, and goals.

When relating to individuals, it is important to recognize and respect the 4 social styles of people as described by Florence Littauer:

Amiable: desires peace; introverted, pessimistic, purpose-driven, and relationship oriented

Analytical: desires perfection; introverted, pessimistic, organized, and goal oriented

Driver: desires power or control; outgoing, outspoken, optimistic, decisive, and goal oriented

Expressive: desires fun; outgoing, outspoken, optimistic, and relationship oriented

To relate well with others, pay attention to people's personalities and meet them where they are. Be sensitive and understanding and have passion and compassion. Set your goals in concrete and your plans in sand.

From the US Peace Corps, I learned that the 3 basic requirements for working effectively in another culture are: knowledge of the local language or access to a good translator, cross-cultural sensitivity, and time for on-the-job orientation and training.

I also learned that when working with volunteers, it is important to build alliances and networks. Over the years, I have developed a simple "3 × 5" approach that works for me. The 3 stands for the 3 Rs: recruit, retain, and recognize. The 5 stands for 5 Is: invite, introduce, induct, indoctrinate, and involve. When recruiting volunteers and prospects that you want to retain over a long period of time, it is important to recognize and celebrate their individual professional and personal achievements. This could be health worker of the month, wedding anniversaries, number of years with the project, family births, birthdays, etc.

When recruiting a new volunteer, invite them to your program's open house and introduce them to new and veteran volunteers and employees so that they can learn about the successful programs and catch the excitement of the team. When inducting them into the program, make this a significant event for them. Follow it up with an orientation or indoctrination session about the program, and lastly, involve them by assigning them a job that best fits their talents and interests. We all know that a square peg does not go in a round hole!

4.4   Capacity Building

In order to work effectively in a community, community readiness is very important. Interviews may need to be conducted to address the following 6 dimensions of the specific health problem. Let's take malaria as an example:

- prevention programs related to malaria

- community knowledge about malaria prevention
- community leadership
- community climate to support malaria prevention
- knowledge about malaria
- resources available for malaria prevention

Hypothetically, in South India for example, the malaria prevention program may consist of burning mosquito coils at bedtime during the rainy season. Such programs can be much more effective if the community is educated to know the importance and changeability of the problem. In other words, how clearly do the data link this behavior (burning mosquito coils) to the health problem (malaria)? And secondly, how much supporting evidence is there to change this behavior?

In order to build capacity in a community, the village leaders will need to be convinced that the anopheles mosquito is the causative vector, and the protective measures that work include attacking the mosquitoes at their breeding grounds by draining or spraying the stagnant pools. Additionally, introducing the proper use of mosquito nets and wearing appropriate clothing after dusk that covers their bodies, including their arms and legs, would be part of the successful intervention.

By creating awareness and interest about malaria you provide knowledge and persuade the target audience to make the decision to first try and then to adopt the intervention that works.

When building capacity, remember you are dealing with volunteers who have to be won over, educated, encouraged, mentored, and recognized as invaluable team members. In Karnataka, India, there is a group of minimally educated, single women, generally of the lowest caste, known as Anganwadis. They serve brilliantly as village health aides, workers alongside visiting doctors, postgraduate medical students, and nurses in pre- and postnatal clinics, polio-plus immunization initiatives, and HIV/AIDS educational campaigns.

4.5 Are We Batting a Thousand?

When conducting health promotion, whether it is in a developed or developing country, it is helpful to remember that rarely do we reach 100% of our target population. In fact, reaching 50% to 84% of your target population is a very laudable goal.

According to Rogers' Diffusion of Innovations theory, it is worth noting that there are 5 groups of people when it comes to adopting a new idea or innovation. He believes that all individuals in a social system do not adopt an innovation at the same time. Instead, they adopt in an overtime sequence, so that individuals can be classified into adopter categories on the basis of when they first begin using a new idea. These 5 categories can be identified on a bell-shaped curve as follows:

Innovators (3%): They are active information seekers and are open to new ideas and ways of doing things differently. The innovator is *venturesome*. They play an important gatekeeping role in the flow of new ideas into a system.

Early Adopters (14%): They are generally the opinion leaders in a community. The early adopter is respected by his or her peers as one who makes wise innovation decisions. Early adopters put their stamp of approval on a new idea by adopting it.

Early Majority (34%): They are cautious and look to early adopters when adopting innovations. The early majority may deliberate for some time before completely adopting a new idea. They follow with willingness in adopting innovations but seldom lead.

Late Majority (34%): They are skeptical and look to their peers and wait until the innovation is established before they adopt it. For this group, peer pressure is necessary to motivate adoption. The uncertainty about the new idea must be removed before the late majority feel that it is safe to adopt.

Laggards (16%): The reference point for this group is the past. Decisions are based on what was done previously, and these individuals interact mainly with those who have traditional values. These are the hard to reach, who are resistant to change and alienated from the mainstream. They tend to be suspicious of innovations and change agents. Their innovation-decision process is relatively lengthy, with adoption and use lagging far behind awareness knowledge of a new idea.

Rogers found that formal education, exposure to mass media, and opinion leadership were variables that were highly related to innovativeness. That is, innovators differed most sharply from laggards on these socioeconomic and communication variables. He also noted that in developing countries, face-to-face communications were important at the knowledge stage in the innovation-decision process.

4.6 Collaboration

Most innovators can identify a need, adapt to change, involve allies, and take risks. Because international health promotion is about nurturing, motivating, mentoring, empowering, and developing leaders, you may want to cultivate partners with leadership potential from the innovator and early adopter groups.

Depending upon the type of local participation you are seeking, it could be any one of the following 4 modes: contractual, consultative, collaborative, or collegiate. Ideally, with the help of key informants, you would be able to identify who among the locals you would have contractual, consultative, collaborative, and/or collegial relationships.

A model of collaboration that I like to use in networking is adapted from one developed by Farquhar et al of Stanford University. The 3 stages include initiation, collaboration, and transformation.

HEALTH PROMOTION IN
DEVELOPING COUNTRIES

Farquhar believes that during the 3 phases of initiation, collaboration, and transformation, the visiting health expert, or *Partner 1*, should play a major leadership role in the initiation and collaboration phases and a decreasing role in the transformation phase. The host, or *Partner 2*, will need encouragement and reassurance during the initiation and collaboration stages until they are self-sufficient and empowered to take over ownership of the project in the transformation phase.

If one can imagine Farquhar's model as a graph, with level of involvement plotted vertically along the y axis and time spent during the 3 phases of initiation, collaboration, and transformation is represented horizontally on the x axis. Then, Partner 1's involvement would resemble a bell-shaped curve skewed toward the left (with heavy involvement during the initiation and collaboration phases) with the right tail of the bell curve tapering off (showing diminishing involvement during the transformation phase).

Likewise, if the level of involvement of Partner 2 were to be plotted over time, the graph would look like an "S" curve, starting from minimal involvement during the initiation stage, climbing to an ever increasing level of involvement in the collaboration stage, then rising to the highest level of involvement in the transformation phase. This model suggests that the runner carrying the baton in a relay race, Partner 1, will only pass the baton to Partner 2 when the receiver is ready and has come up to the same speed as the incoming runner. Until Partner 2 becomes capable, confident, and empowered enough to take on full ownership of the project, Partner 1's level of involvement will continue in a supporting role and gradually diminish to that of a less significant supporting role during the transformation phase.

4.7   Different Research Approaches

In conventional western medical circles, when we try to effect behavior change through health promotion, experimental and quasi-experimental research is the norm. Normally, we conduct a needs assessment to identify the health problem, gather baseline data with a pretest, plan and implement the program with a suitable intervention, and conduct an evaluation by means of a posttest to see if the intervention has made a difference.

Usually, we seek to change knowledge, attitudes, beliefs, and behaviors. Our fix-it approach to health promotion is to do something (a treatment or intervention) for and to the target population that hopefully will eliminate or reduce their health problem. Over time, we have learned that just providing information and knowledge does not necessarily change behavior. For example, if we provide mosquito nets to combat malaria without proper guidance in their use, it may come as a rude awakening when we discover that they were used as fishing nets instead. Or, as Peace Corps volunteers found to their dismay, the outhouses they constructed in Africa were used to keep the fire wood dry.

Ehiri and Prowse (Health Policy Plan 1999;14:1) use the example of infant and childhood diarrhea to show that for a real reduction in mortality and improvements in quality of life to be sustained attention needs to be focused on the environmental and social factors that underlie many of the childhood diseases in the developing world.

Nutbeam (Health Promo Intern 2000;15:259) agrees that in the 19th century, public health action was on the social and environmental determinants of the health of the population, but by the late 20th century there was a shift toward modifying individual risk behavior. He believes that improving health literacy means more than transmitting information and developing skills to be able to read pamphlets and successfully make appointments. By improving people's access to health information and their capacity to use it, he argues that improved health literacy is critical to empowerment.

Whether we use the research of Hochbaum and Rosenstock, which resulted in the Health Belief Model (HBM) as reported by Becker, or the sophisticated Precede-Proceed model of Green and Kreuter as planning models and frameworks for health promotion projects, what seems to work in third world countries is Participatory Research, which is far from easy.

According to Cornwall and Jewkes (Soc Sci Med 1995;11:1), participatory research currently being popularized in health research focuses on a process of sequential reflection and action solicited from and with the local people.

The key difference between participatory research and researcher-directed work is the commitment to involvement of all groups to whom the results apply. In participatory action research, the participants are involved in the following:

- setting the research agenda, including development of the questions to be addressed
- defining how research will be conducted
- creating the change needed by monitoring and evaluating the results.

The researcher's role in this type of work may be as the facilitator but may also be as the expert to provide guidance when the participants request more input.

The advantages of this approach are as follows:

- Participants learn to conduct research.
- Research conducted better meets the needs and interests of the participants.
- Research can continue, and new programs can be developed in the future.

Combining local data with active participation of the targeted community residents provides a powerful approach to sustained development of the specific health program. Local knowledge and perspectives are acknowledged and form the basis for research and planning. The key difference between participatory and conventional methodologies lies in the location of power in the research process. Baseline data may have to be collected through interviews, observations, and focus group discussions, which is time consuming and based on having a good relationship with your volunteers and target audience.

If we decide to use the HBM, the 3 components to consider are individual perceptions, modifying factors, and likelihood of action.

First, an individual's perceptions depend upon his or her perceived susceptibility and severity of the threat, as well as the perceived benefits of preventive action and perceived barriers to prevent action. If the individuals do not perceive that they are susceptible, they will not respond to your plea for behavior change. Neither will the individuals respond if they perceive the severity of the threat as minimal or so great that they are paralyzed to take action.

In designing a program using the HBM, it is important to promote the benefits of the intervention and to minimize or eliminate the barriers. For example, a Native American single mother is persuaded by her friend to have a Pap test. The friend stresses the importance of the procedure in early detection because the subject's mother had died of cervical cancer, making the point that she is susceptible. Thus, if she chooses not to have the Pap, the severity of not doing anything about cervical cancer is serious. Her friend removes the barriers by offering to baby sit the subject's 12-year-old daughter when she comes home from school and by telling her that she can ask to see a female doctor, because she is not comfortable with male doctors. The friend stresses the benefits of the test result being negative, providing peace of mind for the subject and her daughter.

Second are the modifying factors. These would include the perceived threat (of being diagnosed with cervical cancer). The demographic variable is that she is a single mother with a dependent daughter, and the psychosociological variables include the stress of the possibility of losing her job and health benefits, as well as concern for her daughter's future and the question of who will raise her. The cue to action comes from her friend in the form of persuasive communications, information, and a reminder to make the phone call to set the appointment for the Pap test.

Third is the likelihood of action. With the support of the friend, it is more than likely that the subject will take the recommended action.

The Precede-Proceed Model stands for Predisposing, Reinforcing, and Enabling Causes in Educational Diagnosis and Evaluation—Policy, Regulatory, and Organizational Constructs in Educational and Environmental Development. This model is more comprehensive in that the framework considers environmental and organizational factors.

The 7 phases of the Precede framework are as follows:

Phase 1, or social diagnosis, considers the quality of life by assessing problems of concern to the population. Social problems are good barometers of the quality of life.

Phase 2, or epidemiological diagnosis, identifies specific health problems that contribute to the social problems. Four steps that help:

- Determine incidence, prevalence, distribution, intensity, and duration of the problem.
- Note problems with potential for change.
- Ascertain which health problem affects the greatest number and has intervention techniques available.
- Set program goals or objectives by asking who will benefit by how much of what by when.

Phase 3, or behavioral diagnosis, examines the behavioral and nonbehavioral (economic, genetic, and environmental) causes of the health problem. Identify and rank behaviors in terms of importance (how clearly are data linked to the behavior or health problem?) and changeability (what evidence is there to change this behavior?).

Phases 4 and 5, or educational diagnosis, encompasses predisposing, enabling, and reinforcing factors that have potential for affecting health behavior.

Predisposing considers those factors such as knowledge, attitudes, and beliefs that will predispose the person to change his or her behavior. Because perception is more important than reality to individuals, they can relate to the following:

- susceptibility when it is personalized and defined as a range, for example, how likely is it that: I have atherosclerosis; I will have angina pectoris; I will suffer the health consequences of coronary heart disease?
- seriousness of the problem by considering health effects and personal effects, as well as the social implications.

If susceptibility and seriousness levels are both high, this raises fear, and basically people do not take any action. However, they do respond if their susceptibility is high or moderately high, and the seriousness is moderately high or low. For the individual to take action, the program benefits need to exceed the barriers, and the cues to action should be multiple, continual, internal, and external.

Enabling factors are important in initiating the behavior and include availability and accessibility to services and skills in achieving the behavior. For example, by providing a mobile polio-plus immunization service to remote villages in India, the likelihood of mothers bringing their children for the oral vaccine is greatly increased.

Reinforcing factors look at incentives and ways to maintain and sustain the behavioral change. These could be positive or negative reinforcers.

Phase 6, or administrative diagnosis, includes budgeting and analysis of factors that will help or hinder the administration of the program.

Phase 7, or evaluation, should be an integral and continuous part of the entire framework. It is important to state program and behavioral objectives clearly so that standards of acceptability are defined before rather than after the evaluation.

The 4 phases of the Proceed model are as follows:

Phase 1 implementation
Phase 2 process evaluation
Phase 3 impact evaluation
Phase 4 outcome evaluation

For an example of how the Precede-Proceed Model for health promotion planning and evaluation was used in western Australia's Child Pedestrian Injury Prevention Project, see Howatt et al (Inj Prev 1997;3:282).

According to Simons-Morton et al, there are 6 phases in planning a health promotion project. These include the following:

- <u>Needs Assessment:</u> The first phase in identifying their needs is labor intensive, where your participation is as a learner, collaborator, facilitator, and catalyst who interviews key informants, listens and observes, conducts focus groups, etc. As you start this process, you may be perceived as the intimidating expert, and there may be a reluctance to participate on the part of the locals. However, you must resist the temptation to rescue them by identifying their problem for them.

- <u>Goals and Objectives:</u> These must be mutually agreed upon by both you and the local partners. Goals are stated in broad terms such as "the goal is to reduce malaria in Bihar, India."
  - Objectives are stated in more precise, measurable terms. You must be able to spell out who will do what by when, and how will you know it has been done.

- For example "Three hundred Rotarian volunteers from Patna will be paired with 300 medical and nursing students on 5 consecutive Tuesday mornings, April 1, 8, 15, 22, and 29, 2008, and will demonstrate the correct use of and deliver 3000 mosquito nets to village X."

- <u>Intervention/Program Development:</u> This phase in a health promotion project involves program planning. It will involve heavy local input regarding what will work for creating awareness.
  - Here, you help them brainstorm the appropriate intervention. Here, visualization helps immensely. The old adage that "a picture is worth a thousand words" holds true in developing countries. By using pictures, posters, charts, maps, models, slides, PowerPoints, storytelling, puppets, role playing, television, films, and videos, the team can present the problem and the intervention in a manner that is appropriate for the audience.

- <u>Implementation:</u> During this stage, much depends on available funds and resources. For a successful example of a viable and effective comprehensive rural health project in Jamkhed, India, see Mabelle and Rajanikant Arole.

- <u>Evaluation:</u> According to Green and Lewis, there are 3 types of evaluation: process, impact, and outcome evaluation. Although any one of these may be used exclusively under certain conditions, 2 or all 3 are often used in combination. This stage involves wrapping up the project. Here, you want to keep the data collection process simple, and the method of presenting the results should also be simple and easy to understand. Simple pie charts, bar graphs, graphs, and frequency polygons make a more effective impact than paragraphs of narrative.

Process evaluation may include the instructor, the content, methods used, allotted time, and materials used.

Impact evaluation measures knowledge gains, attitude and habit changes, and skill development.

Outcome evaluation examines changes in morbidity and mortality as well as disability and quality of life.

- Review steps for maintaining or terminating the program: This is an opportunity to see what impact the intervention has had.

  If successful, and the locals have the resources and infrastructure to sustain the program, your work is done, and you may only have to make periodic telephonic or electronic checks to monitor the health of the program.

  In a sense, if you have done your job well, congratulations! You have grown another successful health promotion project and worked yourself out of a job and are ready to tackle your next health promotion project in another part of the developing world.

4.8 Bibliography

Arole M, Arole RA. Comprehensive rural health project in Jamkhed (India). In Newell K, ed. *Health by the People*. Geneva: WHO; 1975:70–90.

Becker M. *The Health Belief Model and Personal Health Behaviors*. Thorofare, NJ: Charles B Slack; 1974.

Behrhorst C. The Chimaltenango Development Project in Guatemala. In Newell K, ed. *Health by the People*. Geneva; WHO; 1975:30–52.

Bryant J. *Health and the Developing World*, 2nd printing. Ithaca, NY: Cornell University Press; 1971.

Farquhar J, et al. Education & communication studies. *Oxford Textbook of Public Health*, Vol. 3. London: Oxford University Press; 1985.

Green L, Kreuter M. *Health Promotion Planning: An Educational and Ecological Approach*, 3rd ed. Menlo Park, CA: Mayfield Publishing; 1999.

Green L, Lewis F. *Measurement and Evaluation in Health Education and Promotion*. Palo Alto, CA: Mayfield Publishing; 1986.

Kreuter M, Lezin N, Kreuter M, Green L. *Community Health Promotion Ideas that Work*. Sudbury, MA: Jones and Bartlett; 2003.

Littauer F. *Personality Plus*. Grand Rapids, MI: Revell; 1983.

Newell K, ed. *Health by the People*. Geneva: WHO; 1975.

Rogers E. *Diffusion of Innovations*, 3rd ed. New York: Free Press; 1983.

Simons-Morton B, Greene W. *Introduction to Health Education and Health Promotion*. Gottlieb N. 2nd ed. Prospect Heights, IL: Waveland Press, Inc; 1995.

Chapter 5

Public Health

5.1   Structure and Function of the Health System

(District Health Facilities: Guidelines for Development and
Operations, WHO 1998)

The health systems in most developing countries are a combination of public service and private practice, a mixture that
overlaps with physicians serving both sectors. Doctors may work
at a government clinic in the day and see patients at their home
in the evenings. Or, a surgeon may perform an operation at a
government hospital but still welcome a gratuity from the family
for services.

Government hospitals often have a nominal charge for a
clinic visit or a hospitalization and then require the purchase of
procedures, ie, medicines, IV fluids, X-rays, and dressings. Often a
hospital-operated, fee-for-service pharmacy will fill prescriptions,
and the profits are put back into the hospital budget. Nursing and
ancillary services must be supplemented by the families who will
bathe the patients, help them on the way to diagnostic studies,
cook their food, and sleep at their bedside at night.

Health insurance may be available to government employees
and their families, or special groups may have their own health
system (army, plantation workers, miners). Other special groups
may receive free or subsidized services. "Social diseases" such
as TB, leprosy, and sexually transmitted infections (STIs) may
be treated for free. Maternity and well child health immunization clinics are more often free or heavily subsidized, but the

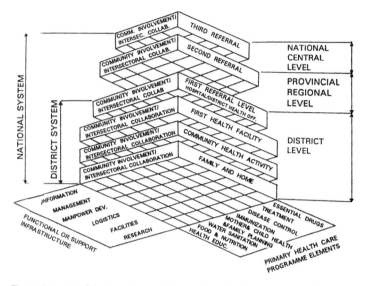

Figure 5.1 Health Care Pyramid. Reproduced with permission of World Health Organization. District Health Facilities: Guidelines for Development and Operations. Western Pacific Series #22, page 6, 1998.

mother still has the burden of arranging transport and childcare and misses the opportunity costs of employment or work in the garden.

Health systems are set up in a pyramidal structure (see Figure 5.1). Primary care is provided at the village or neighborhood level in a rural community or neighborhood health center staffed by community workers. Often nurse aides or health orderlies, they are trained for 1 to 2 years and handle basic health problems from a limited formulary, health education and promotion, sanitation, epidemic surveillance, family planning, and other assigned duties. The backbone upon which the health system is built, aides and orderlies are often poorly and irregularly paid, infrequently supervised, and seldom receive continuing medical education. They may be tasked to supervise volunteer health auxiliaries, a job they often do not find the time or inclination to carry out. Opportunity in private practice is limited; local physicians, traditional healers, and drug sellers in the marketplace win out.

District hospitals or health centers provide the next level of care. Ideally staffed by doctors, they often make do with nurses, midwives, and health aides. This is usually the initial posting of the new medical school graduate. Frequently not a local, he or she may not speak the language or understand the customs. In better financed health systems, the district hospital may have several doctors, even a surgeon or two, who are able to deal with most problems, a laboratory, X-ray, ultrasound, and ancillary staff such as physical therapy. Vertical health systems often have staff posted here for sanitation, water supply, malaria/vector control, maternal-child health (MCH), etc. Several polyclinics and outpatient facilities with specialists may be located in a large district.

One step up is the provincial hospital, which may provide a variety of services depending on the population and geographic area, health finances, and availability of staff. Here, specialists and their residents or registrars may be found along with CT scanners and ventilators. Given their choice and adequate finances, many people prefer to enter the health system here, as services are presumed to be better.

The Provincial (or Regional) Health Office (PHO) supervises the public health services and provides the managerial and budgetary support for all the health services in the area. Section heads for each division operate the vertical programs. Donor agencies (NGOs) usually base their programs here, providing technical and financial support. Depending on the structure of the health system, the PHO may loosely supervise the clinical services, or they may be independent.

National health departments are usually based in the capital city and provide administrative support for the provinces. There are various levels of decentralization of powers and funding to the provinces and districts, which will determine the role of the health headquarters.

In general the national health department performs the following:

- sets goals, objectives, policies, standards, etc.
- supervises medical training
- sets licensing standards through various advisory boards
- conducts health planning and budgeting
- negotiates and coordinates foreign aid programs (NGOs, WHO, UNICEF, etc.)
- operates national specialty hospitals
- provides technical assistance to PHOs
- directs vertical programs: STI; TB; leprosy; environmental, occupational, and social health; acute respiratory infections (ARI); control of diarrheal diseases (CDD); immunization; vector control and health education; nutrition
- collects vital statistics
- enforces quarantine laws
- conducts health research
- purchases capital goods and supplies

Overlying and supervising the health system is the political system led by the Minister of Health. The ministry works closely with the Secretary of Health (usually a civil service position) in setting health priorities and in preparing and defending a budget, which is ultimately approved through a political process. Politicians are also found at the provincial and district levels, and frequently the village health center has a community advisory board.

Table 5.1   Leading Causes of Death

Rank	0–1	1–4	5–9	10–14	15–19	20–24
1	Prematurity	ARI	ARI	ARI	MVA	AIDS
2	Infection	Childhood Diseases	AIDS	MVA	Suicide	MVA
3	Birth injury	Diarrhea	MVA	Drowning	Maternal	Suicide
4	Congenital	Malaria	Childhood diseases	AIDS	ARI	Maternal
5	Tetanus	AIDS	Drowning	Tb	Homicide-war	Homicide-war

5.2   Mortality

The leading causes of death worldwide are still infectious diseases, but in many countries a more developed country pattern is emerging. Leading causes of death are shown in Table 5.1.

Motor vehicle accidents (MVAs) kill 1.2 million people per year and injure another 50 million. Rates are increasing at 5% a year, faster in lower income countries.

Figure 5.2 shows major causes of disability-adjusted life-years and death.

5.3   Primary Healthcare

(Primary Care 1995;22:543)

In 1978 in Alma-Ata, USSR, an International Conference on Primary Health Care issued a declaration that all people were entitled to a level of health that would allow them to live a socially and economically productive existence. The slogan "Health for all by the year 2000" never came about, but the vision that primary healthcare is the best method to obtain this goal remains valid.

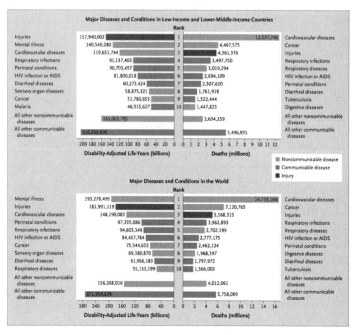

Figure 5.2 Major Cause of Disability Adjusted Life Years and Death. Reproduced with permission. From Anderson GF, Chu E. Expanding Priorities—Confronting Chronic Disease in Countries with Low Income. *N Engl J Med* 2007;356:210. Copyright 2007 Mass. Medical Society. All rights reserved.

In order for primary healthcare (PHC) to succeed, it must provide the following:

- acceptable care delivered at the local level
- accessible to all, geographically, socially, and culturally
- affordable care

- appropriate care to local conditions and requirements
- accountable to community needs

PHC provides preventative, curative, rehabilitative services while promoting a healthy lifestyle through individual and community mobilization. Key components are as follows:

- health education and promotion
- community mobilization and participation
- political will to support healthcare
- safe water and sanitation
- safe food and adequate nutrition
- maternal-child health services including family planning
- immunization programs
- prevention and control of infectious diseases
- treatment of disease and injuries
- provision of essential drugs
- prevention and management of lifestyle diseases

As a medical worker, it is critical that you utilize the PHC approach in every activity you undertake. Each curative service delivered should be accompanied by health promotion and education with consideration of community problems that led to the illness in the first place.

Effective interventions involve changing personal behavior one step at a time. Take the time to build an alliance with your patients, their families, and the community; encourage and support them in bringing about behavior changes and a healthy lifestyle.

5.4 Vaccines

The more common childhood and traveler vaccines are listed in this chapter. Some are available only to certain groups (smallpox) or under certain conditions (cholera). Others are produced locally for specific diseases (anthrax).

Each country will have its own immunization schedule depending on priorities and resources. The WHO recommendations are given here along with those of the United States for comparison. Travelers should consider additional vaccines such as varicella, mumps, rubella, pertussis (DTaP), influenza, and pneumovax depending on their immune status.

At the current time, yellow fever is the only required vaccine for travelers to certain countries and only under limited circumstances. An International Certificate of Vaccination or Prophylaxis is issued when yellow fever vaccine is administered and will need to be carried along with your passport.

Some general rules for immunizations:

- Preserve potency. The cold chain, proper storage of vaccines at 2° to 8°C or frozen is critical for preserving potency.
- Most vaccines have vial temperature monitors and shipping monitor cards to insure storage at the proper temperature.
- Never mix vaccines in the same syringe.
- Give all live vaccines at one visit or space them 1 month apart when possible. But ignore this rule in epidemics.
- Immunize at every opportunity—never pass up a chance to immunize a child. In developing countries, immunize sick and malnourished children.
- Do not give Bacille Calmette-Guerin (BCG) or yellow fever vaccines to symptomatic AIDS infants or children.
- Immunize children on hospital admission if they are eligible.

BCG Vaccine

Disease: M *tuberculosis*

Indications: Residence in area with high prevalence of tuberculosis.

Immunogenicity/Efficacy: Live attenuated vaccine of BCG derived from M *bovis*. Protects > 80% against serious forms (miliary, meningitis) in children (JAMA 1994;271:698). Protection against pulmonary TB in adolescents and adults variable but poor.

Booster: Per country protocol.

Side Effects: Lymphadenitis in neck or axillia 2 to 6 months post vaccination. Most resolve spontaneous over several months. Worsening symptoms or dissemination require standard TB therapy and evaluation for immunodeficiency.

Contraindications: Country policies vary but generally not given to symptomatic AIDS patients. Give to HIV+ in high risk (≥ 5 TB/100 000) countries only.

Dosage and Schedules: Dose 0.05 ml intradermal (ID) newborns to < 3 months, 0.10 ml > 3 months.

Cold Chain: 2°C to 8°C vaccine (but not diluent) may be frozen for long-term storage.

Diphtheria Vaccine

Disease: *Corynebacterium diphtheriae*

Indications: Primary immunization, part of DPT or DaPT vaccine.

Immunogenicity/Efficacy: Killed absorbed onto aluminum salt (adjuvant). Efficacy probably > 95% with 4 doses.

Side Effects: Pain, redness, swelling.

Contraindications: Anaphylactic reaction to previous dose.

Dosage and Schedules: Intramuscular (IM): 0.5 ml, 6, 10, 14, wk as part of DPT.

Booster: WHO: 18 months to 6 yr. United States: every 10 yr with reduced dose "d."

Cold Chain: 2°C to 8°C never frozen. If frozen, will separate into precipitate (discard).

Pertussis Vaccine

Disease: *Bordetella pertussis*

Indications: Primary immunization, part of DPT or DaPT vaccine.

Immunogenicity/Efficacy: Whole cell (P), Acellular (aP) 78% to 85% (after 4th dose).

Side Effects: Fever, local injection site, crying > 3 hr (1% whole cell), hypotonia-hyporesponsive 1:1750 (whole cell).

Contraindications: Anaphylaxis.

Dosage and Schedules: WHO: IM: 0.5 ml; 6, 10, 14 wk as part of DPT; United States: 2, 4, 6, and 18 months.

Booster: WHO: Whole cell 18 months to 6 yr. United States: acellular age 4 to 6 yr, 10 to 12 yr, once as adult.

Cold Chain: 2°C to 8°C never frozen.

Tetanus Toxoid Vaccine

Disease: Tetanus *Clostridium tetani*

Indications: Primary immunization part of DPT or DaPT vaccine. Also given to pregnant women in many countries.

Immunogenicity/Efficacy: Toxin bound to aluminum salt (adjuvant); probably > 95% with 2 doses.

Side Effects: Pain, redness, swelling in up to 50% to 85% of patients, especially with booster doses; 10% fever.

Contraindications: Anaphylaxis.

Dosage and Schedules: IM: 0.5 ml, 6, 10, 14 wk as part of DPT. WHO pregnancy guidelines: first pregnancy #1, 4 wk later #2, 6 months later or next pregnancy #3, 1 yr later or next pregnancy #4, 1 yr later or next pregnancy #5. Safe but not recommended in first trimester.

Booster: WHO: 18 months to 6 yr. United States: 18 months, 4 to 6 yr, 10 to 12 yr, every 10 yr up to age 65 yr. After injury if ≥ 10 yr.

Cold Chain: 2°C to 8°C never frozen, will precipitate. Maintains potency at room temperature for 1 year. Passive immunization with human tetanus immune globulin (HTIG) should be given for those incompletely immunized with tetanus-prone wound.

Polio Vaccine

Disease: Polio

Indications: Routine childhood immunization; booster in travelers to at-risk areas (Africa and S. Asia).

Immunogenicity/Efficacy: Oral vaccine (live virus) OPV 95% to 100%. Inactivated injectable 97% to 100%.

Side Effects: Oral; rare vaccine-associated paralysis $2/10^6$. Injectable; minor local reactions.

Contraindications: IM: allergy to neomycin or polymyxin B. Oral: congenital immunodeficiency.

Dosage and Schedules: Oral: 0, 6, 10, 14 wk, 2 drops. Injectable IM: 0.5 ml, 2, 4, 12 to 18 months, 4 to 6 yr.

Booster: Travelers; endemic countries, OPV, during eradication drives.

Cold Chain: Oral: 2°C to 8°C freeze for long-term storage. Injectable: 2°C to 8°C.

Measles Vaccine

Diseases: *Rubeola*; often given as measles, mumps, rubella vaccine (MMR).

Indications: Routine childhood immunization; anyone without history of disease or born after 1956.

Immunogenicity/Efficacy: Live attenuated > 95% after 2 doses.

Side Effects: Fever 5–15%, rash 5%. Rubella component in MMR may cause arthralgias in 10% to 25% postpubertal females. Mumps component rarely causes parotitis and aseptic meningitis.

Contraindications: Pregnancy, severe immune deficiency (not HIV infection). Not with immune globulins.

Dosage and Schedules: Subcutaneous 0.5 ml; also see chapter 20, measles. WHO: 12 to 15 months and second dose later.

Booster: Second dose required.

Cold Chain: Frozen for long-term storage; 2°C to 8°C after reconstitution. Special diluent must be used.

Hemophilus B Vaccine

Diseases: *Hemophilus influenzae* type B

Indications: Routine childhood.

Immunogenicity/Efficacy: Conjugate-diphtheria protein > 95%.

Side Effects: Minor local, fever 2% to 10%.

Contraindications: Hypersensitivity to vaccine or diphtheria vaccine.

Dosage and Schedules: WHO: IM, 0.5 ml: 6, 10, 14 wk. US: 2, 4, 6 months.

Booster: WHO: none. US: 15 to 71 months once.

Cold Chain: 2°C to 8°C never frozen.

Hepatitis A Vaccine

(MMWR 2006;55:1)

Diseases: Hepatitis A

Indications: Routine childhood immunization in US; travelers to developing countries; anyone with preexisting liver disease.

Immunogenicity/Efficacy: Formalin-inactivated virus 95% to 100%.

Side Effects: Minor local reactions.

Contraindications: None.

Dosage and Schedules: IM, 0.5 ml at 0 and 6 to 12 months. May be given simultaneously with immune globulin (different site).

Booster: None.

Cold Chain: 2°C to 8°C.

Hepatitis B Vaccine

(N Engl J Med 1997;336:196)

Diseases: Hepatitis B

Indications: Routine childhood immunization in most areas.
   Adults: high-risk travelers, healthcare workers, liver disease.

Immunogenicity/Efficacy: Recombinant vaccine; 90% to 95% efficacy after 3 doses.

Side Effects: Minor local reactions.

Contraindications: None.

Dosage and Schedules: IM, 0.5 ml at 0, 1, 6 to 12 months. WHO: 6, 10, 14 wk or birth, 10, 14 wk.

Booster: None recommended.

Cold Chain: 2°C to 8°C, never frozen.

Hepatitis E Vaccine

(N Engl J Med 2007;356:895)

Diseases: Hepatitis E virus

Indications: New vaccine, not commercially available in 2008. Exposure to poor sanitation, uncooked pork products. Travel to S. Asia, Central Asia, NW China.

Immunogenicity/Efficacy: Killed recombinant protein absorbed to aluminum hydroxide; 96% efficacy.

Side Effects: Similar to placebo, pain (82%), redness (24%), swelling (20%) injection site.

Contraindications: Not determined.

Dosage and Schedules: 3 doses, IM, 0.5 ml at 0, 1, 6 months.

Booster: Unknown.

Cold Chain: Unknown.

Meningococcal Vaccine

(J Infect Developing Countries 2007;1:129)

Disease: Acute bacterial infection with meningitis, high morbidity, and mortality; rare in travelers.

Indication: Travel to Sahel (sub-Saharan Africa) or areas with known epidemics where attack rates may reach 1%; check with Centers for Disease Control and Prevention (CDC; 404-332-4559; Meningitis Belt, Lancet 2007;7:797); also consider in patients with splenectomy. Travel to Saudi Arabia.

Vaccine: Quadrivalent single dose vaccine serogroup A, C, Y, W135; purified capsular polysaccharide; no vaccine for serotype B; antibiotic prophylaxis for unimmunized close contacts of infectious cases; no benefit at age < 2. Conjugated meningococcal vaccines may be more effective.

Immunogenicity/Efficacy: Protective efficacy of 70% to 100% for groups A, C; unknown for Y, W135, though both are immunogenic.

Side Effects: Infrequent and mild, localized pain, 1% to 2% mild fever.

Contraindications: Allergic reactions to prior doses (contains thiomersal); category C in pregnancy.

Dosage: Single IM dose.

Booster: Every 3 to 5 yr for adults; revaccinate 2 to 3 yr for children < 4 for polysaccharide; probably same for conjugate but unclear.

Prevent: People-to-people exposure makes prevention difficult; antibiotic prophylaxis (ciprofloxacin 500 mg once, rifampin 300 mg bid × 2 d, or ceftriaxone 125 mg once).

Vaccine: Conjugate serotype A and other combinations available in other countries.

Yellow Fever Vaccine

Disease: Mosquito-borne flavivirus

Indications: Travel to endemic areas in South America and sub-Saharan Africa, also may be required for entry into certain countries in Asia, South America, and Pacific when leaving endemic areas. Check with respective embassy for current details. Must be received at special centers and International Certificate of Vaccination or Prophylaxis (ICVP) required for entry.

Vaccine: Live attenuated virus.

Immunogenicity: ICVP valid 10 d after immunization, > 98%.

Side Effects: Rare, few with low fever. Vaccine associated viscerotropic spread reported.

Contraindications: Pregnancy, egg allergy, active AIDS, immunosuppressed, chronic steroid Rx > 10 mg/d, infants < 9 months old.

Dosage: Single dose 0.5 ml subcutaneous (SQ).

Booster: Every 10 yr, but immunity probably lifelong.

Japanese B Encephalitis Vaccine

(Lancet 1996;348:341)

Disease: Mosquito-borne flavivirus endemic in rural Asia, especially near pig farming areas with associated rice paddies. Most infections asymptomatic (inapparent:apparent disease = 300:1) but serious encephalitis/deaths in up to 40% of symptomatic cases; seasonal transmission.

Indications: Travelers to rural Asia with prolonged (> 1 month) unprotected outdoor activity, especially in summer and autumn in endemic areas with extensive mosquito contact. Disease in travelers is rare (< 2 cases/yr in US travelers/military personnel), and allergic side effects of vaccine make judicious use of vaccine appropriate, especially in persons with multiple allergies.

Vaccine: Formalin inactivated mouse brain derived vaccine JE-VAX: dose adults 1 ml, 3 shot series, 2 doses 1 wk apart gives reasonable short-term protection. A live attenuated vaccine is in use in China.

Immunogenicity/Efficacy: 100% seroconversion by third dose; 80% at second dose.

Risk of Japanese B Encephalitis

Common and Widespread

Bangladesh	Monsoon season	July–December usually
Cambodia	Monsoon season	
India	Monsoon season	(not at high altitude)
Indonesia	Monsoon season	November–March
Laos	May–October	
Malaysia	May–October	
Myanmar	May–October	
Nepal	July–December	(not at high altitude)
Pakistan	June–January	(lowland delta)
P. R. China	April–October	(rural areas)
Philippines	April–January	
Sri Lanka	October–January	(not at high altitude)
	May–June	
Taiwan	April–October	
Thailand	May–October	
Vietnam	May–October	

Sporadic in Australia (Torres Strait and Cape York), Brunei, Hong Kong, Japan, Korea, Papua New Guinea, Russia, and Singapore.

Japanese Encephalitis Vaccine

Doses	Subcutaneous Route (ml)		Comments
	1–2 years of age	≥ 3 years of age	
Primary series 1, 2, and 3	0.5	1.0	Days 0, 7, 30
Booster*	1.0	1.0	1 dose at ≥ 36 months

*In vaccinees who have completed a 3-dose primary series, the full duration of protection is unknown; therefore, definitive recommendations cannot be given. Adapted from Health Information for International Travel, CDC.

Dosage: <1 year not advised, 1–3 years 0.5 ml, >3 years 1.0 ml

Booster: Every 3 yr.

Side Effects:

- Allergic reactions including urticaria 0.5%, local systemic side effects 20%, anaphylaxis can occur.
- Observe for 30 min after immunization; risk of reaction increases with allergy history; in US Marine Corps, reaction rate = 26/10 000 vaccines; 2/3 were urticaria/angioedema; 1/3 were pruritus alone.
- Median time to reaction is < 48 hr dose 1, 96 hr dose 2 (CID 1997;24:265).

Contraindications: Allergic reaction to prior dose; not recommended in pregnancy.

Cold Chain: 2°C to 8°C.

Rabies Vaccine (Pre-exposure)

(N Engl J Med 1993;329:1288)

Disease: An acute fatal viral encephalomyelitis endemic worldwide but with increased risk in South and Central America and parts of Asia and Africa.

Vaccine:

- Pre-exposure vaccination with human diploid cell rabies vaccine (HDCV), purified chick embryo cell vaccine (PCEC), or rabies vaccine adsorbed (RVA).
- Pre-exposure immunization consists of 3 doses of HDCV, PCEC, or RVA, 1.0 ml IM (deltoid area), 1 each on d 0, 7, or 28; only HDCV may be administered by the id dose/route (0.1 ml id on d 0, 7, and 21 or 28).
- The 3-dose HDCV series must be completed before antimalarials are begun if the traveler will be taking chloroquine or mefloquine for malaria chemoprophylaxis; if this is not possible, the IM dose/route should be used.

- Administration of routine booster doses of vaccine depends on exposure risk category.
- Pre-exposure immunization of immunosuppressed persons is not recommended.

Indications: Long-term travelers to endemic areas especially children, those with outdoor occupations, cave explorers, adventure traveling to remote endemic areas; key considerations are duration and remoteness of trip and expected availability of postexposure treatment in the event of exposure. Note that rabies immune globulin is often hard to obtain in many developing countries, which is a key rationale for pre-exposure vaccination (J Travel Med 1999;6:238).

Immunogenicity/Efficacy: 100% antibody formation.

Booster: Often every 2 yr, but check antibody level every yr; if > 30 international units (IU), probably immune for long time. If < 30 IU, will require regular boosting to keep level > 0.5 IU. An alternative more cost-effective approach: boost all at yr 1 and check antibody level 2 wk later. If > 30 IU, no further boosting needed for 20 yr. If < 30 IU, retest in 3 yr (Vaccine 2001;19:1416).

Side Effects: Pain, erythema, itching 3% to 5%, mild systemic symptoms rarely; boosters, 6% type 1 or 3 reaction with repeat use HDCV; can substitute different vaccine in this event.

Prev:

- Travelers must understand need for 2 doses postexposure vaccine in event of bite despite use of pre-exposure regimen; however, immune globulin will not be needed if pre-exposure prophylaxis has been given.
- If rabies exposure overseas, check with embassy regarding reliable source of prescription.
- Note that equine rabies immune globulin is only type available in some countries and can cause serum sickness in 1% and anaphylaxis in 1/40 000.

Typhoid Vaccines

(N Engl J Med 2007;357:11)

Disease: *Salmonella enterica serovar Typhi (S typhi).* 16 to 23 million cases annually, half million deaths (WHO).

Indications: Exposure to poor sanitation, primarily children. Especially S and SE Asia. IM ≥ 2 yr old, oral > 6 yr old.

Immunogenicity/Efficacy: Killed injectable (Vi polysaccharide) 70%; live attenuated oral Ty21a 53% to 96%.

Side Effects: Rare local IM, nausea oral.

Contraindication: Oral not when on antibiotics or proguanil, fever, or acute GI illness.

Dosage and Schedules for Typhoid Fever Vaccination

Vaccination	Age	Dose/Mode of Administration	Number of Doses	Interval Between Doses	Boosting Interval (yr)
Oral Live-Attenuated Ty21a Vaccine					
Primary series	≥ 6 yr	1 capsule*	4	48 hr	5
Vi Capsular Polysaccharide Vaccine					
Primary series	≥ 2 yr	0.5 ml IM	1	—	2
Heat-Phenol-Inactivated Parenteral Vaccine					
Primary series	6 months–10 yr	0.25 ml sc	2	≥ 4 wk	
	≥ 10 yr	0.50 ml sc	2	≥ 4 wk	3

*Administer with cool liquid no warmer than 37°C (98.6°F), 4 doses 1 hr before meals d 1, 3, 5, 7, one wk before exposure.

Common Adverse Reactions to Typhoid Fever Vaccines

| Vaccine | Reactions | | |
	Fever (%)	Headache (%)	Local Reactions
Ty21a*	0–5	0–5	Not applicable
ViCPS	0–1	1.5–3	Erythema or induration ≥ 1 cm: 7%
Parenteral inactivated	6.7–24	9–10	Severe local pain or swelling: 3%–35%

*The side effects of Ty21a are rare and mainly consist of abdominal discomfort, nausea, vomiting, and rash or urticaria. Adapted from Health Information for International Travel, CDC.

Cold Chain: Both 2°C to 8°C storage.

Tick-Borne Encephalitis Vaccine (not available in United States)

Disease: Arboviral encephalitis transmitted by *Ixodes* ticks (sheep ticks) in Eurasia; also by unpasteurized milk.

Indications: For travelers who anticipate extensive exposure to ticks in rural areas endemic for tick-borne encephalitis (ie, persons planning prolonged hiking trips or field biologists, etc.); risk is highly focal. Consult local authorities to assess.

Vaccine:

1. formaldehyde inactivated purified whole virus (FSME; Immune, Immune AG-Austria)
2. similar inactivated purified whole virus (Encepur, FSME vaccine Behring)
3. Russian vaccine, similar (Academy of Medical Sciences, Moscow)

For 1 and 2, give 3 doses; 2 approved for accelerated schedule (0, 7, 21 d).

Efficacy: Estimated at 90% to 95% after 3 doses.

Booster: Every 3 to 5 yr (boost at 12 to 18 months after accelerated schedule).

Side Effects: Local inflammation at injection site, flu-like reactions, allergic reactions.

Contraindications: Increased risk of anaphylaxis in patients prone to allergic reaction. Do not give during acute infections.

Pneumococcal Vaccine

Diseases: *Streptococcus pneumoniae* (Prevnar) types 4, 6B, 9V, 14, 18C, 19F, 23F

Indications: Routine childhood.

Immunogenicity/Efficacy: Conjugate-diphtheria protein protects only against serotypes in vaccine.

Efficacy: Otitis media ~50%.

Side Effects: Minor local, fever 6% to 25%.

Contraindications: Hypersensitivity to vaccine or diphtheria vaccine.

Dosage and Schedules: US: IM, 0.5 ml at 4, 6, 12 to 15 months (up to age 10).

Booster: None.

Cold Chain: 2°C to 8°C.

Cholera Vaccine, Oral (not available in United States)

Disease: Diarrhea caused by *Vibro cholerae*

Indications: Epidemics or anticipated epidemics (Vaccine 2004;22:2444). Not effective against V *cholerae* 0139.

Immunogenicity/Efficacy: Killed (Dukoral) 50% to 86%; parenteral not recommended; live attenuated CVD 103 (Orachol E) 60% to 90%.

Side Effects: Rare GI symptoms.

Contraindications: Live vaccine not advised in pregnancy or during or up to 7 d from antibiotics or immune deficiency. Neither vaccine under age 2, not during acute illness.

Dosage and Schedules:

Killed WC-r BS (Dukoral) Oral Cholera Vaccine	Live Attenuated CVD 103 Hg-R (Orochol E) Oral Cholera Vaccine
2–3 doses orally 10–14 d apart	One orally Not to be given with live typhoid vaccine (Vivotif)
Earliest protection > 20 d; for anticipated epidemics	8 d; for use in ongoing outbreaks

Booster: Yearly.

Cold Chain: 2°C to 8°C, stable 24 hr at 20°C to 25°C. Requires 100–150 ml safe water at time of administration.

Rotavirus Vaccine

(N Engl J Med 2006;354:11,23,75; Lancet 2007;370:302)

Disease: Diarrhea, especially children under 5, causing one-fourth of 1.9 million diarrheal deaths per yr. Risk of death from episode 1:293 (Emerg Infect Dis 2003;9:570).

Indications: Any infant under 12 to 14 wk of age.

Vaccine: RotaTeq pentavalent live oral: given first dose, 6 to 12 wk of age; second dose, 4 to 10 wk later; third dose, 4 to 10 wk later but < 32 wk. Rotarix monovalent live oral: given first dose 6 to 14 wk and second dose 4 wk later but < 24 wk.

Immunogenicity/Efficacy: RotaTeq 3 doses prevented 74% to 98% of mild to serious infections. Rotarix 2 doses 85% to 100% protection against mild to severe infections. Reduction in hospitalization rates for diarrhea of 40% to 60%.

Booster: None.

Side Effects: RotaTeq: diarrhea and vomiting 1% to 3%, Rotarix minor GI. Maximum age of immunization set to decrease risk of intussusception.

Contraindications: OK to immunize with ongoing diarrhea.

Prevention: Breast feeding, clean water, improved sanitation.

Cold Chain: 2°C to 8°C storage.

Cost: Expected to be $3 to $5 in low income countries with GAVI (Global Alliance for Vaccines and Immunizations) assistance.

Cervical Cancer (HPV) Vaccine

Disease: Cervical carcinoma, genital warts, other HPV related cancers, vulva, vagina. Protects against type 16 and 18 cancer and 6 and 11 warts or types 16 and 18 only (bivalent vaccine).

Indications: Adolescents and preadolescents currently not infected with HPV types in vaccine. Licensed US ages 9 to 26 yr.

Vaccines: Gardasil: types 6, 11, 16, 18 recombinant, 0.5 ml IM at 0, 2, 6 months. Types 16 and 18 (bivalent) 0.5 ml IM at 0, 1, 6 months.

Immunogenicity/Efficacy: 30 types of HPV sexually transmitted. Both vaccines 100% effective. Types of HPV vary depending on region, may require different formulations.

Booster: None.

Side Effects: Fever 10%, injection site pain 84%, swelling and redness 25%.

Contraindications: Immunosuppression decreases efficacy. Pregnancy: FDA class B, appears safe (N Engl J Med 2007;356:1915).

Prevention: Condoms, abstinence, one partner.

Cold Chain: 2°C to 8°C storage.

Cost: US dollars (USD) $120/dose.

Smallpox Vaccine

Diseases: Variola (smallpox) also monkeypox and vaccinia (cowpox).

Indications: Not generally available except to special groups such as military.

Immunogenicity/Efficacy: Live vaccinia virus, Dryvax, ACMA 2000; probably 100%.

Booster: Every 5 yr.

Side Effects: Myocarditis 5 to 10/1000, generalized vaccinia, post-vaccine encephalopathy.

Contraindications: Eczema, generalized skin disease, pregnancy, immunosuppressed.

Dosage and Schedules: Intradermal.

Cold Chain: Keep frozen.

Traveler's Diarrhea

(Am Fam Phys 2005;71:2095; Am Fam Phys 2005;72:2525)

Cause: Bacterial (*E coli–Campylobacter, Shigella, Salmonella* species–*Aeromonas*–Vibrios). Parasitic (*Giardia lamblia–Cyclospora, Cryptosporidium cayetonenis–Entamoeba histolytica*). Viral (rotavirus, norovirus, others).

Epidem: 40% to 50% of travelers affected with ≥ 3 loose stools a d with enteric symptoms. Higher risk if low gastric acidity (PPI/H_2 blocker use).

Pathophys: Toxins produced by organisms or direct invasion of bowel wall.

Sx: Diarrhea, fever, nausea, vomiting, cramping, tenesmus, bloody stools.

Si: Abdominal tenderness, hyperactive bowel sounds.

Crs: Usually self-limiting, lasting 3 to 5 d without treatment but varies by etiology; parasitic infections occur later but last longer (weeks).

Lab: Not usually available, but stool culture, antigen tests, and ova and parasites (O & P) examination helpful.

Rx: Prophylaxis with antibiotics not generally indicated, but quinolones are effective (Clin Infect Dis 2002;34:628). Bismuth subsalicylate is 60% effective; it interferes with absorption of doxycycline used for malaria prophylaxis. Dose is about 500 mg 4 times a d. Rifaximin has been useful (> 50% reduction of diarrhea) in Mexico (Ann Intern Med 2005;142:805).

Treatment is disease specific or empiric. When significant diarrhea occurs, increase fluids, start loperide 4 mg with 2 mg after each loose stool (maximum 8 mg/d). Use oral rehydration salts if significant dehydration ensues. Antibiotic choices are region and suspected pathogen specific:

Mexico	rifaximin 200 mg 3×/d for 3 d or ciprofloxacin
Thailand	azithromycin 1000 mg once children 10 mg/kg/d for 3 d
Other areas	ciprofloxacin 500 mg 2×/d for 1–3 d other quinolones effective nalidixic acid 250 mg 4×1 d for 1–3 d
Prolonged symptoms (giardia)	metronidazole 250 mg 3×/d for 5 d or tinidazole 2 grams once

Children and pregnancy: do not use quinolones or bismuth, rifaximin category C, not under age 12.

5.5 Epidemiology

Most of us enjoy treating individual patients or communities. But real progress in morbidity and mortality statistics is made by treating populations, especially in developing countries.

In order to understand and find solutions to public health problems, you need to understand the language. A few key terms used in this book are given below.

Definitions

- *Incidence*: number of new cases of disease/time in a population at risk.
- *Population at risk*: defined group such as children under 5.
- *Prevalence*: number of existing cases in a population at risk at a given point in time.
- *Case fatality*: No. deaths from disease/no. people with disease × 100.

$$\text{Infant mortality rate} = \frac{\text{no. deaths live born infants} < 1 \text{ yr age}}{\text{total \# live births in that yr}} \times 1000$$

$$\text{Child mortality rate} = \frac{\text{no. deaths children 1 to 4 yr}}{\text{total \# children 1 to 4 yr}} \times 1000$$

$$\text{Perinatal mortality rate} = \frac{\text{no. deaths live born infants} < 7 \text{ d age}}{\substack{\text{total \# live births plus} \\ \text{\# fetal deaths} \\ \text{(gestation} \geq 28 \text{ wk) in that yr}}} \times 1000$$

$$\text{Neonatal mortality rate} = \frac{\text{no. deaths infants 0–28 d}}{\text{total no. live births in that yr}}$$

$$\text{Maternal mortality ratio} = \frac{\substack{\text{no. maternal deaths from puerperal} \\ \text{causes within 6 wk postpartum}}}{\text{no. live births in that yr}}$$

- Interpartum case fatality rate (used for births within health facilities = late stillbirths and early (< 24 hr) neonatal deaths/ total deliveries (Lancet 2007;370:1310).

- Puerperal death causes range from ruptured ectopics to postpartum venous thrombosis. Aspiration pneumonia due to eclampsia is a maternal death; the death of a pregnant woman from pneumococcal pneumonia in her third month of pregnancy is not.
- Number live births is used in place of no. deliveries as it is more readily available. Lancet (2007;370:1311) lists individual country maternal mortality ratios.

- Relative risk (risk ratio) = $\dfrac{\text{risk of occurrence of disease among exposed}}{\text{risk in unexposed}}$

- *Confidence interval*: bounds about a population mean in which a value is likely to lie, usually with 95% confidence. Example RR = 5.1 (CI 4.3–6.4) 95%.
- *Primary prevention*: limit incidence of disease by prevention. Example: Penicillin given to children with streptococcal sore throats helps prevent acute rheumatic fever (ARF).
- *Secondary prevention*: reduce complications of disease by early diagnosis and treatment. Example: Children who have had ARF should be registered and receive benzathine penicillin monthly.
- *Tertiary prevention*: reduce the effects or complications of existing disease. Example: Patients with rheumatic heart disease should have access to valve replacement.

Screening

Before instituting any screening program, it is important to consider a number of requirements:

- The disease should be relatively common.
- There should be a long lead time between a positive screening test and overt disease.
- It should be serious if not identified early.

- It must be treatable within the economic means and functional ability of the health system.
- The screening test should be simple, safe, reliable, and acceptable.
- Cost-effectiveness is important.
- Early identification and treatment should reduce morbidity or mortality.
- Reliability of a test is measured by sensitivity and specificity.
- Sensitivity: percent of people with a disease who are correctly identified with a positive test result.
- Specificity: percent of people without disease with a negative test result.

A 2 × 2 table is used to determine the validity of a screening test.

Disease Status

		present	absent
Test Results	positive	a	b
	negative	c	d

Sensitivity = a/(a + c);

Specificity = d/(b + d) Positive predictive value of a test = a/(a + b) = PPV, Negative predictive value of a test = d/(c + d) = NPV. As disease prevalence increases, the sensitivity of a test increases. If you increase the sensitivity of a test, you will decrease specificity.

Commonly used screening tests include HIV testing for blood donors and blood pressure (BP) determination on pregnant women attending antenatal clinic.

A useful concept is the number needed to treat (or test; NNT).

$$NNT = \cfrac{1}{\begin{array}{c}\text{Probability of bad} \\ \text{outcome in control} \\ \text{group}\end{array} - \begin{array}{c}\text{Probability of bad} \\ \text{outcome in treatment} \\ \text{(tested) group}\end{array}}$$

Surveillance

A crucial component of public health activities, surveillance of disease is the responsibility of every clinician. Used for the following:

- recognizing epidemics: example, malaria passive case detection through blood slides on all febrile patients
- maintaining disease registries; rheumatic fever, TB, leprosy
- evaluating control programs; reporting of immunization-preventable diseases
- evaluating health services; monitoring maternal deaths
- targeting health resources

Practical Applications

Immunization coverage is the % of children who have received their complete set of immunizations by a certain age.

WHO coverage includes BCG, 3 doses of diphtheria-tetanus-pertussis vaccine (DTP3), 3 doses polio (Pol3), 3 doses hepatitis B (HepB3), and 1 measles vaccine (MCV). The time period is usually 1 yr of age. Maternal tetanus toxoid and Vitamin A deficiency elimination programs are often monitored by the local MCH team. Other vaccine markers monitored may include DTP1 and Hib3, BCG 1. Each health facility where vaccines are stored and administered should have an immunization coverage chart to monitor their progress on each vaccine goal. An Immunization Monitoring Chart is shown in Figure 5.3.

Blank monitoring chart

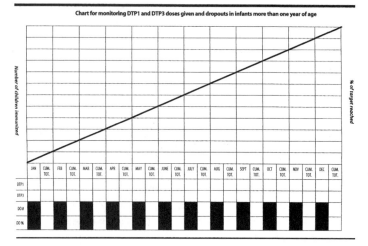

Figure 5.3 Immunization Monitoring Chart. Reproduced with permission of World Health Organization. Immunization in Practice. Chapter 7, page 6.

- number of children under age 1 from the national census adjusted yearly by birth rate minus infant mortality rate
- number of vaccines by adding each month's total of the final vaccine in the series, such as DTP3, administered to infants under 1 yr of age
- ≥ 90% coverage at year's end is a reasonable goal

5.6 Vector Control

Phlebotomine Sand Flies

Agents: *Phlebotomus sp:* old world; *Lutzomyia sp:* new world.

Identification: Small, hairy, 1.5 to 3.5 mm long, hopping movement, hold pointed wings up in a "V" shape. Females require blood for egg production, cutting into skin, drawing visible blood.

Diseases: Leishmaniasis, bartonellosis, sandfly fever.

Ecology: 0 to 2800 m elevation, deserts to rainforest. New world, especially forests. Old world savannahs and urban. Usually night feeders.

Reservoir: Leishmaniasis: rodents, dog, sloth.

Control: Difficult.

- Diethyltoluamide (DEET) for personal protection.
- Residual insecticide spraying of households (some dichloro-diphenyl-trichloroethane [DDT] resistance).
- Untreated bed nets not effective as mesh too large, require fine mesh.
- Window screens not effective due to large mesh.
- Local control of rodents may help.
- Some forest species will not cross open cleared areas around houses.

Mosquitoes

Agents: *Anopheles sp*. Each species has an ecological niche that must be considered in control measures.

A. *gambiae,* A. *arabiensis,* and A. *funestus* important in Africa; A. *albimanus* in Americas; A. *minimus* in SE Asia.

Identification: Specialist needed to identify but in general, spotted wings; hum in flight, difficult to hear. Most rest with proboscis-head-abdomen in straight line at 45° resting upright. Females use blood meal to produce eggs.

Diseases: Malaria, Filariasis (*Wuchereria bancrofti, Brugia timori*), Ross River, O'nyong-nyong, Semliki, Sinbis, VEE, WEE, and other viruses.

Ecology: Night feeders; breed in fresh or brackish water. Some rest in houses after feeding, making them susceptible to residual insecticides, but others have changed biting habits and/or developed insecticide resistance.

Agents: *Culex sp.*
C. pipiens subspecies and *C. quinque fasciatus*. Prefer man and breed domestically; painful bites.

Identification: Specialized; lay eggs to form rafts (other genus lay individual eggs, rest horizontal to surface).

Diseases: *W. bancrofti*, Japanese B, Murray Valley, W. Nile, EEE, WEE, StLE encephalitis, Rift valley fever.

Reservoir: Pigs (JBE), birds for encephalitis, livestock (RVF).

Ecology: Domestic, breeds in polluted waters, rubbish, same as *Aedes aegypti*; may rest indoors during day.

Agents: *Aedes sp.*, *Ae. aegypti* worldwide.

Identification: Specialist required; rest horizontal to surface.

Diseases: Arboviruses: Dengue, Yellow Fever, Chikungunya, Filariasis (*Brugia malayi, W. bancrofti*), Rift Valley fever, Ross River Fever.

Ecology: Mostly seasonal breeders where flooding occurs (monsoons). Important species breed in small water containers, flower pots, rubbish, coconut shells, plant anils (banana). Often day feeders, occasionally nocturnal. May transfer viruses transovarially, from mother to progeny via eggs. Usually limited flight distance.

Reservoir: Monkey for yellow fever, cattle for Rift Valley fever.

Agents: *Mansonia sp.*

Identification: Specialist; egg masses under floating leaves.

Diseases: *W. bancrofti* and *B. malayi*

Ecology: Day (but not in sun) and night feeders (rest outdoors); painful bites.

Reservoir: Leaf monkey, *B. malayi*

Mosquito Control:

- Use DEET for personal protection.
- Treat bed nets, curtains, and window screens.
- Spray residual DDT in homes; safe and effective if species is sensitive to insecticide, and habits include indoor resting after feeding. Other insecticides used include the organophosphates (malathion), organochlorines, carbamates (propoxur), and pyrethroids (permethrin, deltamethrin). Indoor spraying, properly done, avoids most environmental damage. DDT lasts 6 months, other insecticides less. Residual spraying also kills sand flies, house flies, bed bugs, cockroaches, fleas, ticks, and triatomine bugs. A comprehensive monitoring system is necessary for success (Am J Trop Med Hyg 2007;76:1027).
- Treat mosquito nets every 6 months with pyrethroids or lifetime treatment (5 yr) when manufactured (Am J Trop Med Hyg 2003:68, issue on bed net trial in Kenya).
- Toxorhynchites mosquito larvae, predators on other mosquito larvae, in water containers.
- Add temephos to potable water containers.
- Float polystyrene beads in cisterns and pit latrines (Culex larvae).
- Eliminate breeding sites; cover water containers, burn rubbish (especially coconut shells, tires, tin cans), and drain swamps.
- Spray breeding areas with oil, detergents, or biofilms.
- Use insecticidal fogging during evening flights.
- Use larvivorous fish such as *Gambusia affinis* in ponds and cisterns or *Bacillus thuringiensis*, a larvicide, for biological control.
- Repel mosquitoes with certain plants (*Lantana sp. Verbenaceae*; Am J Trop Med Hyg 2002;67:191).

Houseflies

Agents: *Musca domestica* (common housefly), *Muscina stabulans*, *Fannia sp.*, *Stomoxys calcitrans* (blood sucking stable fly).

Diseases: Various bacterial and protozoan diseases especially agents of diarrhea. Trachoma; Protozoa, cestode, and nematode eggs.

Ecology: Breed on excreta, decaying animal and vegetable matter.

Control: Highly resistant to many insecticides.

- deny feeding sites, screen latrines
- sticky traps
- pyrethrin sprays and mists
- paradichlorobenzene (mothballs) 60 gm in garbage cans
- residual insecticide spraying

Triatomine Bugs

Agents: *Triatoma sp.*, *Panstrongylus sp.*, *Rhodnius sp.*; cone nose, assassin, kissing bugs, vinchucas, barbeiros.

Diseases: Chagas' disease.

Ecology: SW United States through S America. Live in cracks in mud houses, chicken houses, peridomestic animal burrows; long lived, up to 2 yr; night biters.

Reservoir: Domestic animals.

Control:

- plaster cracks in wall
- residual insecticide spraying
- beta-cypermethrin impregnated fabric under mattress or roof (Am J Public Health 1999;6:1)

Tsetse Flies

Agents: *Glossina sp.*

       G morsitans group (savannah—E and Central Africa)

       G palpatis group (riverine, W and Central Africa)

Diseases: Trypanosomiasis

Identification: Saber-like proboscis; fold wings scissor like; 7 to 13 mm in size.

Ecology: Tropical Africa in vegetation bordering savannahs or rivers and streams 14°N to 29°S. Rapid flyers; day biters.

Reservoir: Game animals; domestic ungulates (E African); man (W African).

Control:

- residual insecticide sprayed on river-line vegetation
- aerial spraying
- trapping with deltamethrin-impregnated traps
- clear vegetation from river banks
- personal repellents, DEET
- attraction to wood fires and light clothing

Black Flies

Agents: *Simulium sp.*

Diseases: Onchocerciasis

Identification: Small 3.5 mm; clear wings.

Ecology: Live near clear fast-moving streams; day biters. In Africa, prefer biting legs; in C America, head. Seldom enter houses.

Control: Aquatic insecticides such as methoxychlor or temephos (Abate), some resistance.

- DEET less effective
- avoid rivers
- cover skin

Deer Flies

Agents: *Chrysops sp.*

Identification: Only females take blood meals; large 8 to 12 mm.

Diseases: Loa loa, occasionally tularemia.

Ecology: Usually day feeders; painful bites, often several from one encounter. W and Central Africa rainforests, around water sources. Bites usually below knee. Seldom enter houses.

Control: Breeding sites treatment is not possible. Use DEET for personal protection.

Fleas

Agents: *Xenopsylla cheopis* and *X. sp.* (rat fleas).

 Pulex irritans and *Pulex sp.* (man, domestic animals) and others.

Identification: Small, wingless, flat shaped; blood feeders.

Diseases: Plague, murine typhus.

Ecology: Indiscriminate feeders; can live long periods between feeding.

Reservoir: Rodents, mice, domestic animals.

Control:

- insecticide dusts to rodent areas and pets (pyrethrum safe)
- dichlorvos pet collars
- DEET
- flea control before killing/removing preferred host

Lice

Agents: *Pediculus humanus corporis*, *capitis*, and *Pthirus pubis*. Only *P. corporis* transmits diseases.

Identification: Usually by location, body, scalp, and pubic areas.

Disease: Epidemic typhus, trench fever, relapsing fever.

Ecology: Man to man transmission; lice feces infective spread by contact with broken skin, aerosols, or eating nits.

Reservoir: Man.

Control:

- body lice, launder clothing
- residual insecticides (1% lindane, 1% malathion, 10% DDT, others)

- head lice 0.5% malathion, 0.5% carbaryl, 1% lindane (resistance common); remove nits
- pubic lice same as head, may be found in other areas including eyelashes (manual removal)

Chiggers

Agents: *Eutrombicula sp.*, *Leptotrombidium sp.*

Identification: ≤ 1 mm often bright colors.

Disease: Dermatitis, scrub typhus (*Leptotrombidium sp.*)

Ecology: Rare in Africa but found elsewhere. Bites cause reaction noted hours later as pruritis, sometimes with ecchymoses; usually at ankles and legs; where tight clothing, blocks migration, elastic garments. Scrub typhus from India and Himalayas eastward to Oceania. Often localized to a limited area, especially cleared areas, meadows, trails. No skin reaction with scrub typhus vectors.

Reservoir: Rats, small mammals.

Control:
- personal protection, insecticide-treated clothing, DEET
- area cleared of vegetation and mammals

Ticks

Agents: *Ornithodoros sp.* (soft)
Idodes sp., *Demacentor sp.*, *Hyalomma sp.*, *Amblyomma sp.*, and others.

Identification: Expert or field guides.

Diseases: Soft: relapsing fever. Hard: Colorado tick fever, Rocky Mountain fever, tularemia, many others.

Ecology: Household dirt floors and animal shelters for soft ticks; bush, forests.

Control:

- personal protection, DEET; tuck pant legs into stockings
- personal inspection and prompt removal
- permethrins

Chapter 6

Pharmacology

6.1 Model Formularies

The WHO has published a model formulary listing commonly used medications, vaccines, diagnostic agents, and antiseptics. This is available in several languages in a pocketbook, a CD-ROM format, and online at http://www.who.int/medicines/. It includes the standard treatment of common illnesses, drug indications and contraindications, warnings for pregnancy and breastfeeding, and dosage. Drug names are in the British system, and American readers may have a few problems finding common medications.

For instance:

paracetamol = acetaminophen
salbutamol = albuterol
oxytocin = pitocin
methergine (methylergonovine) is used as ergometrine

Drug choices are limited to generics, and some medications are unavailable in the United States. Single dose regimes are preferred to improve compliance. Medical workers on long-term assignments overseas should consider purchasing a copy.

National governments may have their own formulary, often more proscribed than WHO's formulary. Some countries classify drugs by tiers: tier 1 drugs for lower level health workers in primary care health centers; tier 2 drugs for medical officers in district hospitals; and tier 3 drugs with limited distribution to larger hospitals and prescribed only by specialists.

Rational prescribing in developing countries with limited resources requires the following:

- Follow the national formulary.
- Avoid prescribing trade name drugs.
- Keep the number of drugs to a minimum.
- Inquire if the patient can afford to purchase the medications.
- Limit dosing to twice a d or once if possible.
- Communicate with the patient the importance of compliance and finishing the medication.
- Be certain to explain that chronic medications must be taken for a long time and not stopped once the bottle is empty.
- Do not give out large quantities of medications, rather require refills.
- Have the patient carry their medicines to each clinic visit to count pills and verify compliance.
- Consider costs and availability.
- Suggest a reliable provider of medications to insure potency and cost.
- Be sure the patient keeps the medications safely away from children.

6.2   Counterfeit Medications

Fraudulently mislabeled or substandard (inaccurate potency, formulation, or substitution) medicines are a growing problem throughout the world. An estimated $35 billion USD industry, the WHO estimates that 6% to 10% of the world drug market is in counterfeit medicines. Most of us have been spammed with ads for inexpensive Viagra. But, the risks are much higher with fake antimalarial medication (Lancet 2001;357:1948; 2003;362:169).

More than half of all counterfeit medications appear in developing countries, especially SE Asia, where a poorly regulated private health sector exists. In these areas, up to 25% of medications are substandard or fake. The rural poor are most at risk, but there is little to protect the hospital pharmacy from being duped.

Counterfeiters are sophisticated, and many fakes resemble the authentic medication complete with bogus packet holograms and low concentrations of the active drug to subvert unsophisticated testing methods. Artesunate has been a recent target (50% counterfeit in SE Asia) as has human albumin.

Health providers need to be vigilant for the use of counterfeit medications. The treatment failure of a malaria patient could be drug resistance or the use of a substandard drug treatment.

The WHO has a Rapid Alert System to track counterfeit drugs based in their Manila office (http://wpro.who.int).

6.3   Outdated Drugs

Drugs manufactured or distributed in western countries are marked with an expiratory date. These dates are prominently stamped on the bottles or sample packets.

Little is known about the strength, potency, and toxicity of out-of-date drugs for there is little impetus for research on the topic. A Fanconi-like syndrome of vomiting, acidosis, polyuria, glycosuria, and aminoaciduria has been reported with outdated tetracycline. Penicillin G and co-trimoxazole have been reported to lose ~10% of their activity after 90 d at field conditions with temperatures up to 40°C. But no "essential" drug lost > 30% potency after 2 y (Am J Trop Med Hyg 1997;57:31).

Never donate, carry overseas, or distribute outdated drugs. It is usually illegal and potentially dangerous.

Chapter 7
Laboratory

7.1 Using the Laboratory

Laboratory testing is usually available at the district hospital level and occasionally at smaller health facilities. Because most tests are done manually, they take considerable time and trained personnel. Make wise use of laboratory resources and never order tests that are unnecessary or of marginal value. Emergency (or STAT) testing should be kept to a minimum, and such requests are best received and acted upon when accompanied by a personal visit to the laboratory.

This chapter is to help you learn how to conduct your own laboratory examinations when laboratory technicians are unavailable.

7.2 Urinalysis

Urinalysis should be done as soon as possible on a fresh clean catch sample. Often it is easier to obtain the sample by catheterization yourself while conducting a physical examination. Never wait longer than 2 hr to examine unrefrigerated samples or 4 hr for refrigerated urines. Casts and cells will disintegrate.

Note the color:

- pale: dilute
- orange: bilirubin, rifampin, and yellow fruits/vegetables
- green: pseudomonas, biliverdin, kava ingestion

- red/pink: blood, hemoglobin, myoglobin, porphyrins, foods such as beet root
- brown/black: melanin, phenol poisoning, methyldopa, levodopa

Clarity:

- clear: normal
- turbid: cells and casts, bacteria, phosphates (pH > 7, white); urates (pH < 7, pink); mucus
- white: fats

Odor:

- ammonia: bacterial breakdown of urea
- foul: UTI
- fruity: ketones
- fecal: fistula

Foam when shaken:

- small amount: normal
- large amount: protein
- yellow: bilirubin

Specific gravity (SG) may be determined by a urinometer, a refractometer, or reagent test strips. Normal is 1.003 to 1.035. A diseased kidney cannot concentrate urine, and SG approaches 1.010, the SG of plasma. With 12 hr of fluid restriction, the SG should be > 1.020 with normal renal function. A SG > 1.035 usually denotes radiographic media in the urine.

Urine dipsticks are available, and the instructions on the package insert explain their use and false positive and negative results. When strips are not available, several tests can be carried out in a basic laboratory.

Urinary protein (Table 7.1):

- dissolve 70.0 g 5-sulfosalicylic acid in 1 L distilled water
- add 3 ml of the 7% solution to 11 ml centrifuged urine
- mix by inverting twice

Table 7.1   Urine Protein

Result	Protein Concentration mg/dL
clear	< 5
trace turbidity	5–20
1+ milky	30
2+ turbidity milky with granulations	100
3+ turbidity with flocculation	300–500
4+ clumps of precipitate or solid	> 500

If 4+, dilute urine with water 1:1, 1:2, etc, and retest.

- wait 10 min
- mix twice and read against a black background

False positives: radiographic media, high levels penicillin, sulfa drugs, cephalosporins, tolbutamide, tolmetin; these form crystals and not amorphous precipitates.

False negative: highly-buffered alkaline urine. Acidify with HCl and retest.

Reducing sugars can be detected using the copper reduction test. Copper sulfate plus sugar plus alkali (sodium hydroxide) yields a colored solution, which can be read off a scale in the package insert. Besides glucose, a number of other sugars yield a positive result. Commercial tablets are available. Or, you could use ants, which are attracted to urine containing sugar.

Commercial tablet tests are also available for testing of ketones (in urine or blood) and bilirubin. Package inserts offer instructions. Ketones in plasma are useful in monitoring diabetic ketoacidosis; dilutions should be made to quantify the level of ketones.

Microscopic Analysis

A centrifuge is helpful, and a microscope with magnification up to 400× is necessary.

Unspun urine can be examined for bacteria. A single bacteria seen at high power field (HPF) suggests a UTI:

- centrifuge 10 ml urine for 5 min
- set up the microscope while waiting; put the condenser down 1 to 2 mm from the stage; close the diaphragm as necessary to provide contrast
- discard the supernatant
- resuspend the sediment by striking the test tube several times against a hard surface
- place 1 drop on a slide and apply a cover strip
- examine 10 to 15 fields at each power. Low power field (LPF) = 100×, HPF = 400×. Casts are recorded as /LPF; white blood cells (WBC) and red blood cells (RBC) as #/HPF.
- methylene blue stain 1% is a useful counterstain

Red Cells

Biconcave discs, orange-yellow, 7 μm in size. They may appear shrunken and crenated in hypertonic urines. Dysmorphic RBCs are usually of glomerular origin. Hematuria is defined as > 5 RBC/HPF. Sickled RBCs are occasionally seen.

White Blood Cells

Twice the size of RBCs, polymorphonucleocytes have a granular cytoplasm and discrete multilobed nucleus. Degenerate quickly. May "glitter" in dilute urine due to Brownian motion of cytoplasmic granules.

Eosinophils are typically larger with a bilobed nucleus. Seen in drug hypersensitivity. Wright's stain will color the granules red.

Epithelial cells can be differentiated into 3 types.

Squamous cells originate from the trigone and urethra to the vaginal/penile mucosa. Large 30–50 μm with irregular smooth cell wall and a nucleus the size of a RBC. Easily seen under LPF. A clue cell is a squamous epithelial cell covered with coccobacilli and indicative of *Gardnerella vaginalis* vaginitis. The clue cell has a granular appearance and shaggy cell borders. Transitional epithelial cells are large (20–30 μm) with a nucleus the size of a RBC. They are increased in bladder inflammation, infection, and after catheterization. Renal epithelial cells resemble WBCs, often polyhedral in shape. They are 3 to 5 times larger than a RBC with a distinct round nucleus. They have a granular cytoplasm. Large numbers (> 15/HPF) suggest renal disease such as acute tubular necrosis.

Sperm are occasionally seen, their heads 4 to 6 μm long.

Bacteria are seen as contaminates or indicate a UTI. They multiply rapidly in an unrefrigerated sample. Gram stain is useful in planning treatment.

Yeast may be a contaminate or from the bladder, especially in those with diabetes mellitus, or immunosuppression. They are ovoid, smaller than RBCs (5–7 μm), often have buds, and are gram positive. Large mycelia, sometimes branched, with terminal buds are diagnostic.

Trichomonas vaginalis are mobile, pear shaped, 30 μm in size.

Casts result from the compaction and solidification of cells and protein in the renal tubules. Cylindrical in shape with parallel sides and rounded ends, once formed they begin to degenerate, cell walls then granules lyse resulting in an amorphous opaque waxy cast. Casts are sought under LPF and identified in a HPF.

Hyaline Casts: Colorless, homogeneous, hard to visualize, and normal in small numbers < 2/LPF. Made of protein; increased after exercise.

White Blood Cell Casts: Made up of white cells and seen in pyelonephritis. As the WBCs degenerate over time, the cells lose their distinct morphology and become cellular (unable to identify cell type), then granular and eventually waxy.

Renal Tubular Epithelial Cell Cast: Indicate renal tubular damage, often from viral infection or toxins.

Red Cell Casts: Formed from RBCs, usually from the glomeruli. Fragile, yellow to red brown in color, and often seen as fragments.

Usually indicate glomerulonephritis. As the RBC cell walls lyse, it becomes a pigmented cast.

Granular Casts: Normal in small numbers. May be degenerated WBC or renal tubular cells.

Waxy Casts: Rare, associated with severe chronic renal disease or amyloidosis. Homogeneous, refractile, sharp outlines, wider than hyaline casts. Usually broken or cracked. Can be confused with fibers from tissue paper, but waxy casts are almost always accompanied by an abnormal urinalysis.

Crystals are not useful in the diagnosis of most common diseases. They may be absent when renal stones are present. Drugs may form crystals in an acid urine, especially sulfonamides.

7.3 Cerebrospinal Fluid Analysis

Examine for color, clarity, and clotting:

- cloudy usually indicates WBC $> 0.2 \times 10^9/L$
- pink-red RBC $> 0.4 \times 10^9/L$
- xanthochromic after centrifugation and still yellow-pink and indicated central nervous system (CNS) bleed over 2 hr previous
- clotting indicated very high protein level, often TB meningitis

Conduct a cell count and differential in a hemocytometer (counting chamber).

- To count WBCs: rinse a pipette in glacial acetic acid (to lyse RBCs) and dry the outside and tip.
- Draw up 2 cm cerebral spinal fluid (CSF) in the pipette.
- Mix by rotating the pipette.

A Neubauer counting chamber has 2 separate ruled areas each with nine 1 mm × 1 mm squares.

- Use the 10× objective (100 power) to count WBCs.

- Count the number of cells in ten 1 × 1 mm cells. (Conventionally, count 5 cells, the 4 corners, and the middle from each ruled area.)
- Calculate number of cells per μL: # cells in 10 cells = # cells/ μL.
- Determine the type of cells by using 40 power. Neutrophils have segmented nuclei; lymphocytes and monocytes have a round nucleus.
- Wright's stain a spun sample of CSF to differentiate eosinophils from other neutrophils if necessary.

Normals are as follows:

Erythrocytes	0		
Leukocytes	adults	≤ 5	60% lymphocytes, 30% monocytes
	neonates	≤ 30	20% lymphocytes, 70% monocytes

To count RBCs in a Neubauer chamber, do not pretreat the pipette with acetic acid.

- Use the 40× objective.
- Count ten 1 × 1 mm cells.
- Count less cells if many RBCs present or dilute the specimen.
- Use the same formula as for WBCs.
- # cells × dilution factor × volume factor = cells/μL.

7.4 Joint Fluid

The counting chamber may also be used in the analysis of joint fluid. Pretreatment for a few minutes with hyaluronidase will be needed for viscous fluid.

Normal Values for Synovial Fluid

WBC	< 150	Lymphocytes > 75%
RBCs	0	

Abnormal Values for Synovial Fluid

WBC	< 300	neutrophils < 25%	noninflammatory
	300–5000	neutrophils > 70%	noninflammatory
	> 5000	neutrophils > 90%	infectious

Serous fluids (pericardial, pleural, abdominal) and sperm counts are also done in the counting chamber.

7.5 Stool Examination

(Mayo Clin Proc 1994;69:779)

Oval, Larvae, and Cysts

Direct fecal smear.

- Place 2 drops warm saline, one at each end of the slide.
- Apply a small amount of stool with an applicator stick to the drops and mix.
- Stain one side with Lugol's iodine solution.
- Apply cover strip.
- Examine under 10× and 40×.
- Add methylene blue stain or Lugol's iodine to help identify cells.

Lugol's iodine: Potassium iodide 20 mg, iodine 10 gm, distilled water 100 ml.

7.6 Thick Blood Films

Useful for malaria diagnosis, also for trypomastigotes (*trypanosoma*) and spirochetes (*Babesia* and *Leishmania*).

- Place 2 to 3 drops of blood (fresh from a finger stick or anticoagulated tube) on the end of a slide and 1 drop in the middle.
- Quickly smear the middle drop out with the end of a slide feathering out the tail end of the sample.

- Using the end of the same slide, mix the 3 drop sample and spread it into a 1 cm^2 area.
- Allow to dry.
- Do not fix if using Field's stain.

Malaria diagnosis by microscopy requires technical skills beyond those of the novice. (See http://www.rph.wa.gov.au/malaria/diagnosis for practice and quiz.) Dipstick rapid diagnostic tests are available commercially for malaria and trypanosomal antigens.

7.7 Microfilariae

Filariasis can be diagnosed serologically (when available) or by finding the microfilaria in blood, urine, hydrocele fluid, or skin snip preparations. Timing of sample collection is important for some species.

Membrane filtration of anticoagulated blood provides a microfilarial count and is a sensitive test when it is available, or use simple laboratory tests.

For microfilaria in blood:

- Collect blood in a sodium citrate anticoagulant tube.
- Add an equal amount of 2% formalin.
- Mix well.
- Wait 15 min.
- Centrifuge for 20 min.
- Discard the supernate.
- Examine the deposit under a cover slip at 10×.

For microfilaria in urine or hydrocele fluid:

- Collect in a test tube.
- Centrifuge for 5 min.
- Examine deposit as above.

LABORATORY

7.8 Skin Snip for Microfilaria (*Onchocerca volvulus*)

- Identify a pruritic area.
- Collect several small pieces of skin and subcutaneous tissue to 1 mm deep using a scalpel blade and a needle to lift the anesthetized skin.
- Place the skin on a slide with a few drops of saline and a cover slip.
- Wait > 4 hr.
- Examine under 10×.

Slit-skin Smear

Used for leishmaniasis and leprosy.

For leishmaniasis, sample the edge of an ulcer; for leprosy, the edges of active lesions, elbow skin, and ear lobes are fruitful sites.

- Pinch the skin up into a tent, providing a blood-free area.
- Cut the center of this area with a scalpel blade making a 0.5 cm slit, 1 mm deep.
- Turn the blade 90° to scrape out tissue juice and cells.
- Apply to a slide and allow to dry.
- Fix with methanol and stain: Giemsa for leishmaniasis, AFB stains for leprosy.

Leishmania amastigotes are round-oval purple, small 2 to 4 μm, and intramonocytic or extracellular in smears.

7.9 Staining Techniques

Only a few basic stains are commonly used or available in small hospital laboratories.

Gram Stain

For bacteria in sputum, exudates, and urine:

- Fix the slide by passing over a flame.
- Flood the slide with Gram stain while holding it on a slide rack or with a clothes peg.
- Wait 1 min.
- Wash slide with water.
- Flood with Lugol's solution.
- Wait 1 min.
- Tilt slide and decolorize over 5 to 10 seconds using acetone or ethanol.
- Wash with water.
- Counterstain with neutral red for 30 seconds.
- Wash with water.
- Allow to dry by standing vertically.

Ziehl-Neelsen Stain

For acid fast bacilli (AFB) in leprosy and TB. Also *Cryptosporidium* in stool (4–6 μm size)

- Fix slide in flame.
- Flood with carbolfuchsin.
- Heat with flame until it just begins to steam.
- Wait 15 min.
- Wash with water.
- Decolorize with 1% acid alcohol until no color remains.
- Wash with water.
- Counterstain with malachite green for 1 min.
- Wash with water.
- Dry.

AFB stains should be examined for 15 min under 1000× before being declared negative.

7.10 Chemistry

Basic Laboratory Testing

Many district hospitals will have a spectrophotometer (colorimeter) and the reagents necessary for a number of biochemistry tests. Easily performed tests include the following:

Bilirubin	Glucose
Hemoglobin	Alkaline phosphatase
Hemoglobin A_2	Cholesterol
Hemoglobin F (spectrophotometer only)	Uric Acid
AST (SGOT)	CPK
ALT (SGPT)	LDH
Creatinine	BUN

Hemoglobin can also be determined using the hemoglobin color scale (HCS), a laminated card varying from pink to dark red, which corresponds to Hb from 4–14 g/dL. (Int J Epidem 2005;34:1425). but accuracy is variable ± 2 g/dL in 16% of samples (J Clin Path 2005;58:56).

A flame spectrophotometer is difficult to maintain in rural areas. If available, it can test for sodium, potassium, and lithium.

Most rural laboratories can be equipped to do the following:

- Venereal disease research lab (VDRL) with serial dilutions or RPR for syphilis
- HIV screening tests
- Widal
- Rapid malaria antigen testing dipsticks
- Blood type, Rh, and cross match
- Pregnancy tests

Chapter 8

Imaging

8.1 Radiology

Radiologists are seldom found in rural hospitals. Usually a basic X-ray machine is available, along with a technician who knows how to operate it and develop the film. It is recommended that medical providers learn the operation of simple X-ray machines, how to obtain standard views, and the process of developing film. Spend some time with X-ray and ultrasound technicians. (See Am J Trop Med Hyg 1999;60:119 for use of ultrasound in Africa.)

This chapter has lists of X-ray findings and common diagnoses in developing countries. Use it to develop a differential diagnosis. Always read films with company; other providers may know the answer.

Remember that radiographs are expensive and often in short supply. Do not take films to document the obvious or maintain the habit of ordering a PA and lateral chest when a single film will do.

8.2 Differential Diagnosis

Skull

Single osteolytic lesion:

- cholesteatoma in mastoid
- fibrous dysplasia
- depressed skull fracture

- metastasis
- osteomyelitis
- dermal cyst
- secondary syphilis
- TB
- hydatid cyst

Hair on end pattern:

- hemolytic anemia
- cyanotic heart disease (polycythemia)
- iron deficient anemia

Single or multiple intracranial calcifications:

- arterial calcifications
- anatomic structures (arachnoid, choroid, etc)
- healed brain abscess
- cysticercosis
- hydatid cyst
- paragonimiasis
- congenital rubella
- TB
- syphilis, tertiary
- trichinosis
- toxoplasmosis
- cytomegalovirus (CMV)
- hematoma (old)

Bones

Transverse lines in metaphysis

- chronic anemias
- rickets
- severe illness or stress in infants
- scurvy
- TORCH syndromes

- hypercalcemia
- heavy metal poisoning

Aseptic necrosis hip:

- idiopathic Legg-Perthes
- sickle cell
- steroid therapy
- trauma

Bone sclerosis with sequestrum:

- osteomyelitis
- syphilis
- yaws
- TB
- osteoid osteoma
- tropical ulcer

Periosteal reaction/elevation:

- osteomyelitis
- yaws
- arthritis
- fracture
- subperiosteal bleeding
- syphilis, congenital
- hypervitaminosis A
- scurvy
- rickets
- bone infarct in hemolytic anemias
- trauma
- leukemia

Dactylitis:

- osteomyelitis (especially typhoid)
- sickle cell
- leprosy

IMAGING

- TB
- syphilis
- yaws

Heart

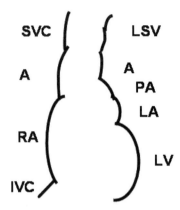

Figure 8.1   Mediastinal Profile

The arcs shown are all vascular: SVC, superior vena cava; LSV, left subclavian vein; PA, pulmonary artery; A, aorta; RA, right atrium; LA, left atrium; LV, left ventricle; IVC, inferior vena cava.

Right atrial enlargement:
- right heart failure
- left to right shunt
- pulmonary stenosis/atresia
- tricuspid regurgitation

Right ventricular enlargement:
- left heart failure, mitral valve disease
- pulmonary hypertension

- left to right shunt
- tetralogy of Fallot

Left atrial enlargement:

- mitral valve disease
- patent ductus arteriosus (PDA)
- ventricular septal defect (VSD)

Left ventricular enlargement:

- aortic valve disease
- coarctation
- congestive heart failure (CHF)
- hypertension
- high output (anemia, beriberi, thyrotoxicosis, etc)

Small ascending aorta:

- atrial septal defect (ASD)
- coarctation
- mitral valve disease
- low output
- VSD

Large ascending aorta:

- aortic aneurysm (syphilis, other)
- aortic insufficiency
- aortic stenosis
- coarctation
- PDA
- tetralogy Fallot
- mass simulating aorta

Chest

Lobar pneumonia: *Strep. pneumococcus*

Lobar collapse:

IMAGING

- bronchial adenoma, tumor
- foreign body
- mucous plug
- pertussis

Recurrent pneumonias:

- aspiration
- bronchial tumors
- bronchiectasis
- foreign body
- parasitic

Acute diffuse alveolar infiltrate:

- pneumonia, viral, bacterial, parasitic
- pulmonary edema
- aspiration

Chronic diffuse alveolar infiltrates:

- sarcoidosis
- TB
- lymphoma
- lymphocytic interstitial pneumonitis (LIP)

Pulmonary edema:

- CHF
- fluid overload
- cerebral: stroke, trauma
- allergic: drugs
- pulmonary embolus
- uremia
- high altitude
- malaria
- transfusion reaction

Miliary nodules:

- TB
- fungal infections
- melioidosis
- sarcoidosis
- metastatic disease
- LIP

Single pulmonary nodule, primary tumor:

- chest wall artifact: nipple
- TB
- metastasis: colon, ovary, testis, Wilms' tumor, choriocarcinoma, sarcoma, hepatoma
- abscess

Multiple pulmonary nodules:

- metastases
- TB
- fungal
- hydatid cysts
- paragonimiasis

Mediastinal lymphadenopathy:

- bronchogenic carcinoma
- TB
- sarcoid
- fungal
- lymphoma
- metastatic disease
- LIP

Abdomen

Nonobstructive ileus with small bowl air-fluid levels:

- drug induced
- hypokalemia
- sentinel loop near inflammation: appendicitis, cholecystitis, pancreatitis
- sepsis and severe illness: pneumonia, myocardial infarction (MI)
- peritonitis
- postoperative
- retroperitoneal hemorrhage
- renal/ureteral calculus
- vascular occlusion
- Chagas' disease

Intestinal obstruction:

- adhesions
- volvulus
- intussusception
- fecal impaction
- malignant lesion
- Crohn's
- parasitic: Chagas, amebiasis, ascaris
- inflammatory mass: TB, diverticulitis
- incarcerated hernia

Toxic megacolon:

- Hirschsprung's disease
- colitis: amebic, cholera, bacillary, typhoid, other
- ischemic

Liver calcifications:

- Hydatid cyst

- granuloma: TB, brucellosis, histoplasmosis
- hepatoma
- liver abscess

Urinary System

Nephrocalcinosis:

- chronic infection including TB
- hyperparathyroidism
- medullary sponge kidney

Bladder calcification:

- schistosomiasis
- TB
- calculus

IMAGING

Chapter 9

Making a Diagnosis

(Good Clinical Diagnostic Practice, WHO 2005:
BMJ.39003.640567.AE)

The task of arriving at a correct diagnosis is considerably
more difficult in developing countries. The clinician has numerous obstacles to surmount.

9.1 History

History of the current illness is a challenge to obtain through
translators. Patients may offer euphemisms. "Sitting on a hot rock
or eating cold rice" indicates a penile discharge in parts of the
Caribbean. Their own preconceptions of the cause of the illness
may cloud the history. See chapter 3.

Consider the patient's following history:

- travel history: contacts with fresh water, malarious area
- occupation: abattoir, fisherman, dump picker, truck driver
- family history: TB, HIV, sickle cell, diabetes mellitus, gout
- immunization history
- sexual practices
- diet: undercooked foods, vegans, water source
- medications: prescription and traditional
- previous treatments, transfusions, and prophylaxis
- bites: animal, insect
- animal contacts
- previous surgery: splenectomy, tattoos
- addictions and habits: alcohol, tobacco, betel nut, kava

- previous illnesses: HIV+, depression: Chagas' disease
- circumstances: refugee camp
- ethnic origin and gender
- housing and economic strata

The physical exam frequently provides the best clues to the diagnosis. Multiple diagnoses are common in patients with little access to medical care. Vital signs are vital and should be obtained carefully. If they appear to be abnormal, do them yourself. Examine every part of the body and hone your skills.

Laboratory tests and X-rays should be used sparingly to conserve resources. Use them to confirm an uncertain diagnosis and not in a "shotgun" manner.

9.2 Weight Loss

A common complaint, often difficult to confirm since there is no baseline weight available. Examination of the patient's belt will often reveal new punctures made for the buckle. If they appear ill and have anorexia, consider the following:

- HIV/AIDS
- TB
- malignancy: hepatoma, cervical carcinoma, lymphoma
- leishmaniasis-visceral
- brucellosis
- schistosomiasis
- renal failure
- anemia

Weight Loss Without Anorexia

- poverty
- stress and depression
- hyperthyroidism (often seen with hydatidiform mole)
- diabetes mellitus

- intestinal helminths and giardia
- chronic malabsorption
- medications

9.3   Fever

Difficult to confirm by history as few patients have a thermometer. An acute onset, a high temperature, and the presence of chills points towards an infectious etiology. The fever pattern may suggest the diagnosis:

- fever every 2 or 3 days: chronic malaria. With acute malaria, the fever is constant as it is in nonimmunes with *P. falciparum*
- biphasic fever, an initial temperature elevation followed by a short afebrile interval with fever returning: dengue, leptospirosis
- undulant fever waxes and wanes over days: brucellosis, visceral leishmaniasis, lymphoma (occasionally with puritis)
- relapsing fevers disappear after several days then recurs
- bradycardia with fever: typhoid, yellow fever, legionnaire's disease, dengue

Acute fevers associated with rashes:

- vesicular: pox virus, disseminated herpes
- maculopapular: measles, dengue/arboviruses, rickettsia, rubella, typhus, primary HIV
- erythematous: scarlet fever, Kawasaki, rheumatic fever, toxic shock
- hemorrhagic: meningococcal, severe chicken pox, hemorrhagic fevers, DIC, severe rickettsia

Acute fevers and hemolytic jaundice:

- malaria
- sickle cell crisis, G6PD crisis
- *Bartonella*

- hemolytic-uremic syndromes
- leptospirosis

Acute fever and jaundice:

- typhoid (mild jaundice)
- cholangitis: occasionally liver fluke, ascaris
- cholecystitis
- viral hepatitis A&E, yellow fever, hemorrhagic fevers, Epstein-Barr virus, cytomegalovirus
- sepsis
- streptococcal pneumonia, pyomyositis, leptospirosis
- alcoholic hepatitis
- malaria

Fever and splenomegaly:

- malaria
- infectious mononucleosis
- cytomegalovirus
- typhoid
- endocarditis
- leptospirosis
- TB
- schistosomiasis
- typhus
- brucellosis
- African trypanosomiasis
- leishmaniasis
- relapsing fever

Fever and eosinophilia: Eosinophilia usually declines with a concurrent bacterial infection. When it is increased, consider the following:

- acute schistosomiasis

- migrating parasites including ascaris, hookworm, trichinosis, fascioliasis, gnathostomiasis, paragonimiasis
- drug hypersensitivity

Chronic fever > 2 weeks:

- TB pulmonary and extrapulmonary
- typhoid
- HIV
- amoebic abscess
- endocarditis
- interabdominal or liver abscess
- visceral leishmaniasis
- non-Hodgkin's lymphoma
- HIV with CMV, pneumocystis pneumonia, atypical mycobacteria, cryptococcus
- brucellosis
- melioidosis

9.4 Lymphadenopathy

Generalized chronic lymphadenopathy

- HIV
- TB disseminated
- secondary syphilis
- brucellosis
- African trypanosomiasis
- Chagas' disease
- visceral leishmaniasis
- sarcoidosis
- toxoplasmosis

Regional chronic lymphadenopathy

- TB

- lymphoma
- filariasis
- metastatic disease
- atypical mycobacteria
- onchocerciasis
- loiasis
- cat scratch disease
- Kawasaki's disease
- lymphogranuloma venereum

Regional acute lymphadenopathy

- plague
- anthrax
- tularemia
- chancroid
- pyogenic adenitis
- primary syphilis
- rickettsia
- diphtheria

9.5   Diarrheas

Chronic diarrhea

- HIV
- giardia
- amebiasis
- TB ileocecal
- strongyloides
- trichinella
- *Capillaria philippinensis*
- chronic pancreatitis
- tropical sprue
- inflammatory bowel disease (IBD)

- lactose intolerance
- medications
- foods: sorbitol
- celiac disease
- schistosomiasis
- bacterial: E coli, shigella

Bloody diarrhea

- shigella
- salmonella
- campylobacter
- E coli
- *Yersinia*
- *Clostridium difficile, perfringens*
- amebiasis
- IBD
- *B. coli*

9.6 Portal Hypertension, Cirrhosis often Associated with Varices

- schistosomiasis
- malaria splenomegaly syndrome
- portal vein occlusion (umbilical cord sepsis common cause)
- hepatoma
- veno-occlusive disease
- Indian childhood cirrhosis
- hemosiderosis
- cardiac disease
- chronic viral hepatitis
- alcohol

MAKING A DIAGNOSIS

Bloody diarrhea

- shigella
- salmonella
- campylobacter
- E coli
- *Yersinia*
- *Clostridium difficile, perfringens*
- amebiasis
- IBD
- *B. coli*

9.6 Portal Hypertension, Cirrhosis often Associated with Varices

- schistosomiasis
- malaria splenomegaly syndrome
- portal vein occlusion (umbilical cord sepsis common cause)
- hepatoma
- veno-occlusive disease
- Indian childhood cirrhosis
- hemosiderosis
- cardiac disease
- chronic viral hepatitis
- alcohol

9.6 *Portal Hypertension, Cirrhosis often Associated with Varices* **121**

Chapter 10

Malaria

(Trans R Soc Trop Med Hyg 2000;94:1; JAMA 2007;297, entire issue on malaria; Management of Severe Malaria, WHO 2000; Am J Trop Med Hyg 2007;77(suppl 6), entire issue on malaria)

Cause: *Plasmodium vivax, ovale, malariae, falciparum, knowlesi.*

Epidem: Life cycle is complex. Transmission via infected female Anopheles mosquito; infected RBCs during transfusion or contaminated needles.

Simplified Life Cycle

- Sporozoites injected from mosquito salivary glands during feeding.
- Enter hepatocytes.
- Multiply via exoerythrocytic schizogony.
- Form merozoites.
- Released 6–16 days later as hepatocyte ruptures. In P. falciparum and malariae, liver infection ends as all merozoites released. In P. vivax and ovale, merozoites may remain in hepatocytes as hypnozoites for years causing relapses.
- Merozoites invade RBCs.
- Evolve into trophozoites (ring forms).
- Grow into schizonts, which mature to:
  - Merozoites, which can infect RBCs and
  - Gametocytes (sexual forms, male and female).
- Gametocytes ingested by mosquito.
- Mate to form zygote.
- Mature to an oocyst in the mosquito stomach.
- Mature and rupture, releasing motile sporozoites.
- Migrate to mosquito salivary gland.

Distribution:

P. falciparum	Africa, Asia, S America, Oceania, Hispaniola
P. vivax	SE Asia, N Africa, Oceania, Central and South America, Middle East
P. ovale	West Africa, uncommon elsewhere
P. malariae	Africa, other areas
P. knowlesi	Malaysia-Sarawak (CID 2008;46:165)

Vector: *Anopheles sp*.

Host Factors: Homozygotes for HgbS and Melanesian ovalocytosis resist RBC invasion. Thalassemias, G6PD, HgbC, HgbE, HgbS trait have reduction of severe infections (JAMA 2007;297:2220). High HgbF seen in thalassemias may be protective. Duffy blood group Fy Fy-absence completely protects from *P. vivax* (N Engl J Med 2000;343:598). Immunity is acquired slowly, probably species specific (Am J Trop Med Hyg 2007;76:997), and is short lived without continued exposure. Pregnant women are more susceptible due to generalized immunosuppression.

Terms:

Hypoendemic: spleen or parasite rate < 10%

Mesoendemic: spleen or parasite rate < 50%

Hyperendemic: spleen or parasite rate < 75%

Holoendemic: spleen or parasite rate > 75%

Spleen rate: % children age 2 to 9 yr with enlarged spleen

Parasite rate: proportion of defined population with microscopically-identified malaria

Transmission index: % < 1 year parasitized

Unstable malaria: variable transmission with low immunity, prone to epidemics

Stable malaria: constant incidence with high transmission and epidemics unlikely

Autochthonous malaria: locally transmitted

Imported malaria: acquired elsewhere

Airport malaria: local introduction of malaria into malaria-free regions, often by human travelers or hitchhiking mosquitoes; causes secondary cases.

Induced malaria: nonmosquito transmission, ie, blood transfusion

Natural index of infection: % mosquitoes infected

Premunition: asymptomatic parasitemia

Pathophys: Results from several factors:

- RBC destruction resulting in anemia
- liberation of RBC and parasitic cell components
- response to lysis with cytokines release such as tumor necrosis factor
- sequestration of infected RBCs causing microvascular obstruction, *P. falciparum*
- immune-mediated damage

   P. falciparum infects all ages of RBCs and releases up to 20 times more merozoites. May have high parasitemia rates.

   P. malariae infects only senescent RBCs.

   P. vivax and *ovale* infect only reticulocytes; parasitemia is low, < 7%.

Sx:

- Mixed infections occur frequently.

	P. falciparum	*vivax*	*ovale*	*malariae*
Incubation period	12 (7–14 d)	13	17	28
	—	may be 6–12 months		
Duration of untreated infection	< 2 yr	< 4	< 4	> 40
Periodicity of attack, hr	none	48	48	72
Duration of attack, hr	16+	8–12	8–12	8–10
Course	potentially fatal	rarely fatal	not fatal	

- Incubation period may be 9 to 12 months in northern areas such as Russia, Korea, China to coincide with onset of summer (N Engl J Med 2003;349:1510).
- Immunity prolongs the incubation period as does partial chemoprophylaxis.

Sx: Dependent on species (*P. falciparum* most severe), host's age, immunity, and pregnancy. Onset resembles influenza with malaise, headache, myalgias, anorexia, and a slight fever. After 2 to 3 d, the fever gradually increases with chills, backache, vomiting, diarrhea, and dry cough frequently seen. Left untreated, a periodic fever becomes established in another 5 to 7 d (not usually *P. falciparum*, where symptoms wax and wane). Paroxysm of periodic fever begin abruptly with a chill; 30 to 60 min later the fever begins with sweating and other symptoms noted above. After 2 to 8 hr, symptoms subside.

Si: Fever, flushed skin, tachycardia, tender hepatosplenomegaly, mental confusion, jaundice.

Crs: In hyper- and holoendemic areas, severe malaria in children (6 months–3 yr) once maternal transferred immunity wanes with splenomegaly and anemia; milder attacks in older children with asymptomatic adults. Asymptomatic malaria in pregnancy but maternal anemia and low birth weight newborns. In areas of less transmission and/or low immunity, severe attacks at any age with cerebral malaria more common.

Cmplc:
- Severe malaria is defined as follows:
  - parasitemia > 5%
  - oliguria
  - jaundice
  - anemia Hb < 5 g/dl
  - reduced level of consciousness

- hypoglycemia < 45 mg/dl (2.5 mmol/liter)
- organ failure
- Cerebral malaria occurs with *P. falciparum*, a frequent cause of mortality. Acute (children) or gradual (adult) onset over several days with fever, delirium, and seizures, progressing to coma. The skin is dry and flushed with good perfusion. Anemia is common; jaundice more often seen in adults. Neurological signs are variable with disconjugate gaze, unequal pupils, reflexes variable, and Babinski's sign in 50%. Hepatospleno-megaly is common. Even with appropriate treatment, mortality is 15% in children up to 50% in pregnancy. Shock suggests a coexistent bacterial sepsis, and a lumbar puncture (LP) is required for any patient in coma. If an LP cannot be done, treat for meningitis also.
- Postcerebral malaria neurological syndrome is common (3% adults, 10–20% children). Almost any neurological find-ing from hemiparesis to blindness may occur. Recovery over several weeks to months in > 90% of patients (JAMA 2007;297:2232).
- Hypoglycemia is common (up to 30%) in children under 3 yr old, in those with coma, convulsions, and with severe hyper-parasitemia (> 10%). It can usually be prevented with a 10% glucose infusion and treated with 5 ml/kg 50% glucose. If IV access is not possible, give by nasogastric (NG) tube.
- Severe anemia (Hb < 5 g/dl) in children and pregnant women; may cause heart failure. Transfusion is indicated if Hb ≤ 4 gm/dl or if Hb ≤ 5 gm/dl and severe symptoms such as shock, heart failure, or hyperparasitemia. Give packed RBCs (10 ml/kg) slowly or whole blood (20 ml/kg). A diuretic is not usually necessary.
- Seizures common in children with high fevers and before the onset of coma in cerebral malaria. Coma should be differenti-ated from status epilepticus. Treat acute convulsions with rectal or IV diazepam (0.5 mg/kg) or paraldehyde rectally or

IM (0.3–0.4 ml/kg). Diazepam may be repeated every 10 min × 3. For persistent seizures, give phenobarbital IV or IM 15 mg/kg. Treat any fever, and do an LP.

- Shock is treated with 20 ml/kg normal saline over 30 min or with whole blood.
- Aspiration pneumonia is common.
- Typhoid fever, bacterial sepsis, and meningitis are often confused clinically.

Lab:

- CBC is useful for anemia, leukocytosis.
- Thrombocytopenia is common.
- Protime (PT) and partial thromboplastin times are prolonged in severe infections.
- Disseminated intravascular coagulation (DIC) is unusual.
- Hemoglobinurinia can occur with hemolysis (Blackwater fever).
- Elevated bilirubin is expected.
- Acidosis is primarily due to elevated lactate.
- Hypoglycemia.
- Renal impairment occurs.
- Diagnosis is by thick and thin blood smear. Giemsa's stain is best (> 30 min preparation). Field's stain quicker. Parasite counting and speciation can be done.
- Rapid antigen tests are available with sensitivity and specificity in the 90% range (Am J Trop Med Hyg 2007;76:481).
- If the lab test is negative, there is probably no need to treat. If you are not going to believe the results, do not waste the time and money!

Rx: Treatment of malaria involves a number of considerations;

- The disease: *P. falciparum* is deadly in the nonimmune and partially immune. Hospital admission is frequently necessary. Uncomplicated *P. vivax*, *ovale*, and *malariae* can usually be treated as outpatients.

- The patient: Pregnant women are at special risk. Coexisting illness may be present. Meningitis often precipitates an attack of malaria.
- Available drugs, laboratory facilities, and parasite resistance. Presumptive treatment is often necessary.
- National drug policy.

Chloroquine (300 mg base = 500 mg salt) is the drug of choice for *P. ovale* and *P. malariae*. It is effective against most *P. vivax* infections (rare resistance in Oceania, Americas, Indonesia, Myanmar, and India). It is curative of *P. falciparum* acquired in Mexico, west of the Panama Canal, Hispaniola, Mauritius, and most of the Middle East and Egypt. Chloroquine resistance in *P. falciparum* is common elsewhere, and it should not be used alone.

Oral Dosage	Adult	Child
Initial	600 mg base	10 mg/kg
6 hr	300 mg	5 mg/kg
24 hr	300 mg	5 mg/kg
48 hr	300 mg	5 mg/kg

IM dosage should be reserved for those unable to take medications by mouth. Give 2.5 mg/kg every 4 hr until a total of 25 mg/kg is administered.

IV dosage must be given slowly over at least 8 hr. Initial dose is 10 mg/kg followed by 5 mg/kg until a total of 25 mg/kg is given.

Change to oral dosage as soon as possible.

- Do not give chloroquine with artemether, quinine, and lumefantrine (ventricular arrhythmias) or mefloquine (convulsions). Take with food if possible.
- Mixed infections of *P. falciparum* with another species of malaria are common and may be deadly if the patient's blood smear is misread and a chloroquine-resistant *P. falciparum* infection is missed.
- Safe in pregnancy.

MALARIA

- When used for prophylaxis (adult 300 mg base/wk, child 5 mg/kg wk; given daily in Francophone areas). Avoid in those with seizure disorder, psoriasis, myasthenia gravis, or G6PD deficiency.
- Overdose: use IV diazepam.
- Quinine treatment of severe chloroquine-resistant P. *falciparum* infection. Quinine is the drug of choice except in areas where quinine resistance is common (SE Asia, Amazon basin).
- Give quinine orally when possible.
- Unattended IV therapy can be deadly; use IM instead.

Oral Dosage	Adult	Children
Quinine sulfate	600 mg/8 hr	10 mg/kg/8 hr

IV Dosage
Quinine dihydrochloride diluted in 10 ml/kg IV fluid (D5W)

Initial	20 mg/kg over 4 hr	20 mg/kg over 4 hr
Every 8 hr	10 mg/kg over 2–4 hr	10 mg/kg over 2–4 hr
Maximum dose	1800 mg/d	

If the IV rate cannot be monitored, it is not safe; give quinine IM but divide initial dose into 2 parts of 10 mg/kg every 4 hr. Dilute parenteral solution with sterile water.

- Give 50% dose initially if patient has been taking quinine, quinidine, or mefloquine during the last 12 hr.
- Repeat oral dose if any dose vomited in < 1 hr.
- Various quinine salts may be available: Quinidine gluconate loading dose 10 mg/kg over 1 to 2 hr (maximum 600 mg), then continuous infusion 0.02 mg/kg/min.
- Quinine sulfate 300 mg = Quinine disulfate 215 mg.
- Reduce IV quinidine or quinine doses 50% after 48 hr therapy to 3.75 to 5 mg/kg/8 hr or 5–7 mg/kg/8 hr, respectively.
- Change to oral dosing as soon as possible but do not reduce dose.

- Treat for 3 to 10 d depending on local conditions.
- Cardiac monitoring is advised for IV dosing. Watch for conduction delays and heart block. Will accelerate atrial fibrillation and elevate digoxin levels.
- Quinine causes hypoglycemia by increasing insulin release.
- Reversible cinchonism with tinnitus and high frequency hearing loss is to be expected; warn patients.
- Steroid treatment increases mortality (N Engl J Med 1982;306:313).
- Use when necessary in pregnancy.

Quinine therapy is often combined with a second drug such as IM artemether, IV artesunate, sulfadoxine-pyrimethamine (SP), tetracycline, doxycycline, or clindamycin, depending on availability and local patterns of resistance.

For severe malaria treated with quinine add the following:

- IM artemether 3.2 mg/kg IM on first d, then 1.6 mg/kg IM daily until able to take artesunate orally 2 mg/kg/d for a total treatment of 7 d; or
- IM or IV artesunate 2.4 mg/kg IM or IV on first d, then 1.2 mg/kg IM or IV in 12 hr, then 1.2 mg/kg IM or IV every 24 hr until able to take artesunate orally as above; or
- Artemisinin suppositories 40 mg/kg rectally on first d, then 20 mg/kg daily until able to take oral artesunate; or
- Sulfadoxine-pyrimethamine (500 mg/25 mg tabs); single dose at end of quinine treatment; adults 3 tablets.

Children

5–10 kg	½ tablet
11–20 kg	1 tablet
21–30 kg	1½ tablets
31–45 kg	2 tablets
> 45 kg	3 tablets

Only used if malaria sensitive to SP; or

- Clindamycin;

Dosage	Adults	Child > 1 month
Oral	300 mg/6 hr	3–6 mg/kg/6 hr
IM or IV	600 mg/6 hr	4–10 mg/kg/6 hr

or

- Doxycycline 100 mg po twice daily for 7 to 10 d; not for pregnant women or children under 9 yr of age.
- Artesunate IV available from CDC; see Web site for telephone numbers.

Outpatient Treatment of Malaria

Chloroquine is acceptable in areas with sensitive *P. falciparum* malaria and for confirmed *P. vivax, ovale,* and *malariae.* Beware mixed infection with missed *P. falciparum.*

Sulfadoxine-pyrimethamine resistance is common in the Amazon basin, SE Asia, and parts of Sub-Saharan Africa. See previous page for dose. Slow acting cure. No longer recommended for prophylaxis in travelers. Used for intermittent prophylaxis in pregnancy but not in last 4 wk prior to delivery. Dose for prophylaxis (nonpregnant) is 1 tablet weekly.

Amodiaquine (153 mg base = 200 mg salt) similar to chloroquine but sometimes effective against chloroquine-resistant *P. falciparum.*

Agranulocytosis in 1:2000 limits its use (Lancet 1986;1:411). More palatable than chloroquine and therefore used occasionally in children.

For treatment (one option):

Oral Dosage	Adults	Children
Initial	400 mg twice daily	7.5 mg/kg twice daily
Next 2 d	400 mg twice daily	5 mg/kg twice daily
Prophylaxis	400 mg weekly	5 mg/kg weekly

WHO Approved Treatment Regimes

Shown as Tables 10.1 through 10.7.

Table 10.1   Artemether/lumefantrine (20/120 mg tabs)

	Adult (≥ 35 kg)	Child		
		10–14 kg	15–24 kg	25–34 kg
Initial	4 tabs	1	2	3
8 hr	4 tabs	1	2	3
24 hr	4 tabs	1	2	3
36 hr	4 tabs	1	2	3
48 hr	4 tabs	1	2	3
60 hr	4 tabs	1	2	3

Take with food. Most effective Rx in Uganda (JAMA 2007;297:2210). Prolongs QT interval on EKG.

Table 10.2   Artesunate (50 mg) plus amodiaquine (153 mg)

	Adult	Child
Artesunate	4 mg/kg/d for 3 d	
Amodiaquine	4 daily for 3 d	< 10 kg ½ daily for 3 d
		> 10 kg 1 daily for 3 d

Table 10.3   Artesunate (50 mg) plus sulfadoxine/pyrimethamine (SP 500/25 mg)

	Adult	Child
Artesunate	As above	
SP	See previous	

Table 10.4   Artesunate (50 mg) plus mefloquine (250 mg)

	Adult	Child
Artesunate	As above	
Mefloquine		< 15 kg not recommended
Initial	750 mg	12.5 mg/kg
6–8 hr later	500 mg	12.5 mg/kg

Table 10.5   Amodiaquine (153 mg) plus SP (500/25 mg)

	Adult	Child
Amodiaquine	As above	
SP	As above	

Table 10.6   Atovaquone/Proguanil Malarone® (250/100 mg) and (62.5/25 mg) pediatric dose

	Adult	Child
Treatment	4 tablets daily for 3 d	11–20 kg 1 tablet (250/100 mg) for 3 d
		21–30 kg 2 tablets for 3 d
		31–40 kg 3 tablets for 3 d
Prophylaxis	1 tablet daily	11–20 kg 1 tablet (62.5/25 daily)
		21–30 kg 2 tablets (62.5/25 daily)
		31–40 kg 3 tablets (62.5/25 daily)

Take 1–2 d before exposure and 7 d after for prophylaxis.

Table 10.7   Mefloquine (250 mg tablets)

	Adult	Child
Treatment		< 15 kg not recommended
Initial	750 mg	12.5 mg/kg
6–8 hr later	500 mg	12.5 mg/kg
Prophylaxis	250 mg weekly	5 mg/kg wk

Take 1–3 wk before exposure and 4 wk after. No excess neuropsychiatric symptoms (JAMA 2007;297:2251). Not with epilepsy, pregnancy, or infants; OK with breast feeding. Not for malaria contracted on Thai-Myanmar-China, Thai-Cambodia, or Cambodia-Vietnam borders (40% resistance; CDC Traveler's Health Yellow Book).

- Doxycycline (100 mg tablet): Not for single drug treatment. Prophylaxis 100 mg/d adult, child over 8 yr 1.5 mg/kg/d. Start day before exposure and continue 4 wk after.
- Chlorproguanil/dapsone (2/2.5 mg/kg/d): Effective against *P. vivax* (JAMA 2007;297:2201).

Adult	Child
2/2.5 mg/kg/d for 3 d	2/2.5 mg/kg/d for 3 d

- Emergency treatment of malaria in travelers; standby emergency self-treatment (SBET).
- Medical workers and travelers to remote malaria-endemic areas should consider carrying a SBET kit for presumptive treatment. This avoids seeking emergency treatment in possibly substandard facilities or purchasing inappropriate or counterfeit medications. Suitable regimens include the following:
  - chloroquine (where no resistance)
  - mefloquine
  - quinine ± doxycycline
  - artemether/lumefantrine (not available in United States)
  - atovaquone/proguanil
  - quinine + clindamycin (in pregnancy)

- Primaquine (15 mg base tablets): Used to eradicate long-lived hypnozoites in liver in *P. ovale* and *P. vivax* to bring about a radical cure. Also highly gametocytocidal against all species and used to prevent mosquito infection in epidemics. It can be used for prophylaxis at 0.5 mg/kg/d with food, adult 30 mg.
- Unless hypnozoites are destroyed; *P. vivax* and *P. ovale* have a tendency to recur. In areas of high parasite densities, radical cure is not practical unless the patient can leave the malarious area and prevent reinfection. Radical cure is usually reserved for patients with proven previous infection with susceptible species or those with presumed infection and continued suppression of clinical symptoms by taking a prophylactic drug.
  - Before treating for radical cure, test the patient for G6PD deficiency.
  - Eradicate any merozoites with standard chloroquine therapy.
  - Treat with 250 μgm/kg daily in children or 15 mg in adults for 14 d taken with food. A higher dose of 15 mg twice a day may be necessary with resistant strains (Clin Infect Dis 2004;39:1336).
  - Gametocytocidal treatment of *P. falciparum* (adult 30 mg, child 500–750 μg/kg) single dose; G6PD testing not required. Avoid in pregnancy and breast feeding.
- Tafenoquine is a long lasting 8-aminoquinoline similar to primaquine. Dosage is 600 mg orally once (Clin Infect Dis 2004;39:1095). G6PD should be checked and the drug avoided if there is an enzyme deficiency and in pregnancy. Longer treatments have been effective for primaquine resistant *P. vivax*: 200 mg daily for 3 d, then 200 mg weekly × 8 (Am J Trop Med Hyg 2007;76:494).
- An alternative is to suppress the *P. vivax* or *P. ovale* malaria with weekly chloroquine. Treatment may need to be continued 3 to 4 yr to prevent relapse.
- Transfusion-acquired malaria does not have a liver stage so no radical cure is necessary.

Supportive measures in the treatment of severe malaria:

- Insert NG tube and elevate head of bed in comatose to avoid aspiration.
- Careful monitoring of fluid intake and output.
- Treat fever.
- Give oxygen for respiratory distress.
- Monitor for hypoglycemia, especially with quinine therapy.
- Control seizures and watch for status epilepticus.
- Transfusions for anemia.
- Watch for signs of DIC; give vitamin K, clotting factors, whole blood.
- Avoid bed sores by frequent turning.
- Rule out meningitis with an LP.
- Monitor parasite count frequently.
- Consider exchange transfusion when parasitemia > 10%; goal is < 5%.
- Dexamethasone and steroids do not reduce mortality.

Prev: Three billion people are at risk for contracting malaria with 300 million episodes per year and more than 1 million deaths, most of them children. The Roll Back Malaria Partnership has set a goal of reducing malaria-associated mortality by 50% by 2010 (from 2000 levels), a lofty target that will require a sustained and coordinated community and health system effort for generations to come.

The current effort to fight malaria is the second worldwide program in recent memory. The first, started after World War II and centered around residual Dichloro-Diphenyl-Trichloroethane (DDT) spraying and prompt treatment, failed in many less developed countries but did succeed in N America, Europe, Australia, and Taiwan.

Current options include the following:

- Patient centered
  - chemoprophylaxis

- presumptive treatment of disease
- protection, repellents, treated bed nets
- prevention of transmission
- future vaccines
- Mosquito centered
  - residual insecticide spraying
  - larvicides
- Environmental
  - control of breeding sites
  - alternative living situations

See chapter 5.6 for vector control.

Protection by repellents is an ancient method. Living in a smoky house is one alternative, but respiratory problems are the price paid for an insect-free environment. Mosquito coils, dwelling screens, repellents such as picaridin or DEET, and insecticide-treated clothing or soap (permethrin or DEET) offer some protection but are often too expensive and not effective enough for local application. In holoendemic areas, 30 bites per d from infective mosquitoes is not unusual.

Chemoprophylaxis regimes are effective but inconvenient, expensive, and when used improperly with irregular or sub-therapeutic dosing, promote drug resistance. An exception is in pregnant women.

The dihydrofolate reductase-thymidylate synthase (DHFR) inhibitors, such as pyrimethamine, chloroproquanil, and atovaquone, inhibit the parasite's liver and RBC stages (causal prophylaxis) and development in the mosquito (sporontocidal).

Chloroquine and mefloquine inhibit asexual RBC development but are not effective against the liver stage (suppressive prophylaxis).

All these drugs are gametocidal, except against *P. falciparum*.

Primaquine is active against the liver stage and gametocytes of all species. Tetracyclines are active against liver and asexual blood stages but do not cause a radical cure of *P. vivax*.

Drugs that are effective against the liver stage of the parasite can be stopped soon after leaving a malarious area. Those that are not should be continued 4 wk to allow the liver stage of *P. falciparum* to clear.

Amodiaquine (toxicity), quinine (ineffective), and artemisinin drugs (save for Rx) should not be used for prophylaxis.

In areas with active malaria transmission, pregnant women should receive prophylaxis. Chloroquine should be given weekly if there is no resistance or preventive intermittent treatment given in the second and third trimesters with sulfadoxine-pyrimethamine (500–25 mg), 3 tablets (Am J Trop Med Hyg 2001;64:28). Tetracyclines and primaquine should not be used in pregnancy.

Chemoprophylaxis has been successfully used in children (Lancet 1988;1:1121), but this will delay the acquisition of immunity.

Gametocidal drugs such as primaquine and DHFR inhibitors will prevent human-to-mosquito transmission. They are useful to halt extension of epidemics in nonimmunes. Artemisinin derivatives also reduce gametocyte carriage.

Presumptive treatment of malaria is used in areas when diagnostic facilities are unavailable. The rationale behind this policy is that patients with fever, particularly children and pregnant women, may have malaria, which could be fatal and should therefore be treated, even if the diagnosis of malaria cannot be confirmed. However, from 1/3 to over 90% of febrile patients are inappropriately treated (JAMA 2007;297:2227). Outpatients often fail to complete their 3-day course and save the remaining medication thus encouraging resistance. Artemether-based antimalarial drugs are expensive ($1/course). As much as possible, the presumptive treatment of malaria should be replaced by laboratory investigative and targeted treatment of those actually infected.

Insecticide-treated bed nets (ITNs) are effective in reducing childhood malaria mortality 60% (Lancet 1991;337:1499), but introduction of ITNs has been slow (JAMA 2007;297:2241). Retreatment with deltamethrin every 6 to 12 months is necessary with older nets, but new technology allows a single treatment effective for the life of the net. Costs ($~5/net) are currently being covered by donors in many areas. Effectiveness is somewhat limited by human practices (being under nets during mosquito biting periods) (Am J Trop Med Hyg 2007;76:1100), mosquito habits (peak biting times), and emerging resistance to insecticides.

Epidemics of malaria in nonimmune populations are best prevented by careful monitoring of rainfall, temperature, population migration, and rapid assessment measures such as school or clinic attendance. Management involves mass drug therapy including primaquine to kill gametocytes (Emerg Infect Dis 2007;13:681).

Chapter 11

Leprosy

(Infolep Leprosy Services http://www.infolep.org, http://www.ilep.org.uk, http://www.leprosy.org; Am Fam Phys. 1995;52:172)

Cause: Caused by the acid-fast bacilli *Mycobacterium leprae*.

Epidem: Hansen's disease has been targeted by the WHO for "elimination as a public health problem." Worldwide prevalence has decreased from about 12 million in 1982 to an incidence of approximately 700 000 newly diagnosed cases annually.

Found in 122 countries, 10 have 96% of cases: India, Brazil, Indonesia, D R Congo, Bangladesh, Nigeria, Ethiopia, Mozambique, Nepal, and Tanzania. The United States has about 5000 active cases, incidence ~100/yr.

Pathophys: Highly infectious with a low pathogenicity and virulence; most people are resistant and self-cure; certain populations susceptible to develop clinical disease (Pacific Islanders). Incubation period 2 to 12 yrs (2 months–40 yr) spread by nasal secretions and open lesions; the bacilli resist drying and grow best in cool areas of the body: skin, nose, ear, testes, anterior chamber of the eye, and peripheral nerves.

Sx/Si: Diagnosis is primarily clinical and often missed due to clinician's inexperience and patient's reticence to call attention to signs of a stigmatizing disease.

- hypopigmented or red colored, anesthetic to light touch, macular skin lesions
- peripheral nerve thickening with loss of sensation
- skin smears positive for AFB

Table 11.1   Ridley Jopling Scale

Indeterminate (depigmented skin macule ± anesthesia) 80–90% Self-Cure or Progress to Clinical Leprosy				
Multibacillary			**Paucibacillary**	
LL	**BL**	**BB**	**BT**	**TT**
Lepromatous	borderline lepromatous	borderline	borderline tuberculoid	tuberculoid
Diffuse skin lesions			Distinct skin lesions	
Skin smear +			Skin smear often negative Use skin biopsy	

Patients with all 3 signs have a 97% diagnostic sensitivity of having leprosy. One finding will make the diagnosis in experienced hands. A pure neuritic form exists (with no skin lesions); prevalence varies from 0.5% in Ethiopia to 8.7% in Nepal. Multibacillary disease patients may not have macular skin lesions. Skin smears are 100% specific but only 50% sensitive, most frequently in multibacillary or relapsed disease. They can be obtained and processed in any district hospital that can do acid-fast staining.

Classification is important for treatment. Use the Ridley-Jopling scale (Table 11.1) or the WHO scale.

WHO Classification:

1 lesion = indeterminate

< 5 lesions = paucibacillary (PB); usually tuberculoid (leprosy; TT), borderline tuberculoid (leprosy; BT)

≥ 5 lesions or + skin smear = multibacillary (MB); borderline (leprosy; BB), borderline lepromatous (leprosy; BL), Lepromatous (leprosy; LL)

Other signs: LL: multiple ill defined, symmetrical macules, plaques, nodules in skin, face, legs, and buttocks. Loss of eyebrows, thickened ear lobes, leonine face (thick furrowed forehead), xerosis legs, thickened nerves (radial cutaneous, median at wrist, great auricular, ulnar, perineal), bone resorption, stocking-glove anesthesia, and iritis.

TT: few symmetric papules or plaques with distinct borders, depressed center, anesthetic, hairless, and do not perspire. Usually < 10 cm. Occur on cooler areas of the skin; less common in the midline, inguinal area and axilla. Muscle weakness in arms, legs, and eyelids. Painless wounds or burns.

Diagnosis may require referral for expert opinion or re-examination in 6 months when skin lesions will become anesthetic (because of sensory overlap, facial lesions may not readily demonstrate anesthesia). Because of social stigma, do not make the diagnosis without a careful physical examination and some certainty.

Cmplc: Differential diagnosis includes cutaneous leishmaniasis, dyspigmentation and keratitis of onchocerciasis, hyperkeratosis of yaws, and tinea versicolor. Granuloma multiforme, discoid lupus, and sarcoid resemble TT and BT. Cutaneous TB causes more tissue destruction. Sarcoidosis in the skin is not anesthetic and often there are systemic lesions.

Lab: Making a skin smear, see laboratory chapter. Biopsy of the edge of an active lesion may be necessary.

Tip: Mucus blown by a LL patient into a tissue and smeared directly onto a slide will demonstrate infectiousness and keep your laboratory technicians on their toes!

Rx: Treatment begins with referral or reporting to the public health authorities. They may manage the patient and treatment and/or follow-up, or it may be left to local health workers. Multidrug therapy (MDT) depends on classification. Blister packs for MB, PB (adults and children) of drugs containing 4 wk of medicine are usually available.

MB (adult, 12-month course)

LEPROSY

- Rifampin 600 mg once a month
- Clofazimine 300 mg once a month and 50 mg daily
- Dapsone 100 mg daily

  MB (children ages 10–14 yr, 12-month course)

- Rifampin 450 mg once a month
- Clofazimine 150 mg once a month and 50 mg every other day
- Dapsone 50 mg daily

  PB (adult, 6-month course)

- Rifampin 600 mg once a month
- Dapsone 100 mg daily

  PB (Children ages 10–14 yr, 6-month course)

- Rifampin 450 mg once a month
- Dapsone 50 mg daily

  Children under 10 yr use these doses and the appropriate MB or PB schedule:

- Rifampin 10 mg/kg/dose
- Clofazimine 1 mg/kg/d and 6 mg/kg/month
- Dapsone 2 mg/kg/d

  Indeterminate leprosy (1 lesion) will usually self cure, or you can use a WHO recommended treatment of rifampin 600 mg + ofloxacin 400 mg + minocycline 100 mg once. Because of the uncertainty of the cure, the patient will need to be followed closely for 10 yr.

  Controversies exist among leprosy experts as to the effectiveness of the WHO MDT regime (Trop Med Intern Health 2006;11:268; J Am Acad Dermatol 2004;51:417).

  Side effects of treatment are hemolytic anemia in G6PD-deficient patients treated with dapsone, reddish-brown skin discoloration with clofazimine and orange coloration of secretions, liver toxicity and interaction of HIV/AIDS drugs with rifampin.

Other drugs with activity against leprosy that may be recommended by an expert include ofloxacin, pefloxacin, clarithromycin, ansamycins, streptomycin, and minocycline.

Cmplc: Reversal reactions are hypersensitivity reactions to leprosy bacillus antigens. They may occur before, during (usual), or after drug treatment.

Type 1 reactions occur in paucibacillary disease (BB, BT, BL). It is characterized by tender swollen nerves with loss of sensory and motor function and redness and swelling of the skin lesions. Onset can occur overnight. Continue MDT and add analgesics; start prednisone 30 to 80 mg per d, decreasing 5 mg every 2 to 4 wk after the symptoms improve; 3 to 6 months of therapy is required, longer (up to 20 months) in BL patients. Follow the neuropathy signs; occasionally a silent neuropathy occurs or follows a painful type I reaction. Expect a 60% to 70% improvement in nerve function. Continue to follow for nerve damage for several years after drug therapy stops (Am J Trop Med Hyg 2007;77:829).

Type 2 reactions (Erythema Nodosum Leprosum, ENL) occur in 20% LL and 10% BL patients with a high bacteria load. The patient is systemically ill with fever, erythema nodosum, and perhaps iritis, neuritis, orchitis, dactylitis, arthritis, lymphadenitis, and bone pain anywhere the bacilli are numerous. Steroids are the mainstay of therapy; a shorter course of 1 to 2 mg/kg prednisone with a rapid reduction in dose is effective (2–3 wk). Increase or restart steroids if symptoms reappear. Increase clofazimine to 300 mg daily for several months or longer (for its anti-inflammatory properties). Thalidomide (400 mg daily) is the drug of choice when available, but precautions are necessary in women of child-bearing age because it causes birth defects. Treat iritis with ocular steroids and cycloplegics (see ophthalmology).

Relapse after treatment occurs, perhaps at the rate of 0.1% per yr. It may be difficult to differentiate from a reaction.

LEPROSY

Relapses usually occur more than 3 yr after treatment. Skin lesions appear in new areas, and the onset is insidious. Classify the patient and treat with the same MDT.

Pregnancy worsens disease and increases Type 1 and 2 reactions. MDT is safe and should be continued.

Unlike TB, HIV/AIDS does not seem to worsen the course of leprosy, although Type 1 reactions may be common (Lancet Infect Dis 2006;6:350).

Leprosy causes disability through nerve damage (paralysis, anesthesia, and autonomic dysfunction).

Autonomic nerve injury leads to loss of sweating and skin dryness, resulting in skin cracking and fissuring with a greater susceptibility to infection. Loss of vascular tone causes increased bruising and impaired oxygenation.

Paralysis leads to disuse, atrophy, and contractures, causing abnormal pressure points.

Anesthesia allows injuries and ulcers to go unnoticed and untreated. The problem is similar to diabetic neuropathy and treated in the same manner.

Leprosy reactions may cause inflammatory injury to the eye, joints, and bone leading to blindness, contractures, and bony destruction.

Direct invasion by the bacilli in LL causes sterility, bone thinning with fractures, and the heavy antigen load which may lead to amyloidosis.

Prev: BCG vaccine provides some incomplete protection. Single dose rifampicin has been studied as a chemoprophylaxis agent in the COLEP study in Bangladesh (Br Med J 2008). It was effective in preventing disease at 2 yr but with no further protection over 4 yr after high risk exposure (NNT 297). Long-term dapsone alone provides some protection as does BCG immunization. A medical worker is unlikely to develop clinical leprosy even after prolonged contact with patients.

Chapter 12

Tuberculosis

(Am J Respir Crit Care Med 2003;167:603; TB/HIV A Clinical Manual, 2nd ed, WHO; 2004; Am Fam Physician 2005;72:1761, 2225; Core Curriculum on Tuberculosis 2004, http://www.cdc.gov)

Cause: Caused by *Mycobacterium tuberculosis*, occasionally M *bovis*, rarely M *africanum*. Sources are patients with active pulmonary tuberculosis (respiratory) and milk (bovine TB).

Epidem: The TB and HIV epidemic are intertwined. The lifetime risk of developing TB is 5% to 10% in immunocompetent individuals and 50% in those HIV+. Conversely, 75% of TB patients in Sub-Saharan Africa are HIV+. Nearly 2 billion people are infected with tuberculosis; 9 million have active disease, and 2 million die each year (25% of preventable adult deaths in developing countries). Multidrug-resistant TB (MDR TB) makes up about 5% of cases, and it infects a half million people per year. About 10% of these are XDR-TB (extensively drug resistant).

Pathophys: Primary infection is usually pulmonary (PTB) with TB multiplication in the lower lungs and hilar lymph nodes, development of a delayed hypersensitivity and cellular immune response, and no clinical disease in 90% of healthy adults. Milk-borne TB multiplies in the cervical lymph nodes as scrofula or in the abdominal lymph nodes.

Sx/Si: Unchecked by the immune system, TB may progress in the lung to cause a progressive pneumonia, cavitation, upper lobe infiltrates, pleural effusions, and rarely empyema. Cough, weight loss, hemoptysis, and night sweats are common.

It may disseminate, especially in children < 5 yr and in the immunosuppressed. Common areas of spread include the cervical lymph nodes, CNS (meningitis and tuberculoma), pericardium, GI tract (ileocecal and peritoneal), bone (thoracic-lumbar spine and joints). Less common are the kidney, adrenal, testis and epididymis, ovary and endometrium, skin, disseminated miliary, spleen and liver, and breast.

Alternatively, the immune system can suppress infection and allow a latent state to follow for months or years until the disease reactivates when immunity wanes, as in HIV infection or cancer.

Diagnosis of pulmonary infection is initially clinical. Given a suggestive history of cough, sputum production, and weight loss, obtain an AFB smear: if positive, register the patient and start therapy. If smear is negative, treat for bronchitis/pneumonia per country protocol (doxycycline 100 mg bid for 7–10 d is one option). Do not use fluoroquinolones, as they are effective against TB (N Engl J Med 2006;354:1729). See the patient back in 3 wk, reassess, do another sputum for AFB if indicated, and obtain a chest X-ray (CXR) if necessary. If the CXR looks like TB, register and treat. If diagnosis uncertain but the patient is still ill, repeat the cycle of bronchitis treatment and close follow-up. Examine carefully for a lesion to biopsy. A purified protein derivative (Mantoux; PPD) skin test is not helpful in adults in an area with high TB prevalence. In low-risk populations and children, inject 0.1 ml tuberculin intradermally and read in 48 to 72 hr. See Table 12.1.

Tips:

- Weight loss and fever more common in HIV+.
- Cough and hemoptysis more common in HIV–.
- Pulmonary TB and sputum+: 90% have cough.
- Three samples of sputum should be collected; early morning is best.

Table 12.1   Interpretation of Tuberculin Skin Tests

Size Induration	Population	Interpretation
≥ 5 mm	HIV+, immunosuppressed	Positive
	Close contacts, CXR suggests old TB	Positive
	IV drug users (HIV status unknown)	Positive
≥ 10 mm	IV drug users (HIV negative), born in high risk area, living in residential community, poor, < 4 yr old, other illnesses such as diabetes	Positive
≥ 15 mm	No risk	Positive

Ignore old BCG immunizations in interpretation.

- Mitral stenosis with CHF will be short of breath (SOB), cough, hemoptysis.
- Cavitary TB > 90% AFB slide+.
- M. *tuberculosis* cultures require sophisticated laboratory facilities; take too long for practical use and may be false + in a poorly supervised lab.
- In children, smear negative PTB is the most common type then extrapulmonary. Cavitation < 6 yr old is unusual.
- Gastric aspiration for AFB is not useful for microscopic examination but can be sent for culture.
- Intestinal TB is usually ileocecal.
- Needle biopsy of hepatic nodules for TB vs hepatoma, hepatic abscesses for bacteria and amoeba.
- Urine AFB stains for TB are often falsely + due to AFB in smegma.

Extrapulmonary TB is common in young children and HIV+ individuals. Suspicion of extrapulmonary TB should always prompt re-evaluation for pulmonary TB.

Lymph node infection progresses from discrete adenopathy to matted fluctuant nodes, then abscesses and drainage.

Differential diagnosis is lymphoma, Kaposi's sarcoma, metastasis, sarcoid, and drug reaction, and in children, lymphoid interstitial pneumonitis with persistent generalized lymphadenopathy, pyogenic and viral infection, and Burkitt's lymphoma.

Lab: To diagnose TB adenopathy, obtain a needle aspirate of lymph node tissue, or better yet, a biopsy. Look for caseation on the bisected node or needle biopsy specimen and do an AFB smear. Sensitivity is 70% to 80%. The node should be sent to pathology.

Miliary TB is widespread dissemination of TB. Fever and wasting are usual; respiratory symptoms may or may not be present. CXR shows multiple small "millet" seed shadows of infection. Hepatomegaly and tubercles in the optic fundi may be seen. Positive AFB smears can be sought in the blood, sputum, CSF, liver biopsy, or bone marrow. Differential includes HIV wasting, bacteremia, disseminated carcinoma and atypical mycobacteria, trypanosomiasis (Africa), and rarely connective tissue disease.

Serous effusions of the pericardium, pleura, and peritoneum (ascites) are more common in primary TB disease, HIV+ adults, and children. Aspirates usually are negative by AFB stains. The bacilli live on the serous surfaces, not in the fluid.

Pleural effusion: tap when identified; do not wait.

While listening to the chest with a stethoscope, shake the patient.

A succession splash indicates a pyopneumothorax. Confirm with a CXR and treat with a chest tube.

If it is a simple pleural effusion, do a thoracentesis.

If the fluid forms fine web-like clots, it is an exudate.

Or calculate the difference between the pleural fluid and the serum albumin. A pleural fluid or ascites albumin minus the serum albumin < 11 g/l (1.1 mg/dl) is an exudate.

If you drain pus and not pleural fluid, send it to the lab for AFB and Gram stain and culture. Place a chest tube (see surgery chapter).

A pericardial effusion from TB is painless. Differential is mycotic infection, uremic pericarditis, CHF, cirrhosis, myxedema, chronic constrictive pericarditis (chronic TB), Kaposi's sarcoma, ruptured hepatic amoebic abscess. Sonography is diagnostic; CXR and EKG (low voltage, electrical alternans) are helpful. Unless there is cardiac tamponade, it is usually better to avoid drainage as anti-TB drugs and oral steroids (prednisone 40 mg daily for 1 wk or 2, then weaned slowly) will cause resolution.

Tubercular ascites may present as wasting with palpable mesenteric lymph nodes, bowel obstruction, or fistulas. Ultrasound will identify the adenopathy and a pocket of fluid to tap.

The fluid is usually yellow but occasionally thick or bloody, an exudate, with > 300 WBC/mm^3, mostly lymphocytes. AFB stains are negative. Laparotomy or laparoscopy to obtain peritoneal lesions or nodes is diagnostic.

Other causes of exudative peritoneal fluid: malignancy and peritonitis.

Tubercular meningitis has a gradual onset with headache progressing to decreased consciousness, Kernig's sign, cranial nerve palsies, and seizures. Rule out increased intracranial pressure (CT or funduscopic exam for papilledema). If safe, do an LP and look for:

- high opening pressure
- clear or cloudy
- protein high (may clot in tube)
- glucose low
- WBC usually < 500, mostly lymphocytes
- centrifuge 10 ml CSF for 30 min and then look for AFB for 30 min
- gram stain and India Ink for cryptococcal disease
- HIV+ patient may have normal glucose (15%), protein (40%), WBC (10%)

A scoring system for HIV negative patients awarded points for age ≥ 36 yr (2), blood WBC > 15,000 (4), duration of illness ≥ 6 d (–5), CSF-WBC ≥ 900 (3), and CSF % neutrophils ≥ 75% (4). Scores ≤ 4 are tuberculosis with a sensitivity of 97%. Scores 5 and above are bacterial meningitis, sensitivity 81% (Am J Trop Med Hyg 2007;77:55).

Extrapulmonary sites of TB are listed in Table 12.2.

Table 12.2   TB Extrapulmonary Sites

Renal, bladder	Hematuria Sterile pyuria Frequency Flank pain	Culture IVP Sonogram
Adrenal	Addison's disease	Abdominal film Calcification Sonogram
Female genital	Infertility PID, ectopic	Sonogram Biopsy Exam
Male genital	Epididymitis	Exam
Liver	Pain, mass	Sonogram Biopsy
Breast	Solitary painless mass, matted with axillary spread and fistula	Biopsy
Spine (Pott's disease)	Back pain Deformity (usually T-10 to L-1) Psoas abscess Spinal cord compression	X-ray Vertebral body erosions Disc narrowing
Bone	Osteomyelitis	Biopsy
Joints	Especially hip, knee	Biopsy
Intestine	Diarrhea Obstruction	Biopsy Barium enema

Rx: Before you can treat TB successfully, you need to classify the patient and ensure adequate follow-up.

Category 1

- new smear+ pulmonary
- new smear– pulmonary and CXR extensive disease
- new+ extrapulmonary
- severely ill and HIV+

Category 2

- previously treated smear+ pulmonary
- relapse
- defaulter restarting treatment
- treatment failure

Category 3

- new smear–, CXR limited disease, HIV–; new less severe extrapulmonary: lymph node, unilateral pleural effusion, bone, joint, adrenal
- HIV–

Category 4: chronic and MDR (multidrug resistant)

- smear positive: 2 AFB+, or 1 AFB+ and CXR+ or 1 AFB+ and culture+
- severe extrapulmonary: miliary, meningitis, pericarditis, peritonitis, intestinal, genitourinary (GU), spinal, bilateral pleural effusions

TB culture and sensitivity take ≥ 4 wk when available. They should be obtained in category 2 and 4 patients.

Drugs and dosages (Table 12.3) will vary by country program. Public health officials must always be notified when treatment is started; a national standard treatment should be used unless there is an excellent reason to deviate from the country's plan and you or your organization are able and willing to super-

Table 12.3 Standard Drug Dosage

Drug	Daily Dose	Intermittent Dose 3× Wk
Isoniazid (H)	5 mg/kg (300 mg max)	10–15 mg/kg (900 mg max)
Rifampicin (R)	10 mg/kg (600 mg max)	10 mg (600 mg max)
Pyrazinamide (Z)	25 mg/kg range 15–30 mg/kg (2000 mg max)	35 mg/kg (2000 mg max)
Streptomycin (S)	15 mg/kg (1000 mg max)	15 mg/kg (1000 mg max)
Ethambutol (E)	15 mg/kg (1000 mg max)	20–30 mg/kg (2400 mg max)
Thioacetazone (T)	2.5 mg/kg	must be given daily

vise ongoing care of the patient and ensure an affordable and constant supply of medications.

Treatment regimens are abbreviated in a standard manner. Numbers signify the months of therapy, a backslash (/) a change in therapy, and a subscript the number of doses/wk.

Example:

2 SHRZ/4 HR: 2 months of streptomycin (S), isoniazid (H), rifampin (R), and pyrazinamide (Z), then 4 months of isoniazid and rifampin. All given daily.

2 SHRZ/4 H_3R_3: 2 months SHRZ and 4 months of H and R given 3 times/wk. Directly observed therapy (DOT): health worker sees patient take drug. Table 12.4 shows a common treatment plan.

Treatment tips:

- In TB meningitis, use streptomycin over ethambutol.
- Ethambutol (E) may be omitted in Category 3 smear negative, pulmonary, HIV−, and children with primary disease.

Table 12.4   Treatment Regime

TB category	Initial phase	Continuation phase
1	2 HRZE or 2 HRZS	4 HR or 6 HE
2	1 HRZES then 1 HRZE	5 HRE
3	2 HRZE	4 HR or 6 HE
4	Individualized by country guidelines or expert advice	

- Thioacetazone (T) must be given daily, never to HIV+.
- DOT is essential, especially during the first 2 months of therapy and when rifampin is used (to prevent R resistance).
- Streptomycin injections hurt.
- Hearing tests weekly while on streptomycin.
- Color vision should be checked regularly on E.
- Fixed drug combinations (FDC) should be used when possible to prevent dosage errors.
- Streptomycin cannot be used in pregnancy (deafness in newborn).
- All drugs are compatible with breast feeding, but none provide therapeutic levels for an infected infant.
- Renal failure: give pyridoxine with H, avoid S and E or reduce dose and increase interval; never use T. The safest regimen 2 HRZ/4 HR.
- Liver disease: never Z, H, and R, potentially toxic; watch carefully. Safest: 2 SRHE/6 HE or 2 SHE/10 HE.
- Steroid treatment can be lifesaving.
- R is a potent hepatic enzyme inducer. Increase drug doses, ie, steroids, anticonvulsants, oral contraceptives as appropriate.
- Pyridoxine 10 mg/d with H if HIV+, alcoholic, and whenever available.
- One drug should never be added to a failing combination.
- Rifabutin (dose varies) can be substituted for R for HIV+ patients on protease inhibitors or nonnucleoside reverse transcriptase inhibitors (NNRTI).

- *M. bovis* is resistant to P.
- E and T are bacteriostatic; use T only if E cannot be used.
- H, R, Z, and S are bacteriocidal.

Drug reactions are common; some are absolute contraindications to restarting again:

S: hearing loss, vertigo

T: severe rash, agranulocytosis

E: visual acuity/color loss (test monthly)

R: renal failure, shock, thrombocytopenia

P: hepatitis

Hepatitis may be caused by TB drugs in descending order of frequency: H>P>R>T>S>E. Try to rule out other causes of hepatitis. If drug-induced hepatitis is suspected, stop all drugs, wait 2 wk after the jaundice has cleared or until liver tests are normal, and resume the previous regime but start H, P, and R slowly, increasing each one separately over 3 d. Seriously ill patients should be started on, or continued on, S and E during the drug holiday. Add ofloxacin 300 mg/d if life-threatening illness is present.

Prednisone/prednisolone are indicated for inflammatory reactions to infection that are life threatening, such as: decreased consciousness or neurological defects in meningitis; adrenal disease with hypotension; renal TB (prevent obstruction); large effusions; or lymphadenopathy, which compromises function. Give 1 to 2 mg/kg/d for 1 to 4 wk, then wean over several more weeks. Use the higher dose when R is part of the regimen or in children (1–3 mg/kg/d).

Monitor treatment with sputum if patient is sputum+, otherwise clinically. Do not use CXR to monitor therapy; it wastes films. Sputum for AFB should be checked at prescribed frequencies as shown in Table 12.5.

Table 12.5   Monitoring Sputum+ AFB Patients Category 1 & 2

Time (Months)	Regime	Sputum	Treatment
0	Diagnosis	+	2 HRZE, 2 HRZES, or 1 HRZE
1	Check 1 HRZE	+	Maintain HRZE
		–	Start continuation 5 HRE
2	Check 1 HRZE and 2 HRZES	+	Maintain therapy, check compliance
		–	Start continuation 4 HR, or 6 HE
3	Recheck 1 HRZE sputum positive	+	Maintain therapy, check compliance
		–	Start continuation 5 HRE
4	Recheck those sputum positive at 2 months	+	Start continuation therapy
		–	appropriate to category
5	Check all groups	+	Treatment failure
		–	continuation therapy
6	Check during last month of therapy	+	Treatment failure
		–	cure
7	Check during last month of therapy		Treatment failure
			cure
8	Check during last month of therapy	+	Treatment failure
		–	cure

Those in Category 1 who fail treatment move to Category 2 and start that drug regimen. Those in Category 2 who fail move to Category 4.

Outcome classification is as follows:

- cure (2 negative sputums at 5 months and last month of therapy)
- treatment completed
- treatment failure
- died
- defaulted
- transferred out

Drugs for Category 4, MDR and XDR TB:

MDR TB is resistant to at least H and R. XDR TB is resistant to H, R, any fluoroquinolone plus at least one second-line injectable drug. See below (MMWR 2006;55:301,1176.) Treatment is longer, more expensive, and should be done in consultation with an expert and the national TB program. It is important not to use second-line TB drugs for other purposes (unless no other drug is appropriate) to avoid development of TB resistance in the community. An estimated 5% to 25% of new TB patients are MDR. XDR TB has been reported from 45 countries (WHO [news release] February 26, 2008).

Second-line drugs (SLDs):

- Aminoglycosides other than streptomycin (injectable kanamycin and amikacin)
- Capreomycin (injectable)
- Fluoroquinolones (ofloxacin, ciprofloxacin, levofloxacin, and moxifloxacin)
- Thioamides (prothioamide and ethionamide)
- Serine analogs (cycloserine and terizidone)
- Salicylic derivatives (para-amino salicylic acid, PAS)
- Clofazimine is occasionally used as are rifampin analogs

MDR TB is treated with 4 to 6 drugs to which the bacilli is sensitive. The same recommendation holds for XDR TB, but this may not be possible (Emerg Infect Dis 2007;13:380). Unfortunately, cross resistance between H-E and kanamycin-E are common. Resistance to kanamycin and amikacin is universally shared. Treatment duration is usually 24 months.

Control of MDR TB and XDR TB is difficult. It requires sophisticated microbiology laboratory support and an efficiently functioning health system. A DOTS-Plus program promoted by WHO is one approach. Judicious use of potential TB drugs, treatment of concomitant HIV/AIDs, and support of national TB control programs are essential.

Prevention: Primary prevention includes the following:

- BCG vaccine (see immunizations)
- Isolation of infective individuals, especially those with MDR TB
- Isolate HIV+ from potential TB patients

    Secondary prevention:

- Give isoniazid (H) to recent PPD converters, any PPD+ HIV+ patients, breastfed infants of mothers with pulmonary TB, children < 5 living in household with smear + pulmonary TB.
- Give H dose 10 to 15 mg/kg/d up to 300 mg maximum for 6 to 9 months.
- Consider H for high-risk HIV+ patients: prisoners, miners, close contacts.

    Tips:

- Rifampin daily for 4 months is an alternative to H.
- Rifampin plus pyrazinamide for 2 months (MMWR 2001;50:1) is dangerous and not advised.

TUBERCULOSIS

Chapter 13

Sexually Transmitted Infections

(TB/HIV A Clinical Manual 2nd ed, WHO, 2004; Guidelines for the management of STI, WHO, 2003; Am Fam Physician 2007;76:1827; MMWR 2006;55:997)

13.1   Syndromic Management

The evaluation and treatment decision making of STIs is based on syndromic management. STI are classified here into 4 common syndromes easily displayed on flow sheets and practical for implementation in any health facility. Syndromic management is rapid, straightforward, does not require laboratory backup, or follow-up visits. This simplicity allows easy reporting although overdiagnosis, overtreatment, and missed diagnosis of asymptomatic STIs remains a problem.

13.2   Urethral Discharge and Cervicitis

Cause: *Neisseria gonorrhea* (GC), *Chlamydia trachomatis*, occasionally *Ureaplasma sp.*, *Mycoplasma sp.*, rarely *Trichomonas vaginalis*.

Epidem: Most common syndrome. Gonorrhea may disseminate (0.5–2%). Mixed infections common.

Sx: Males: urethral discharge (most infections asymptomatic)
Females: dysuria, cervicitis

Crs: 2 to 7 d incubation period for GC, 1 to 3 wk for chlamydia.

Cmplc: GC: epididymis, abscess and fistulas, urethral strictures, sterility, purulent conjunctivitis, dissemination with arthritis, tenosynovitis, skin lesions. In females: Skene's and Bartholin's gland infections, pelvic inflammatory disease (PID), endometritis with uterine bleeding, neonatal infection.

Chlamydia: Males: epididymo-orchitis and urethral stricture. Females: cervicitis, endometritis, perihepatitis, neonatal infection.

Lab: Gram stain in GC shows intracellular gram-negative diplococci, sensitivity > 95% in males and 67% in females. Polymerase chain reaction (PCR) tests available for GC and chlamydia.

Rx: Treatment will vary depending on national guidelines and drug availability. For urethral discharge or cervicitis without specific diagnosis use azithromycin 2 grams and ciprofloxacin 500 mg (not in pregnancy) orally single dose.

Other single dose options for GC:

- ceftriaxone 250 mg IM
- cefixime 400 mg orally
- spectinomycin 2 gm IM
- trimethoprim/sulfamethoxazole 80 mg/400 mg 10 tablets orally
- gentamicin 240 mg IM

For chlamydia, a 7-day course of the following:

- doxycycline 100 mg orally twice/d
- erythromycin 500 mg orally 4 times/d
- tetracycline 500 mg orally 4 times/d
- amoxicillin 500 mg orally 3 times/d (pregnant)
- For persistent symptoms, consider *T. vaginalis*, resistant GC, or reinfection.

13.3 Vaginal Discharge

Cause: *Trichomonas vaginalis*, *Candida sp.*, *Gardnerella vaginalis* (BV), often GC and *Chlamydia trachomatis*, especially with mucopurulent cervicitis.

Epidem: In areas of high prevalence of GC and chlamydia, treat for these also.

Sx/Si: Vaginal discharge, watery, fishy smell, no dyspareunia suggests gardnerella; diabetes, HIV+, dyspareunia, vulvar rash; cottage cheese-like discharge that scrapes off in candida; dyspareunia, watery, bubbly yellow-greenish with punctate hemorrhages on cervix with trichomoniasis.

Lab: Wet mount microscopic examination shows: pseudohyphae (use 10% KOH on second slide) in candida; motile flagellated parasites (50–80% sensitive) in trichomoniasis; clue cells (100% sensitive) in BV.

Rx: Candidiasis: nystatin 100 000 IU vaginally (pv) daily for 14 d or miconazole or clotrimazole 200 mg pv daily for 3 d or clotrimazole 500 mg pv once.

Fluconazole 150 mg orally once.

Trichomonas and BV: metronidazole or tinidazole 2 gm orally once.

Consider treatment for GC or chlamydia cervicitis.

13.4 Genital Ulcers

Cause: *Treponema pallidum* (syphilis), *Haemophilus ducreyi* (chancroid), *Herpes simplex*, *Klebsiella (Calymmatobacterium) granulomatis* (Donovanosis).

Epidem: Common in sex workers. Previous infection with yaws may be protective of syphilis, Donovanosis in India, Papua New

Guinea, Brazil, and S Africa. Local epidemiology guides diagnosis of chancroid, granuloma inguinale, and LGV (see section 13.5).

Sx/Si: Chancroid: Papule evolves to painful purulent dirty, undermined ulcer(s), bleeds easily with tender inguinal adenopathy.

Syphilis: Papule evolves to painless, indurated, clean-based ulcer, usually single; does not bleed and not undermined. Painless hard adenopathy. Note: Clinical diagnosis alone is not reliable.

Herpes: Vesicles evolve to small ulcers that crust over and resolve without scar; painful lymphadenopathy especially with first attack. Ulcers intractable in HIV+.

Donovanosis: Papule ruptures and evolves to raised red-purple granuloma that is painless and bleeds easily. Extends along skin folds.

Cmplc: Chancroid: Will locally spread and may cause extensive destruction.

Syphilis: Chancre will resolve in 3 to 6 wk when secondary rash and disseminated disease will appear. Spread to fetus common ~80%.

Herpes: Recurs in outbreaks; may be transmitted at time of birth.

Donovanosis: Primarily spreads along the skin but may be extragenital (especially face) and extend into the pelvis resembling TB (1–5%). Rarely systemic spread.

Lab: Chancroid: Gram stain low sensitivity and specificity. Culture possible, 80% sensitive.

Syphilis: Dark-field microscopy seldom available. Reagin tests (VDRL, RPR), can do titers with VDRL, 1° 75% positive, 2° 100%. False+ in yaws, pinta, occasionally leprosy, sarcoid, malaria, mononucleosis. TPHA and fluorescent treponemal antigen (FTA) more specific, remain positive for life.

Herpes: Can be diagnosed clinically.

Donovanosis: Giemsa stain of tissue smear shows intracellular bipolar organisms.

Rx: Syndromic treatment for primary syphilis:

> Benzathine penicillin 2.4 million units IM or Procaine penicillin G 1.2 million units IM daily × 10 or

> If allergic to penicillin:

Tetracycline 500 mg orally 4 times a day or
Doxycycline 100 mg orally twice a day or
Erythromycin 500 mg orally 4 times a day, all for 15 d

> Plus treatment for chancroid:

Azithromycin 1 gm orally once (20 mg/kg)
Ciprofloxacin 500 mg orally twice a day × 3 d or
Ceftriaxone 250 mg IM once or
Erythromycin 500 mg orally 3 times a day × 7 d or
Trimethoprin and sulfamethoxazole (TMP/SMX) 80 mg/400 mg,
   2 tablets orally twice a day for 7 d

> Note: A single dose of 1 gm azithromycin cures both (Ann Intern Med 1990;131:434); 2 grams suggested (N Engl J Med 2005;353:1236). Follow up titer for syphilis suggested.

> Herpes simplex: Acyclovir 200 to 400 mg orally 5 times a day for 7 to 10 d (primary) or 5 d (recurrent) or until healed (HIV+). Famciclovir 1 gm orally twice a day for 1 d for recurrent disease.

> Donovanosis: Azithromycin 1 gm orally once then 500 mg daily × 14 (preferred) or streptomycin 1 gm IM daily × 14 or tetracycline 500 mg orally 4 times a day × 14 or TMP/SMX 80 mg/400 mg, 2 tablets twice daily for 14 d. Erythromycin and doxycycline also effective; longer therapy required for disseminated disease and HIV+. Consider streptomycin or gentamicin in addition to oral antibiotic in HIV+.

13.5   Inguinal Bubo

Cause: *Haemophilis ducreyi* (chancroid) and *Chlamydia trachomatis* serotypes L1, 2, 3 (lymphogranuloma venereum [LGV]).

Epidem: Clinically more common in men 5:1. Up to 20% prevalence at some STI clinics. Primarily tropical.

Sx/Si: LGV primary lesion small, 5 mm painless papule that heals in a few days and is usually not detected. Secondary stage days to months later with lymphadenopathy usually unilateral (two-thirds) then lymphadenitis with painful matted, fluctuant nodes. Rupture and sinus tracts occur.

Cmplc: LGV: elephantiasis, rectal fistulas, fibrosis, rarely systemic spread. Late malignancy.

Rx: Syndromic management of bubos without ulcers (LGV):

Doxycycline 100 mg orally twice a day, or
Tetracycline 500 mg orally 4 × daily, or
Erythromycin 500 mg orally 4 × daily, or
Sulfadiazine 1 gm orally 4 × daily, all for 14 to 21 d.

13.6   Syphilis

Secondary Syphilis

Primary syphilis is covered under genital ulcers; secondary syphilis is a generalized disease with protean manifestations. Secondary syphilis may appear as the primary lesion is healing (25%) or after a latency of 2 wk to 6 months.

Pathophys: Bacteremia occurs with a contagious period ranging from 2 to 4 yr, up to 10 yr to the fetus.

Sx/Si: Skin: Usually generalized and symmetrical with macular or macular-papular rash, occasionally follicular, psoriasiform, or crusting pustular. Involves palms and soles. In warm and moist areas, lesions are hypertrophied, confluent, and flattened as condyloma lata. These are highly infectious. Rarely pruritic, the rash clears in 1 to 3 months. Mucous membranes show circular or oval mucous patches of shallow erosions and "snail tract" ulcers. Lymphadenopathy is nontender, mobile, discrete, and rubbery. Hair may be lost as patchy alopecia. Periostitis with periosteal elevation and bone pain, iritis, glomerulonephritis, hepatitis, epididymitis, parotitis, and meningitis may occur.

Crs: Relapse occurs within 2 yr in 25% of untreated patients, the remainder self-cure. Relapse is hard to tell from reinfection. After secondary stage, latency begins.

Cmplc: Yaws and pinta give positive serological tests for syphilis.

Lab: Dark-field microscopy is positive on moist lesions (avoid oral lesions as false positives). All serological tests are positive. CSF 30% positive tests, elevated protein and lymphocytes.

Rx: For primary, secondary and latent < 2 yr (see genital ulcers).

Tertiary Syphilis

After secondary syphilis, the disease enters a latent phase. After several years lesions may reappear.

Pathophys: Probably a hypersensitivity reaction with only a few organisms present.

Sx/Si: Skin or subcutaneous nodules, painless, indurated, often ulcerate then heal in the center with a serpentinous form. Usually over the buttocks, sternum, head, and legs. 75% of gummas are cutaneous. Mucosal ulcerations with destruction of palate, nasal septum, macroglossia, painful leukoplakia. Bone is involved in 10% with painful periostitis and osteitis. Cardiovascular 10% to 15% occurs late, 10 to 40 yr after infection. Aortitis with insufficiency due to aneurysm and coronary ostial occlusion with angina are the usual manifestations.

Neurosyphilis may be as follows:

- Meningovascular of the brain (stroke) or spinal cord (spastic paraplegia) occurs early 2 yr after infection.
- General paralysis (paresis) of the insane occurs after 10 to 20 yr. Psychosis, dementia, tremors, Argyll Robertson pupils (small, unequal, constrict with accommodation but not light).
- Tabes dorsalis occurs late with lightning pains of the legs, paresthesias, loss of position, vibration sense, and reflexes; ataxia with high stepping gait is common.

Labs: HIV+ patients: tests often positive as infection accelerates time of onset of presentation. VDRL or RPR positive in 75% on CSF, FTA-ABS 98%. CSF protein and cells usually elevated with neurological symptoms.

Rx: For late latent syphilis > 2 yr duration:

Benzathine penicillin G 2.4 million units IM weekly × 3, or
Procaine penicillin G 600 000 units IM daily × 15 d, or
Procaine penicillin G 1.2 million units (50,000 units/kg) IM daily × 10 d, or
Second choice doxycycline 100 mg orally twice daily × 4 wk

Neurological or cardiovascular syphilis:

Penicillin G (benzylpenicillin) 3 to 4 million units IV every 4 hr for 2 wk, or
Procaine penicillin G 2.4 million units 4 times a day for 2 wk, plus
Probenecid 500 mg orally 4 times a day.

If penicillin allergy:
28 days of doxycycline as above or erythromycin or tetracycline 500 mg orally 4 times a day
Follow-up after treatment of latent and late syphilis:

- Test titers with VDRL at 3, 6, 12 months and yearly.
- Expect titers to stop decreasing about 1:8.
- Retreat if no change or increasing.

- Retest CSF titers at 6, 12, 24 months until negative. Cell count should be < 10 at 6 months; if not retreat.

Congenital Syphilis

Cause: Transmission from mother, highest risk in primary, secondary, and early latent

Epidem: Rates up to 25% reported in some areas.

Pathophys: Spirochete crosses placenta early, but fetal immunity develops in second trimester and results in pathological changes.

Sx: Nasal discharge and obstruction (snuffles), pallor.

Si: Hepatomegaly (90%) with prolonged severe jaundice (50%), low birth weight, bullous rash (30%), anemia (60%), painful joint swelling, bone changes on X-ray (95%), metaphyseal destruction, periosteal elevation especially about knee and wrist.

Crs: May appear normal at birth but failure to thrive by 3 months with secondary syphilis-like rash or years later with deafness, corneal keratitis, bone and teeth changes, or neurosyphilis.

Cmplc: Stillbirth 25%, neonatal death 15%. Guidelines for diagnosis (Clin Trop Med Commun Dis 1987;2:124).

Lab: Screen mother and baby with VDRL or RPR. If one or other positive, best to treat, as false negatives common in newborn. CSF cell count and protein elevated in 40%.

Xray: Metaphyseal dystrophy with areas of increased calcification and/or porosity (95%), periosteal changes (40%), normal (5%).

Rx: Penicillin G 50,000 units/kg IM or IV every 8 hr × 10 d, or Procaine penicillin 50,000 units/kg IM daily × 10.

For older children: Benzathine penicillin 50,000 units/kg IM (max 2.4 million units) once if CSF negative; × 3 weekly if CSF positive or unknown.

Prevention of Jarisch-Herxheimer Reaction

A generalized reaction to killed treponemas of syphilis occurs 3 to 12 hr after initial treatment. The patient develops a syndrome of myalgias, headache, fever, chills, and arthralgias, and the rash may become more pronounced. Most frequently seen (70–90%) in secondary syphilis treated with penicillin; the patient should be warned and pretreated with aspirin. Also seen in leptospirosis.

13.7　STI Counseling and Control

All STI patients should do as follows if possible:

- Be tested for HIV.
- Receive counseling and education.
- Receive condoms and promotion.
- Be offered other forms of contraception.
- Have their sexual contacts managed.
- Be reported to public health authorities for contact tracing.
- Be told to return in 1 wk or sooner if not improved.
- Receive single dose observed therapy when possible, with 100% efficacy in high risk groups such as sex workers.

Chapter 14

HIV/AIDS

Donn Colby & Dimitri Prybylski

(Bartlett JG, Gallant JE. Medical Management of HIV Infection. 2007)
(Lancet 2006;368:489; WHO TB/HIV A Clinical Manual (2nd Ed) 2004; WHO HIV/AIDS Guidelines http://www.who.int/hiv/pub/guidelines/en/)

14.1 Introduction

Cause: The etiological agent, HIV, is a retrovirus that can lead to acquired immunodeficiency syndrome (AIDS), a late-stage condition in which the immune system fails, leading to life-threatening opportunistic infections. There are 2 types: type 1 (HIV-1) and type 2 (HIV-2). These viruses share similar epidemiological characteristics although they are relatively distinct serologically and geographically. Worldwide, the predominant virus is HIV-1, which is more pathogenic than HIV-2. The relatively uncommon HIV-2 type is concentrated in West Africa and is rarely found elsewhere.

Epidem: AIDS is one of the most destructive pandemics in recorded history, killing more than 25 million people since it was first recognized in 1981. By the end of 2007, an estimated 33.2 (30.6–36.1) million adults and children were living with HIV globally (Table 14.1). The staggering burden of the pandemic masks its epidemiological heterogeneity as related to its geographic distribution, magnitude, and mode of transmission.

Even at the country level there are wide variations in infection levels between different areas. Sub-Saharan Africa remains the epicenter of the pandemic and is by far the worst affected region, accounting for over two-thirds (68%) of worldwide infections. The average life expectancy in the 35 African nations with the highest HIV prevalence is 48.3 yr—6.5 yr less than it is estimated to be without the disease (UNAIDS, 2006). Nearly 90% of children infected with HIV live in Sub-Saharan Africa.

It is estimated that 15.4 (13.9–16.6 million) women were living with HIV worldwide in 2007, and this comprised half (50%) of all infections. In Sub-Saharan Africa, the proportion of women who are infected has increased over time and almost 61% of adults living with HIV are women. Globally, the number of children (< 15 yr of age) living with HIV was estimated to be 2.5 million (2.2–2.6 million) in 2007.

The HIV/AIDS pandemic has 2 main regional epidemiological patterns:

1. Generalized epidemics sustained in the general populations of many Sub-Saharan countries, especially in southern Africa.
2. Epidemics in the rest of the world concentrated among subpopulations that practice high-risk behaviors such as sex workers and their partners, injecting drug users, and men who have sex with men.

HIV is transmitted from person to person through transfer of infected bodily fluids, namely blood, semen, vaginal fluid and pre-ejaculate, or breast milk. The 3 main transmission modes are unprotected sexual intercourse, contaminated needles and syringes, and transmission from an infected mother to her baby. Screening of blood products for HIV has largely eliminated transmission via blood transfusion or blood products throughout the world. The primary mode of HIV transmission worldwide is heterosexual transmission, which accounts for 85% of all infections, although there is considerable geographic diversity in this regard (see Table 14.1).

Table 14.1   Regional Summary of Key HIV Epidemiological Characteristics, 2007

Region	Adults and Children Living with HIV	Adult Prevalence (%)	Main HIV Transmission Modes
Sub-Saharan Africa	22.5 million (20–24.3 million)	5.0% (4.6–5.5%)	HSex
North Africa and Middle East	380 000 (270 000–400 000)	0.3% (0.2–0.4%)	HSex, IDU
South and South-East Asia	4.0 million (3.3–5.1 million)	0.3% (0.2–0.4%)	HSex, IDU
East Asia	800 000 (620 000–960 000)	0.1% (< 0.2%)	HSex, IDU, MSM
Oceania	75 000 (53 000–120 000)	0.4% (0.3–0.7%)	MSM
Latin America	1.6 million (1.4–1.9 million)	0.5% (0.4–0.6%)	HSex, MSM, IDU
Caribbean	230 000 (210 000–270 000)	1.0% (0.9–1.2%)	HSex, MSM
Eastern Europe and Central Asia	1.6 million (1.2–2.1 million)	0.9% (0.7–1.2%)	IDU
Western and Central Europe	760 000 (600 000–1.1 million)	0.3% (0.1–0.3%)	MSM, IDU
North America	1.3 million (390 000–1.6 million)	0.6% (0.5–0.9%)	HSex, MSM, IDU

HSex = heterosexual sex; IDU = injecting drug use; MSM = men who have sex with men.

HIV transmission and acquisition are enhanced in the presence of concurrent sexually transmitted infections (especially when ulcerative in nature), concurrent sexual partnerships, high rates of partner change, macro-level issues such as population mobility for economic and other reasons (eg, natural disasters, wars), and recreational drug or alcohol use.

Pathophys: HIV enters macrophages and CD4+ T lymphocytes. The spikes on the surface of the virus particle allow the viral envelope to attach to and fuse with the cell membrane. The contents of the HIV virus are then released into the cell where the HIV enzyme reverse transcriptase converts the viral RNA to DNA. This DNA is transported to the cell's nucleus and spliced into the human DNA by the HIV enzyme integrase. Once integrated, the HIV DNA is known as provirus. HIV provirus may lie dormant within a cell for a long time, but when the cell becomes activated, it treats HIV genes in much the same way as human genes. First, it converts them into messenger RNA (using human enzymes), then the messenger RNA is transported outside the nucleus and is used as a blueprint for producing new HIV proteins and enzymes. The HIV protease enzyme processes proteins for final assembly into a new viral particle.

How HIV damages the immune system: In the process of replication, the virus destroys increasing numbers of T lymphocytes. This causes a progressive decline in immunity that leaves the body open to opportunistic infections (OI).

Sx/Si/Crs:

Acute HIV Infection (Acute Retroviral Syndrome): During the acute or primary HIV infection, typically 2 to 4 wk postexposure, most persons (50–90% in developed countries, but little data exist in the developing world) develop a 1 to 2 wk mononucleosis-like illness: fever, lymphadenopathy, pharyngitis, rash, arthralgia, myalgia, and malaise. Infrequently acute neurological symptoms occur, which are typically self-limiting. These include meningitis, peripheral neuropathy, encephalitis, and myelitis.

Tips:

• Acute retroviral syndrome is often not diagnosed due to the nonspecific clinical features and because HIV serological tests do not become positive until 4 to 12 wk after infection.

- Viral load testing can diagnose HIV infection during the acute symptomatic stage. Viral load peaks at 3 to 4 wk after infection and a result of > 50,000 copies/ml is diagnostic.

Asymptomatic HIV Infection

- Adults: There is a long, variable, latent period from HIV infection to the onset of HIV-related disease and AIDS. A person infected with HIV may be asymptomatic for many years— typically 5 to 10 yr with a range 2 to 20 yr.
- Children: The vast majority of children are infected during the perinatal period, and the asymptomatic infection is typically shorter than in adults. Most children start to become ill before 2 yr of age, but clinical latency can last longer.

Progression from HIV Infection to HIV-Related Disease and AIDS: If left untreated, the vast majority (if not all) HIV-infected persons will eventually develop HIV-related disease and AIDS. The rate of progression depends on virus and host factors.

- Virus factors: HIV-1 progresses faster than HIV-2
- Host factors: age < 5 yr, age > 40 yr, concurrent infections, and genetic factors can lead to faster progression

The WHO Clinical Staging and Disease Classification System shown as Table 14.2 (revised in 2006) can be used readily in resource-constrained settings without access to CD4 cell count laboratory testing.

Tip: Clinical stage is important as a key criterion for evaluating immune status, providing medications to prevent OI, and initiating antiretroviral therapy (ART).

Lab:

HIV Testing

- HIV infection is usually diagnosed through the detection of antibodies to the virus in serum or plasma using

Table 14.2 WHO Clinical Staging (Modified from: WHO Case definitions of HIV for surveillance and revised clinical staging and immunological classification of HIV-related disease in adults and children, 2006)

Adults and Adolescents	Children < 15 yr old
Clinical Stage 1	
Asymptomatic	Asymptomatic
Persistent generalized lymphade-nopathy	Persistent generalized lymphadenopathy
Clinical Stage 2	
Weight loss (< 10%)	Unexplained persistent hepatospleno-megaly
Recurrent upper respiratory tract infections	Recurrent upper respiratory tract infections
Herpes zoster	Herpes zoster
Angular cheilitis	Lineal gingival erythema
Recurrent oral ulceration	Recurrent oral ulcerations
Papular pruritic eruptions	Unexplained persistent parotid enlargement
Seborrhoeic dermatitis	Papular pruritic eruptions
Fungal nail infections	Extensive warts or molluscum contagiosum
	Fungal nail infections
Clinical Stage 3	
Weight loss (> 10%)	Moderate malnutrition
Unexplained chronic diarrhea > 1 month	Unexplained persistent diarrhea > 14 d
	Unexplained persistent fever > 1 month
Unexplained persistent fever > 1 month	Oral candidiasis (after first 6–8 wk of life)
Oral candidiasis	Oral hairy leukoplakia
Oral hairy leukoplakia	Acute necrotizing ulcerative gingivitis or periodontitis
Acute necrotizing ulcerative stoma-titis, gingivitis or periodontitis	Pulmonary or lymph node tuberculosis
Pulmonary tuberculosis	Recurrent bacterial pneumonia or bronchiectasis
Severe bacterial infections	Symptomatic lymphoid interstitial pneumonitis
Unexplained anemia (< 8 g/dL), neutropenia (< 500/mL) and/or thrombocytopenia (< 50 000/mm^3)	Unexplained anemia (< 8 g/dL), neutropenia (< 500/mL) and/or thrombocytopenia (< 50 000/mm^3)

Table 14.2   Continued

Adults and Adolescents	Children < 15 yr old

Clinical Stage 4

Adults and Adolescents	Children < 15 yr old
HIV wasting syndrome	Severe wasting, stunting or severe malnutrition
Pneumocystis pneumonia	Pneumocystis pneumonia
Recurrent severe bacterial pneumonia	Recurrent severe bacterial infections
Chronic herpes simplex infection > 1 month	Chronic herpes simplex infection > 1 month
Esophageal candidiasis	Esophageal candidiasis
Extrapulmonary tuberculosis	Extrapulmonary tuberculosis
Kaposi's sarcoma	Kaposi sarcoma
Cytomegalovirus infection	Cytomegalovirus infection
Central nervous system toxoplasmosis	Central nervous system toxoplasmosis
HIV encephalopathy	HIV encephalopathy
Extrapulmonary cryptococcosis (ie, meningitis)	Extrapulmonary cryptococcosis (ie, meningitis)
Disseminated non-TB mycobacterial infection	Disseminated non-TB mycobacterial infection
Progressive multifocal leukoencephalopathy (PML)	Disseminated mycosis (histoplasmosis, coccidiomycosis)
Chronic cryptosporidiosis	Chronic cryptosporidiosis
Chronic isosporiasis	Chronic isosporiasis
Disseminated mycosis (histoplasmosis, coccidiomycosis)	Cerebral or B-cell non-Hodgkin lymphoma
Recurrent septicaemia	Progressive multifocal leukoencephalopathy
Cerebral or B-cell non-Hodgkin lymphoma	HIV-associated nephropathy, cardiomyopathy
Invasive cervical carcinoma	
Atypical disseminated leishmaniasis	
HIV-associated nephropathy, cardiomyopathy	

enzyme immunoassays (EIA), rapid test kits, Western blot, immunofluorescence assay (IFA), or particle agglutination.

- Production of HIV-specific antibodies typically begins 3 to 8 wk after infection. New infections during the "window period," before HIV antibodies are detectable, can only be diagnosed by more technically difficult and expensive tests that detect virus directly (eg, viral RNA, p24 antigen), which are not widely available in resource-constrained settings. These direct methods are also needed to detect HIV infection in infants < 18 months of age who might still bear maternal HIV-antibodies.

Standard HIV Diagnostic Testing Algorithm:

- The use of a multiple test algorithm is recommended for diagnostic purposes in order to increase testing accuracy (UNAIDS/WHO, 2001).
- If the initial screening HIV test result using EIA or a WHO-approved rapid test is nonreactive, the specimen is considered HIV negative.
- Specimens with reactive EIA or rapid test results are retested. If the result of this test is reactive, further confirmatory testing is recommended with a more specific supplemental test (eg, Western blot, IFA, or latest generation EIA or rapid test). Only specimens that are repeatedly reactive are considered HIV+.

Tips:

- Serological tests are available that test for both HIV-1 and HIV-2, but it is important to check the packaging material to determine the specifications.
- If the HIV test is negative but there has been any high-risk behavior in the past 3 months, the patient could be in the window period. Repeat HIV testing in 3 months.

Rapid HIV tests: Many commercial HIV antibody test kits are available that equal the performance of EIA testing and are ideal for use in resource-constrained settings. They do not require special equipment, reagents or highly trained staff. There are 4 main types of rapid test types: agglutination, comb/dipstick, flow-through membrane, and lateral-flow membrane. These rapid test assays can be done on plasma, serum, whole blood, or saliva and can provide results within 10 to 20 min. In most formats, a simple visual-based format is used in which a line or dot indicates a positive test result.

Tips:

- Make sure that test kits are WHO-approved. It is important to also check the expiration date and storage requirements.
- The use of HIV rapid tests has the strong advantage of allowing same day results to be given to persons along with pre- and post-test counseling.

Clinical Testing

Laboratory testing will depend on local availability. WHO guidelines allow for ART in the absence of laboratory testing. At the minimum, a complete blood count (CBC) with calculation of total lymphocyte count (TLC) should be done. In endemic areas, there should be a very low threshold for TB screening on all HIV-positive patients.

Routine laboratory evaluation for the initial evaluation of HIV patients:

- HIV: confirm positive test if not already done
- CBC: calculate TLC (white blood cell count × % lymphocytes)
- TB screen: CXR, sputum for AFB stain
- CD4: if available. (The CD4 count is the best available laboratory test to evaluate immune function, assess the risk for OI, and to make decisions on when to initiate prophylactic medications and ART.)
- Liver function: ALT (SGPT), AST (SGOT)

HIV/AIDS

- Hepatitis: HAV, HBsAg, HBsAb, HCV (especially for injection drug use [IDU])
- Pregnancy: for females before use of Efavirenz (EFV)
- Others: Cr, BUN, glucose, VDRL/RPR, PAP smear (females), STI screening (if indicated)

CD4 count: Normal range is 500 to 1500 cells/mm^3. See Table 14.3. Test reproducibility is only about 30%, meaning that a test result of 200 could represent a true value of 140 to 260. CD4 percentage is preferred for children < 5 yr old, who have higher and more variable CD4 counts. CD4 should be measured at baseline and then every 3 to 6 months before and while on ART. On treatment, CD4 should rise by > 50 in the first 1 to 2 months and then by 50 to 100 per yr thereafter.

Viral Load (VL) can be used to diagnose acute HIV infection and is the gold standard for determining treatment failure. Higher VL correlates with increased infectivity. Result is reported in copies/ml or the $\log_{10}$ c/ml. Changes of ≥ 0.3 $\log_{10}$ are significant. On ART, VL should decrease by > 0.5–1.0 $\log_{10}$ at 4 wk, by > 1–2 $\log_{10}$ at 8 wk, and to undetectable at 6 months. In developed countries, any sustained detectable VL is considered evidence of treatment failure. WHO guidelines (2006) recommend VL > 10,000 copies/ml (> 4.0 $\log_{10}$) as evidence of treatment failure in developing countries, where second-line and salvage ART regimens may be limited or unavailable.

Table 14.3   CD4 Count/Percentage and Immune Suppression

Immunological Status	CD4 ct (cells/mm^3)	CD4 %
Normal	> 500	> 29%
Mild immunosuppression	350–499	21–28%
Moderate immunosuppression	200–349	14–20%
Severe immunosuppression	< 200	< 14%

Resistance testing can assist with treatment decisions in patients with virological failure on ART. Many guidelines also recommend resistance testing in primary HIV infection, to detect transmission of resistant HIV. In general, a VL of at least 500 to 1000 copies/ml is required. Tests detect resistance only if present in > 20% of circulating HIV. Patients with treatment failure should be taking ART when the test is performed, because stopping ART allows wild-type virus to reemerge and predominate. HIV strains resistant to discontinued drugs can be "archived" and may not be identified on resistance testing but will quickly reemerge if the drug is started again. Two factors limit the usefulness of resistance testing in developing countries: (1) genotype testing was developed in western countries where HIV subtype B is common, and it has not been validated for the subtypes that circulate in other areas, and (2) the limited availability (or lack) of second-line ART.

There are 2 types of resistance tests. Genotype assays are less expensive and more widely available. Sequencing of the viral genome detects mutations expressed in amino acid substitutions that are known to confer resistance to specific drugs. Assistance for interpretation of genotype test results can be found at http://hivdb.stanford.edu or http://www.iasusa.org. Phenotype assays are more expensive and are performed in only a few commercial laboratories. The assay is similar to antimicrobial sensitivity testing in which virus is grown in the presence of various concentrations of antiviral drugs. The virtual phenotype uses the genotype assay to predict a phenotype based on comparison of the mutations identified with a database containing tens of thousands of HIV isolates.

Rx: It may seem that poor healthcare facilities, lack of trained medical personnel, and unavailability of diagnostic testing would make proper HIV care next to impossible in developing countries. However, relatively simple procedures, such as early HIV diagnosis, attention to hygiene and nutrition, co-trimoxazole prophylaxis, and the prompt diagnosis and treatment of OIs such as tuberculosis, can lead to substantial improvements in morbidity and mortality in even the most remote locations. In addition, the availability of ART is increasing rapidly in the developing world as the prices for medications decline and treatment programs expand.

Tips:

- The care of the HIV-infected patient should be undertaken as a multidisciplinary team approach. The team may include a doctor, nurse, counselor, pharmacist, and/or social worker.
- Involve the patient, family and caregivers in making treatment decisions as much as possible. This will engage them in the treatment process and improve adherence to medications and follow-up appointments.

Prophylaxis for OIs

Co-trimoxazole (CTX) is a combination medication containing TMP and SMX. It is inexpensive, well tolerated, and simple to take. It is an integral part of pre-ART treatment and chronic care for the HIV patient.

Prophylactic Dose:

Adults: 960 mg daily (TMP 160 mg + SMX 800 mg)
Children: 5 to 8 mg/kg (of TMP component) once daily

When to start:

Adults and children ≥ 5 yr: any of the following criteria:
- CD4 < 200
- WHO clinical stage 3 or 4, regardless of CD4 count.
- WHO clinical stage 2 and CD4 testing not available.
- WHO recommends CTX prophylaxis for patients with CD4 < 350 in resource-limited settings where malaria and bacterial infections are prevalent.

Children ≤ 5 yr:

- HIV exposed infants (born to HIV+ mother): start CTX at 4 to 6 wk and continue until 6 wk after cessation of breastfeeding and HIV infection is excluded by testing.
- HIV+ infants < 1 yr: all regardless of CD4 count. Once started, continue CTX until 5 yr of age.
- HIV+ infants 1 to 4 yr: WHO clinical stage 2, 3, 4 or CD4 < 25%.

When to stop:

Adults and children ≥ 5 yr:

- On ART with CD4 > 200 for at least 3 to 6 months.
- If CD4 testing not available: patient on ART with good adherence and no new WHO clinical stage 2, 3, 4 events for 1 yr.
- In settings where malaria and bacterial infections are common, consider continuing CTX until CD4 > 350 for 3 to 6 months.

Children < 5 years:

- HIV exposed: confirmed HIV-negative testing performed at least 6 wk after complete cessation of breast feeding.
- HIV+ children: once started, continue CTX until 5 yr of age, then follow adult guidelines.

Benefits of co-trimoxazole prophylaxis:

- Prevention of infections: PCP, toxoplasmosis, malaria, *Isospora belli* (diarrhea), *Nocardia asteroids*, bacterial infections (*S. pneumoniae, Salmonella, Shigella, E. coli, S. aureus, H. influenzae*).
- Other benefits: decreased mortality, decreased hospital admissions, decreased morbidity and mortality among HIV-uninfected family members (AIDS 2005;19:1035).

Risks and side effects:

- Rash (less common in Asia and Africa than in western countries).

- GI intolerance, increased liver function test (LFT), bone marrow suppression.

  Desensitization (see Table 14.4):

- Can be safely administered to most patients with history of previous hypersensitivity.
- Do not give to patients with history of severe reaction to CTX or other sulfa drugs.
- Give antihistamines daily throughout desensitization.
- Repeat the same dose daily until stable for mild reactions.
- Stop CTX for severe or worsening reactions.

Alternative Prophylactic Regimens for PCP:

- Alternative drugs are less effective than CTX at preventing PCP and do not prevent other OI.
- Dapsone 100 mg/d is inexpensive and available in most countries.
- Aerosolized pentamidine 300 mg/month or atovaquone 1500 mg/d are expensive and rarely available in developing countries.

Table 14.4   WHO Co-trimoxazole Desensitization Schedule (Modified from WHO, Guidelines on co-trimoxazole prophylaxis for HIV-related infections among children, adolescents and adults in resource-limited settings, 2006)

Day	Dose
1	80 mg SMX + 16 mg TMP (2 ml oral susp)
2	160 mg SMX + 32 mg TMP (4 ml oral susp)
3	240 mg SMX + 48 mg TMP (6 ml oral susp)
4	320 mg SMX + 64 mg TMP (8 ml oral susp)
5	400 mg SMX + 80 mg TMP (1 SS tablet)
6+	800 mg SMX + 160 mg TMP (1 DS tablet)

Mycobacterium Tuberculosis (see also Chapter 12)

Preferred prophylactic regimens:

- INH 300 mg + pyridoxine 50 mg daily × 9 months
- INH 900 mg + pyridoxine 100 mg 2×/wk times 9 months

Alternative prophylactic regimen:

- Rifampin 600 mg/d × 4 months

Indications:

- Positive PPD ≥ 5 mm without previous treatment.
- Recent contact with active TB case.
- In settings where PPD testing is not available, consider treatment for all HIV+ patients with high risk for TB infection: prisoners, miners, populations with estimated high prevalence (> 30%).
- Active TB must be excluded before treatment is started to prevent development of drug resistance.

Fungal Infections

Prophylactic regimens:

- Fluconazole 400 mg/wk or 200 mg 3×/wk
- Itraconazole 200 mg/d

Indications:

- Generally not recommended in developed countries
- Primary prevention of cryptococcal meningitis in areas of high prevalence (SE Asia) for patients with CD4 < 100
- Stop when CD4 > 100 for at least 3 months

Mycobacterium Avium Complex (MAC)

Prophylactic regimens:

- Azithromycin 1200 mg/wk (preferred)
- Clarithromycin 500 mg 2×/d
- Rifabutin 300 mg/d (expensive, not available in most developing countries)

Indications:

- CD4 < 50.
- Recommended in most developed countries.
- Recommended in Thailand national guidelines, but cost and low incidence of MAC in many developing countries preclude widespread use.
- Stop when CD4 > 100 for at least 3 months.

Antiretroviral Therapy (ART)

Indications for ART:

- Based on clinical and immunological (CD4) criteria.
- Screen and treat OI **before** initiating ART.
- Adherence to ART is crucial for treatment success and to prevent the emergence of resistant virus. Many programs in developing countries provide counseling and education, often mandatory, to patients before provision of ART.
- Best treatment results are achieved when adherence to ART is > 95%.
- Specific indications for ART in adults and children are listed in Tables 14.5 and 14.6, respectively.

Table 14.5   Criteria for Starting ART in Adults and Adolescents (Modified from WHO, Antiretroviral therapy for HIV infection in adults and adolescents in resource-limited settings, 2006)

WHO Clinical Stage	CD4 Not Available	CD4 Available
1	No ART	ART if CD4 < 200
2	No ART	ART if CD4 < 200
3	ART	Consider ART if CD4 < 350. Start before CD4 falls below 200
4	ART	ART

Table 14.6 Criteria for Starting ART in Children (Modified from WHO, Antiretroviral therapy of HIV infection in infants and children in resource-limited settings, 2006)

WHO Clinical Stage	CD4 Not Available	CD4 Available
1	No ART	Use CD4 criteria*
2	Use TLC criteria*	Use CD4 criteria*
3	ART	≤ 11 months: ART
		≥ 12 months: use CD4 criteria*
4	ART	ART

* TLC and CD4 criteria listed in Table 14.7.

Table 14.7 CD4 and TLC Criteria for Severe Immunodeficiency in Children < 5 Yr Old (Modified from WHO, Antiretroviral therapy of HIV infection in infants and children in resource-limited settings, 2006)

Test	Age-Specific Criteria to Initiate ART		
	≤ 11 months	12–35 Months	36–59 Months
CD4 % (preferred)	< 25%	< 20%	< 15%
CD4 count (cells/mm³)	< 1500	< 750	< 350
TLC (cells/mm³)	< 4000	< 3000	< 2500

Tip: CD4 testing, where available, should be done before ART. However, the unavailability of CD4 testing should not delay the initiation of ART in patients with clinical criteria for treatment.

First-line ARV regimens in developing countries (see Figure 14-1):

• See Table 14.8 for ARV medications, abbreviations, doses, and common side effects.

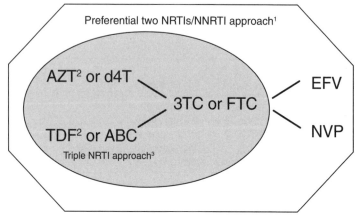

Figure 14.1 First-line ARV Regimens. (From WHO. Antiretroviral therapy for HIV infection in Adults and Adolescents in Resource-Limited Settings: Towards Universal Access, 2006)

- Highly active anti-retroviral therapy (HAART) consists of treatment with 3 different antiretroviral medications. Mono- or dual-drug therapy leads to the rapid development of drug resistance and should never be given.
- In general, first line regimens in developing countries include 2 NRTI + 1 NNRTI (see Figure 14.1 for the WHO preferential approach to first-line ART). Protease inhibitors (PI) are much more expensive and, where available, are reserved for second-line regimens.
- Most ART programs use 5 drugs: 3 NRTI (D4T, AZT, 3TC) and 2 NNRTI (NVP, EFV) from which 4 different first-line regimens can be provided: D4T/3TC/NVP, AZT/3TC/NVP, D4T/3TC/EFV, AZT/3TC/EFV.
- The most common first-line regimen used in developing countries is D4T/3TC/NVP, due to its low cost and availability in a triple combination pill.

Table 14.8 ART Medications: Abbreviations, Doses, Adverse Effects

ARV Drug	Usual Dose (Adult/Pediatric)	Notes & Common Adverse Effects (AE)
NRTI (Nucleoside/Nucleotide Reverse Transcriptase Inhibitors)		
All NRTI	**Lactic Acidosis/Hepatic Steatosis:** rare but potentially fatal	
Abacavir (ABC)	**A:** 300 mg ×2/d, OR 600 mg/d **P:** 8 mg/kg ×2/d	AE: headache, nausea, vomiting, diarrhea, fatigue **Hypersensitivity Reaction** 4–8%, may be less in Africa and Asia: symptoms include fever, fatigue, GI sx, respiratory sx, rash. If suspected, stop abacavir and **never use again. Re-use of Abacavir in hypersensitive pts can be fatal.**
Didanosine (DDI)	**A:** < 60 kg: 250 mg/d > 60 kg: 400 mg/d **P:** 90–120 mg/m² ×2/d*	Take 30 min before or 2 hr after meals. AE: Peripheral neuropathy, pancreatitis, headache, nausea, diarrhea. ↑ AE if taken with D4T or TDF. **Pregnant women: do not use D4T+DDI due to risk of fatal lactic acidosis/ hepatitis.**
Emtricitabine (FTC)	**A:** 200 mg/d **P:** 6 mg/kg/d	Similar adverse effect profile and hepatitis B activity as Lamivudine.
Lamivudine (3TC)	**A:** 150 mg ×2/d, OR 300 mg/d **P:** 4 mg/kg ×2/d	Usually very well tolerated with few side effects: headache, nausea, diarrhea, insomnia, abdominal pain. **Active against HBV: patients with co-infection may have exacerbation of hepatitis when stopping 3TC.**
Stavudine (D4T)	**A:** 30 mg ×2/d **P:** 1 mg/kg ×2/d	AE: Peripheral neuropathy 15–50%; lactic acidosis, pancreatitis, diarrhea, nausea, vomiting, headache, lipoatrophy/fat redistribution. D4T+DDI ↑ AE. **Pregnant women: do not use D4T+DDI due to risk of fatal lactic acidosis/ hepatitis**

(Continued)

Table 14.8 Continued

ARV Drug	Usual Dose (Adult/Pediatric)	Notes & Common Adverse Effects (AE)
Tenofovir (TDF)	A: 300 mg/d P: 8 mg/kg/d	Usually very well tolerated with few side effects: diarrhea, nausea, vomiting, renal toxicity. ↑ AE if taken with DDI. **Peds: risk of ↓ bone mineral density**
Zidovudine (AZT, ZDV)	A: 250–300 mg ×2/d P: 180–240 mg/m² ×2/d*	AE: nausea, vomiting, headache, fatigue, myalgia/myopathy, anemia, neutropenia.

NNRTI (Non-Nucleoside Reverse Transcriptase Inhibitors)

ARV Drug	Usual Dose (Adult/Pediatric)	Notes & Common Adverse Effects (AE)
Efavirenz (EFV)	A: 600 mg/day P: 10–15 kg: 200 mg/d 15–20 kg: 250 mg/d 20–25 kg: 300 mg/d 25–30 kg: 350 mg/d 30–40 kg: 400 mg/d > 40 kg: adult dose	Central nervous system: dizziness, insomnia, fatigue, bad dreams, depression. CNS symptoms usually resolve after 1–4 wk. Rash: 10–30%, usually mild. Rare Stevens-Johnson syndrome. Hepatitis: transient ↑ LFT, severe hepatitis less common than with NVP. **Teratogenic: Contra-Indicated in first trimester pregnancy. Women on EFV must use effective birth control.** **Peds: do not use in patients < 3 yr old or < 10 kg.**
Nevirapine (NVP)	Induction Dose (First 2 wks) A: 200 mg/d P: 160–200 mg/m²/d* Maintenance Dose A: 200 mg ×2/d P: 160–200 mg/m² ×2/d*	Rash common (15–30%) in first 2–6 wk. Mild rash resolves with continuation of NVP and antihistamines. Stop NVP for severe rash (1–7%), blisters, fever, systemic symptoms, or mucous membrane involvement. Stevens-Johnson Syndrome rare but potentially fatal. Hepatitis: transient elevation of LFT common, but < 5% stop due to hepatitis. ↑ risk with pre-ART LFT elevation, HBV or HCV. **Peds: use higher dose range (200 mg/m²) in children < 8 yr.**

PI (Protease Inhibitors)

ARV Drug	Usual Dose (Adult/Pediatric)	Notes & Common Adverse Effects (AE)
All PI		Hyperglycemia, abnormal lipids, fat redistribution.

ARV Drug	Usual Dose (Adult/Pediatric)	Notes & Common Adverse Effects (AE)
Atazanavir (ATV)	Unboosted: **A:** 400 mg/d Ritonavir-boosted: **A:** 300/100 mg/d **P:** not recommended	Take with food, requires gastric acidity for absorption. ATV/r preferred. Do not use unboosted ATV in treatment-experienced patients or with TDF, EFV, NVP. Better GI tolerance than other PI; little risk for insulin resistance and hyperlipidemia. ↑ indirect bilirubin common, jaundice 5–9%.
Fosamprenavir (FPV)	Unboosted: **A:** 1400 mg ×2/d Ritonavir-boosted: **A:** 1400/200 mg/d 700/100 mg ×2/d	Take with or without food. PI-experienced pts should take boosted, twice daily regimen. AE: rash, GI intolerance, hepatitis. No dose recommendations for children.
Indinavir (IDV)	Unboosted **A:** 800 mg ×3/d **P:** 500 mg/m² ×3/d* Ritonavir-boosted: **A:** 800/100 mg ×2/d **P:** 500/100 mg/m² ×2/d*	Take without food (unboosted); no food restrictions for IDV/r. AE: nausea, vomiting, diarrhea, ↑ indirect bilirubin, dry skin, dry hair, kidney stones (12% adults, ↑ in children), prevent by drinking > 2 liters water per day.
Nelfinavir (NFV)	**A:** 1250 mg ×2/d **P:** < 10 kg: 75 mg/kg ×2/d > 10 kg: 60 mg/kg ×2/d	Diarrhea 30–40%. Manufacturing problems led to recalls in 2007.

(Continued)

Table 14.8 Continued

ARV Drug	Usual Dose (Adult/Pediatric)	Notes & Common Adverse Effects (AE)
Lopinavir/Ritona-vir (LPV/r)	**A:** 400/100 mg ×2/d **P:** (LPV target per dose, given ×2/d) 5–7.9 kg: 16 mg/kg 8–9.9 kg: 14 mg/kg 10–13.9 kg: 12 mg/kg 14–39.9 kg: 10 mg/kg	Supplied only in combination boosted formulation. Storage: tablets (Aluvia) stable at room temp, oral solution and capsules (Kaletra) should be refrigerated, but can be stored at up to 25°C for 2 months. AE: Diarrhea, nausea, vomiting, hepatitis, hyperlipidemia. hypertriglyceridemia, insulin resistance. ↑ absorption with food.
Saquinavir (SQV)	Use boosted only: **A:** 1000/100 mg ×2/d 2000/100 mg/day **P:** > 25 kg: adult dose	Take within 2 hr of meal for ↑ absorption. Do not use unboosted SQV. Not licensed for use in children < 16 years or < 25 kg. AE: GI intolerance, headache, hepatitis, fat accumulation, insulin resistance, hyperlipidemia.
Tipranavir (TPV)	Use boosted only: **A:** 500/200 mg ×2/day **P:** not recommended	Storage: Refrigerated but can be stored at up to 25°C for 2 months. Take with food. AE: GI intolerance, rash, hyperlipidemia. Fatalities due to hepatitis and intracranial bleeding have been reported.

*Estimated Body Surface Area (m²) = square root of [weight(kg) × height(cm)/3600]; A = adult; P = pediatric; AE = adverse events.

- EFV may be used in place of nevirapine (NVP) in case of allergic rash, hepatitis, or concurrent use of rifampin for TB.
- The triple-NRTI option is less effective and should only be used for patients with contraindications to using both NNRTI and PI.

Response to ART:

- Immune reconstitution inflammatory syndrome (IRIS) is the paradoxical appearance or worsening of symptoms of OI after initiation of ART, despite the improvement in laboratory parameters such as CD4 and VL. IRIS can represent: (1) the emergence of a dormant or previously unrecognized OI, or (2) the heightened immune response to a previously or currently treated OI. Up to 25% of pts in developing countries develop IRIS within the first 1 wk to 6 months of ART, most commonly related to TB. Treatment of IRIS includes the following:
  - Diagnose and treat any new or recurrent OI.
  - Continue ART unless symptoms are life-threatening.
  - Give nonsteroidal anti-inflammatory drugs (NSAIDs) for fever or pain.
  - Use steroids for severe symptoms.
- Signs of treatment success: weight gain, improvement in OI, increase in CD4, decrease in VL.
- Treatment failure criteria (WHO, 2006): In general, patients should be taking ART with good adherence for at least 6 months before diagnosing treatment failure.
  - Clinical criteria: new or recurrent WHO clinical stage 4 condition (see Table 14.2).
  - Immunologic: CD4 falls to or below pretreatment level, declines > 50% from on-treatment peak, or persistently < 100 after 12 months of ART.
  - Virological: VL > 10 000.

HIV/AIDS

Stopping and changing ART:

- For toxicity or intolerance, single-drug substitutions can be made.
- For treatment failure, switch to 3 new drugs. Never add 1 drug to a failing regimen, which could lead to resistance to the new drug.

Second-line ART regimens:

- Usually consist of 2 new NRTI + PI.
- Second-line NRTI include ABC, TDF, DDI.
- Avoid the combination of TDF + DDI due to increased toxicity and decreased efficacy.
- 3TC retains residual antiviral activity despite the presence of resistance mutations and can be considered for continued use.
- AZT may be added to prevent or delay mutations to second-line NRTI.
- Ritonavir-boosted PI (PI/r) are preferred due to better pharmacokinetic profiles and better treatment outcomes. The choice of PI will largely be based on local availability.
- Common second-line regimens: DDI/ABC/PI, TDF/3TC/PI, TDF/ABC/PI, TDF/3TC/AZT/PI.

14.2   Diagnosis and Treatment of Common Opportunistic Infections (OI)

Candida

Si/Sx: Oral thrush, esophagitis (odynophagia), dermatitis, vaginitis.

Lab: Usually clinical diagnosis, endoscopy (esophagitis), wet prep (vaginitis or dermatitis).

Rx:

- Oral thrush (7–14 d)
  - Clotrimazole troches 10 mg ×5/d

- Nystatin susp 4 to 6 ml or 1 to 2 flavored pastilles × 4–5/d
- Fluconazole 100 mg/d
- Itraconazole oral susp 200 mg/d
- Esophagitis (14–21 d)
  - Fluconazole 100 to 400 mg/d
  - Itraconazole susp 200 mg/d
  - Ampho B 0.3 to 0.7 IV mg/kg/d
- Vaginitis: same as HIV negative (see Chapter 15)

Secondary prophylaxis: Usually not necessary, consider fluconazole 100 to 200 mg/d for recurrent esophagitis.

Cryptococcus neoformans

Cause: Common cause of meningitis when CD4 < 100. Can also cause fungemia and skin lesions.

Si/Sx: Meningeal signs, fever, delirium.

Lab: Cryptococcal culture or Ag from blood or CSF, India Ink prep (CSF).

Rx:

- Ampho B 0.7 IV mg/kg/d × 14 d, then fluconazole 400 mg/d × 8 wk.
- Flucytosine (5-FC) 100 mg/kg/d should be added for the first 2 wk, if available (expensive and often not available in developing countries).
- Fluconazole 400 to 800 mg/d can be substituted for Ampho B in first 2 wk for patients with mild sx and otherwise stable.
- Elevated intracranial pressure: treat with repeat LP every 1 to 2 d, lumbar drain, or shunt.

Secondary prophylaxis: Fluconazole 200 mg/d until CD4 > 100 × 3 to 6 months.

Cytomegalovirus (CMV)

Cause: Most common manifestation is retinitis when CD4 < 50. Less
common: esophagitis, colitis.

Si/Sx: Decreased visual acuity, floaters, scotomata, odynophagia,
diarrhea.

Lab: Typical appearance on fundoscopic exam, endoscopy with biopsy
for GI disease.

Rx: (Retinitis):

- Ganciclovir 5 mg/kg IV every 12 hrs × 2 to 3 wk, then 5/mg/kg/d.
- Valganciclovir 900 mg orally every 12 hrs × 2–3 weeks, then
  900 mg/d.
- Foscarnet 90 mg/kg IV every 12 hrs × 2 to 3 wk, then 90 to 120
  mg/kg/d IV.
- Cidofovir 5 mg/kg IV weekly × 2, then 5 mg/kg every other wk.
- Ganciclovir intraocular implant every 6 months.
- All of the above are very expensive. An alternative treatment
  for CMV retinitis in developing countries is intravitreal injections of ganciclovir 2 mg twice weekly for 2 wk, then weekly
  (Comm Eye Health 2003;16:38). The cost is a small fraction
  of systemic therapy, but does not prevent extraocular disease or
  spread to the other eye.
- Esophagitis or colitis: systemic therapy with ganciclovir, valganciclovir, or foscarnet at the acute doses above for 3 to 4 wk.
  Maintenance or secondary prophylaxis not necessary except for
  relapses.

Secondary prophylaxis: Retinitis: continue maintenance until CD4
> 100 × 3 to 6 months.

Histoplasma capsulatum

Cause: Disseminated disease when CD4 < 150.

Si/Sx: Fever, weight loss, fatigue.

Lab: Culture of blood, sputum, CSF, or skin lesion; tissue stain; Ag test of urine or blood.

Rx:

- Ampho B 0.7 IV mg/kg/d × 3 to 10 d (until clinical improvement).
- Then: Itraconazole 200 mg × 2/d × 12 wk.
- Itraconazole 200 mg × 2 to 3/d can be substituted for Ampho B in less severe cases without meningitis.

Secondary prophylaxis: Itraconazole 200 mg/d or fluconazole 800 mg/d indefinitely.

Mycobacterium avium Complex (MAC)

Cause: Disseminated infection when CD4 < 50 to 100.

Si/Sx: Fever, night sweats, weight loss, abdominal pain, diarrhea.

Lab: Blood culture > 90% sensitive, lymph node or bone marrow biopsy.

Rx:

- Clarithromycin 500 mg 2×/d + ethambutol 15 to 25 mg/kg/d.
- Can substitute Azithromycin 500 to 600 mg/d for clarithromycin.
- Consider third drug: levofloxacin 500 mg/d, ofloxacin 400 mg ×2/d, ciprofloxacin 500 to 750 mg ×2/d, rifabutin 300 mg/d, amikacin 7.5 to 15 IV mg/kg/d.

Secondary prophylaxis: Continue treatment for at least 1 yr and until CD4 > 100 for 3 to 6 months.

Mycobacterium tuberculosis (See Chapter 12)

Penicillium marneffei (Penicilliosis)

Cause: Disseminated disease in SE Asia when CD4 < 50 to 100.

Si/Sx: Fever, weight loss, wasting, papular rash.

Lab: Wright's stain of skin lesion or node aspirate, culture of blood, node, or skin scraping. Clinical diagnosis of characteristic skin lesions in endemic areas.

Rx:

- Ampho B 0.7 IV mg/kg/d × 14 d.
- Then: itraconazole 200 mg ×2/d × 10 wk.
- Itraconazole 200 mg ×2/d can be substituted for Ampho B in mild-moderate cases.

Secondary prophylaxis: Itraconazole 200 mg/d until CD4 > 200 × 6 months.

Pneumocystis jiroveci

Cause: Formerly called Pneumocystis carinii pneumonia, still referred to as PCP. Causes pneumonia when CD4 < 200.

Si/Sx: Subacute onset nonproductive cough, dyspnea, fever, tachycardia, chest pain.

Lab: CXR shows diffuse interstitial infiltrates but may be normal in up to 25%.

Xray: Elevated LDH, hypoxia. Stain of induced sputum or Broncho-Alveolar Lavage (BAL).

Rx: (all 21 d):

- TMP/SMX 15–20 mg/kg/d (of TMP component) divided 2 to 4×/d.
- Moderate-severe cases with hypoxia (PaO_2 < 70 mmHg): add prednisone 40 mg twice a day × 5 d, then 40 mg/d × 5 d, then 20 mg/d × 11 d.
- Alternatives: TMP 15 mg/kg/d + dapsone 100 mg/d; clindamycin IV 600 mg every 8 hrs; clindamycin PO 300 to 450 mg every 6 hrs + primaquine PO 15 to 30 mg/d.

Secondary prophylaxis: TMP/SMX 960 mg/d until CD4 > 200 × 3 months.

Toxoplasma gondii

Cause: Reactivation of latent cysts causes encephalitis when CD4 < 100.

Si/Sx: Fever, headache, focal neurologic deficits.

Lab: Toxoplasma serology.

Xray: Multiple ring-enhancing lesions on computerized tomography (CT) or magnetic resonance imaging (MRI).

Rx: (4–6 wk):

- Pyrimethamine 200 mg PO × 1 dose, then 50 to 75 mg/kg/d + sulfadiazine 1–1.5 gm PO every 6 hrs + folinic acid 10 to 20 mg/d.
- Alternatives:
  - TMP/SMX 10 mg/kg/d (of TMP component) divided twice/d.
  - pyrimethamine + folinic acid (doses above) + 1 of: clindamycin IV/PO 600 mg every 6 hrs; clarithromycin PO 1 gm every 12 hrs; azithromycin 1 to 1.5 g/d; or dapsone 100 mg/d.

Secondary prophylaxis: Pyrimethamine + folinic acid + sulfadiazine at one-half of treatment dose: also protects against PCP. Pyrimethamine + folinic acid + clindamycin at half the treatment dose prevents recurrent toxoplasma but not PCP.

Preventing sexual transmission of HIV

Safe sex prevention methods aim to limit the exposure of infected bodily fluids between sexual partners.

Behavior aims for HIV prevention include the following:

- correct and consistent condom use
- abstinence and delayed sexual debut for young people
- monogamy within relationships
- reduction in the number of partners

Effective HIV prevention involves openly discussing sexual behavior in a nonjudgmental manner, which, in many settings, may challenge deeply held societal norms, traditions, and religious beliefs regarding human sexuality. It is critical to be aware of this larger context to appropriately customize behavioral interventions at the individual level.

Condoms: For sexually active populations, condoms represent a key prevention method. When used correctly and consistently male condoms reduce the risk of HIV transmission by 80% to 90%, and female condoms also offer strong protection against HIV infection (UNAIDS, 2006). In addition to stressing the importance of condom use in high-risk commercial sex transactions, prevention efforts should prioritize encouraging condom use for all sexually active adults, especially in countries with generalized epidemics.

HIV Testing and Counseling (HTC): The vast majority of persons living with HIV worldwide do not know their serostatus. Once diagnosed with HIV in the context of proper counseling, most individuals take steps to avoid transmitting HIV to others (UNAIDS 2006; Lancet 2000;356:113). As a result, UNAIDS/ WHO currently recommend an approach to HIV testing that involves enhanced diagnostic HIV testing in routine health service settings. HTC is also a critical entry point to further prevention, treatment, and support services.

• Preventing Sexually Transmitted Infections:

The presence of untreated STIs is a strong cofactor for HIV transmission, and the prompt diagnosis and treatment of STIs is an important HIV prevention strategy.

Tip: In settings where diagnostic testing is not possible, the syndromic treatment of STIs may be necessary. WHO's guidelines for the management of STIs in resource-constrained settings is available at http://www.who.int/reproductive-health/

publications/rhr_01_10_mngt_stis/index.html (see Chapter 13).

Adult male circumcision:

Found to be protective against HIV transmission and has been endorsed recently as an intervention to reduce the risk of heterosexually acquired HIV infection in men (UNAIDS/WHO, 2007).

Recommended for consideration in countries with high HIV prevalence, generalized heterosexual HIV epidemics and low existing rates of male circumcision.

Preventing Unsafe Injection Drug Use

Effective interventions targeting injection drug users involve the following 2 major strategies:

- providing uncontaminated injection equipment and teaching safe injection practices.
- treating the underlying chemical dependency thereby eliminating the route of exposure.

Reducing exposure to contaminated needles via needle and syringe exchange programs is a highly effective method (WHO/UNODC/UNAIDS, 2004). These programs should be integrated with community-based outreach and risk-reduction programs.

Drug dependency treatment, particularly substitution treatment (eg, methadone maintenance) is also effective, albeit more technically and logistically intensive (WHO/UNODC/UNAIDS, 2004).

It is strongly recommended that such interventions also include information and counseling on reducing high-risk behavior, safe injection practices, and primary healthcare such as hepatitis B vaccination and vein care. IDUs should be accessing voluntary HIV testing and counseling, condoms, prevention, and treatment of STIs.

Safe injections and universal precautions in the healthcare setting: Effective prevention measures to prevent blood-borne HIV transmission in healthcare settings involve the following strategies:

- Universal precautions that involve the routine use of gloves and other protective equipment to prevent occupational exposure and safe disposal of sharps. For further guidance see http://www.cdc.gov/ncidod/dhqp/bp_universal_precautions.html.
- The use of low-cost auto-disable syringes eliminates the risk of inadvertent needlestick injuries by making the reuse of injection equipment impossible (WHO, 2004).
- Timely administration of postexposure prophylaxis (PEP) of a combination of antiretroviral drugs for all workers potentially exposed to HIV through a needlestick or other occupational injury. For further guidance see the Occupational PEP section in this chapter.

Prevention of mother-to-child transmission (PMTCT): Effective PMTCT interventions involve a comprehensive approach using the following strategies:

- primary prevention of HIV transmission for women
- prevention of unintended pregnancies in HIV+ women
- prevention of HIV transmission from HIV+ women to their infants
- care, treatment, and support for mothers living with HIV, their children, and families

Without intervention, the risk of an HIV+ mother passing HIV to her child during pregnancy, birth, or through breast feeding is 20% to 45%. With use of ART, elective cesarean section and complete avoidance of breast milk, the risk can be < 2%.

Principles of ART for PMTCT (see Table 14.9):

- AZT is safe in pregnancy and effective at preventing HIV transmission.

Table 14.9 Recommendations for ARV in PMTCT (Modified from WHO, Antiretroviral drugs for treating pregnant women and preventing HIV infection in infants in resource-limited settings, 2006)

Situation	Mother			Child[4]
	Pregnancy	Labor	Postpartum	
Mother has criteria for ART and CD4 < 250	AZT/3TC/NVP[1]			Sd-NVP + AZT × 7 d
Mother does not have criteria for ART	AZT[1]	Sd-NVP[2] + AZT/3TC[3]	AZT/3TC[1] × 7 days	Sd-NVP + AZT × 7 d
Mother presents in labor	—	Sd-NVP[2] + AZT/3TC[3]	AZT/3TC[1] × 7 days	Sd-NVP + AZT × 28 d
Mother receives no ART	—	—	—	Sd-NVP + AZT × 28 d

Doses: [1]Standard adult dosing.
[2]Adult: Sd-NVP 200 mg single dose at onset of labor.
[3]Intralabor: AZT 300 mg every 3 hrs + 3TC 150 mg every 12 hrs.
[4]Pediatric: Sd-NVP 2/mg/kg or 6 mg immediately after birth or within 72 hrs + AZT 4 mg/kg twice a d.

- NVP is safe if the pretreatment CD4 < 250. At higher CD4 counts, pregnant women are at risk for potentially fatal hepatotoxicity.
- EFV is contraindicated during the first trimester due to teratogenicity.
- There is little data on the use of PI in pregnancy, but SQV/r and NFV appear to be safe and effective at standard doses.
- Specific recommendations in Table 14.9. More detailed information available in the WHO publication *Antiretroviral Drugs for Treating Pregnant Women and Preventing HIV Infection in Infants in Resource-Limited Settings* (available at http://www. who.int/hiv/pub/guidelines/pmtct/en/index.html).

Occupational Postexposure Prophylaxis (see Table 14.10):

- Risk from single occupational needlestick to healthcare worker (HCW) is 0.3% (Ann Intern Med 1990;113;740). Risk with mucosal exposure 0.09%. No risk from exposure to intact skin.
- ↑ risk with deep injury, visible blood on needle, needle used in vein or artery, or source patient in late-stage AIDS .
- AZT prophylaxis can ↓ risk by 79% (N Engl J Med 1997;337:1485).
- Principles of PEP:
  - Rapid testing can be done with counseling and consent if HIV status of the source pt is unknown.

Table 14.10   Occupational PEP Recommendations (Modified from MMWR 2005;54;RR-9:1)

Exposure Category	Source Status (HIV+)	
	Low Risk: *asymptomatic or VL < 1,500*	High Risk: *symptomatic, acute seroconversion, or VL > 1,500*
Percutaneous Injury		
Mild -*superficial, solid needle*	2-drug PEP	3-drug PEP
Severe -*hollow needle, deep injury, visible blood, needle in artery/vein*	3-drug PEP	3-drug PEP
Mucous Membrane or non-intact skin exposure		
Mild -*few drops*	Consider 2-drug PEP	2-drug PEP
Severe -*large volume*	2-drug PEP	3-drug PEP

- PEP should be started as soon as possible, if indicated, preferably with 1 to 2 hrs and up to 72 hrs and continued for 4 wk at standard treatment doses.
- Exposed HCW should have HIV testing at baseline, 1 month, 3 months, and 6 months.
- NVP or ABC should not be used due to risk of adverse effects.
- EFV and TDF should be avoided in pregnant women.
- Risk and PEP regimen should be determined.
- 2-drug regimens: AZT/3TC, D4T/3TC, TDF/3TC, AZT/FTC, D4T/FTC, TDF/FTC.
- 3-drug regimens: 2 NRTI (above) + (LPV/r or EFV)
  - Alternative PI: SQV/r, ATV/r, ATV, IDV/r.

Nonoccupational Postexposure Prophylaxis (nPEP):

- Estimated risk from single exposure to HIV+ source (N Engl J Med 1997;336:1072):
  - IDU 0.67%.
  - Sexual contact 0.05% to 0.5% (↑ risk for receptive partner, anal sex > vaginal sex, oral sex has minimal risk).
- nPEP should be considered if there is significant genital, mucosal, subcutaneous, or nonintact skin exposure to blood, semen, vaginal secretions, breast milk, or body fluid from a source likely to be HIV infected and the time from exposure is < 72 hrs (MMWR 2005;54;RR-2:1).
- Choice of ART (4 wk):
  - Preferred regimens:
    - (AZT or TDF) + (3TC or FTC) + EFV.
    - AZT + (3TC or FTC) + LPV/r.
  - Alternative regimens/notes:
    - 2 NRTI + (EFV or PI).
    - Triple NRTI (AZT + 3TC + ABC).
    - Do not use EFV for pregnant women.
    - Do not use NVP (toxicity).

14.3 Bibliography

UNAIDS. *AIDS Epidemic Update: 2007*. Available at http://www.unaids.org/en/KnowledgeCentre/HIVData/EpiUpdate/EpiUpdArchive/2007/

UNAIDS. *Global AIDS Report*. 2006. Available at http://www.unaids.org/en/KnowledgeCentre/HIVData/GlobalReport/2006/

UNAIDS. *Joint UNAIDS Statement on HIV Prevention and Care Strategies for Drug Users*. 2005. Available at http://data.unaids.org/UNA-docs/CCO_IDUPolicy_en.pdf

UNAIDS/WHO Working Group on Global HIV/AIDS/STI Surveillance. *Guidelines for Using HIV Testing Technologies in Surveillance*. 2001. Available at http://www.who.int/hiv/pub/surveillance/guidelinesforUsingHIVTestingTechs

UNAIDS/WHO. *WHO and UNAIDS Announce Recommendations from Expert Consultation on Male Circumcision for HIV Prevention*. 2007. Available at http://www.who.int/hiv/mediacentre/news68/en/index.html

WHO. *Case Definitions of HIV for Surveillance and Revised Clinical Staging and Immunological Classification of HIV-Related Disease in Adults and Children*. 2006 revision. Available at http://www.who.int/hiv/pub/guidelines/en/

WHO. *Guidelines on Co-trimoxazole Prophylaxis for HIV-Related Infections Among Children, Adolescents and Adults in Resource-Limited Settings*. 2006. Available at http://www.who.int/hiv/pub/guidelines/ctx/en/index.html

WHO. *Antiretroviral Drugs for Treating Pregnant Women and Preventing HIV Infection in Infants in Resource-Limited Settings*. 2006. Available at http://www.who.int/hiv/pub/guidelines/pmtct/en/index.html

WHO. *Antiretroviral Therapy for HIV Infection in Adults and Adolescents in Resource-Limited Settings, 2006*. Available at http://www.who.int/hiv/pub/guidelines/adult/en/index.html

WHO. *Guidelines for the Management of Sexually Transmitted Infections*. 2003. Available at http://www.who.int/reproductive-health/publications/mngt_stis/index.html

WHO/UNODC/UNAIDS. *Evidence for Action on HIV/AIDS and injecting drug use: Policy Briefs.* 2004. Available at http://www.who.int/hiv/pub/idu/idupolicybriefs/en/

WHO. *Guiding Principles to Ensure Injection Device Safety.* 2004. Available at http://www.who.int/injection_safety/WHOGuidPrinciples InjEquipFinal.pdf

HIV/AIDS

Chapter 15

Diarrhea

15.1 Viral Gastroenteritis

Causes: A growing list, in order of frequency: rotavirus (multiple groups, subgroups), calicivirus (Norwalk, Novo), adenovirus coronavirus, astrovirus, others.

Epidem: Peak incidence in developing countries ages 6 months to 1 yr. Rotavirus most serious; 20% of childhood deaths; has reservoirs in domestic animals. Incubation 1 to 3 d. Oral-fecal and water borne spread with massive and prolonged fecal shedding after diarrhea clears.

Sx/Si: Watery diarrhea lasting 6 d (2–23) for rotavirus, vomiting (especially caliciviruses) usually precedes diarrhea. No fever.

Lab: Antigen testing available for rotavirus.

Rx: See treatment section, Tables 15.1 and 15.2.

Prev: Rotavirus vaccine available.

15.2 Noninflammatory Bacterial Diarrheas

Causes: Enterotoxigenic and enteropathogenic *E. coli*, *V. cholerae* O1 and O139, *V. parahaemolyticus*, *Bacillus cereus*, less commonly *Campylobacter spp.*, *Salmonella spp.*, *Plesiomonas*, *Clostridium perfringens*.

Epidem: Common causes of traveler's diarrhea. Fecal-oral, water, and food borne spread. 95% of cholera occurs in Sub-Saharan Africa.

Pathophys: Osmotic or secretory toxins in small intestine.

Sx/Si: Voluminous watery diarrhea with cramping, nausea, vomiting. Severe abdominal pain and fever unusual. Blood and white cells not present in stool.

Crs: Most will recover in 5 to 7 d without treatment, 5% > 30 d. Cholera case fatality rate 1.8% in Africa but up to 10% in some outbreaks (Am J Trop Med Hyg 2007;77:705).

Lab: Stool culture may identify, ova and parasites (O&P), specific antigen tests.

Rx:

- Supportive, see treatment section.
- Early treatment with Ciprofloxacin 250 to 500 mg orally twice a day d for 1 to 3 d; other floxacins also effective.
- Azithromycin 500 mg orally once, then 250 mg daily for 1 to 2 d; pediatric dose 10 mg/kg once, then 5 mg/kg daily.
- Cholera responds to the above or tetracycline, doxycycline, erythromycin, co-trimoxazole, chloramphenicol for 3 d. A single dose of 300 mg doxycycline is also adequate.
- Antisecretory drugs, such as loperamide 4 mg, with first diarrheal stool then 2 mg with subsequent ones (max 16 mg) are frequently used by travelers but not on the WHO model formulary.

Prev: Cholera vaccine available only in special circumstances.

15.3   Inflammatory Bacterial Diarrheas

Cause: Enteroinvasive, enterohemorrhagic, and enteroaggregative *E. coli*; *Campylobacter spp.*, *Salmonella spp.*, *Shigella spp.*, *Clostridium difficile*, *Aeromonas*, *Yersinia enterocolitica*.

Epidem: Often in outbreaks, occasionally point sources and sporadic. Incubation period 1 to 5 d *Shigella*, *Campylobacter*; 1 to 2 d *E. coli*;

1 to 11 d *Yersinia* and *Salmonella* (longer in typhoid fever). During or following (often weeks) antibiotic therapy with C. *difficile*.

Sx/Si: Frequent, small volume bloody diarrhea with white cells in stool. Abdominal pain, cramping, tenesmus, fever. Distal ileum and colon invasion with mucosal death.

Cmplc: Bacteremia with spread, perforation.

Hemolytic-uremic syndrome with E. *coli* 0157:H7 and *Sh. dysenteriae*.

Relapse common 10% to 35% with C. *difficile* and *Campylobacter*.

Reiter's syndrome 1% to 2% with *Shigella*, *Campylobacter*, *Yersinia*.

Lab: Stool culture, stool white cells, and gram negative rods.

Immunoassays in C. *difficile*, E. *coli* 0157:H7 antigen testing.

Rx: Supportive

E. *coli*: 0157:H7, no antibiotics or loperide

E. *coli*: other types, no antibiotics

C. *difficile*: Stop antibiotics, no loperide. If very ill, give metronidazole 250 to 500 mg orally or IV 3 × daily for 7 to 10 d. Vancomycin orally is effective but cost prohibitive, 125 mg 4 × a d. It does not work IV.

Campylobacter: No antibiotics unless seriously ill, then erythromycin 250 mg orally 4×/ d for 5 d or azithromycin. Quinolone resistance common.

Yersinia: If very ill, tetracycline, chloramphenicol, trimethoprim/sulfamethoxazole.

Shigella: Antibiotics shorten illness but resistance is common; local sensitivity studies essential. Treatment may be reserved for those hospitalized and the most seriously ill, the young, old, and malnourished. Ciprofloxacin 500 mg orally daily × 5 d, Azithromycin 500 mg orally d 1 then 250 mg for 4 d, Nalidixic acid 1 gram orally every 6 hr for 5 d (children over 3 months 15 mg/kg every 6 hr). Ofloxacin 15 mg/kg orally (Trans R

DIARRHEA

Soc Trop Med Hyg 2000;94:323). Pivmecillinam orally 20 mg/kg (400 mg maximum) every 6 hr for 5 d.

Salmonella: No treatment for mild-moderate illness. TMP/ SMX 160/800 mg orally twice a day or ciprofloxacin 500 mg orally twice a day or another floxacin for 5 to 7 d. 1% will become carriers; may be treated with prolonged course (1 month) of antibiotics if necessary. (See Typhoid Fever Chapter 19.)

15.4   Parasitic Causes of Diarrhea

Giardiasis

Cause: *Giardia lamblia.*

Epidem: Common protozoan enteropathogen, in some areas universal at some point during childhood, prevalence rates 20% to 45% in children, which declines in adolescence. Animal reservoirs, especially dogs. Worse with IgA deficiency. Incubation 1 to 3 wk. Most infections asymptomatic.

Pathophys: Lives in duodenum and ileum. No invasion but disrupts mucosal border.

Sx: Diarrhea, weakness, weight loss, abdominal pain, nausea, steator-rhea, vomiting, fever < 20%.

Si: Abdominal distention.

Crs: Recovery usual in 2 to 4 wk; 25% have chronic symptoms with malabsorption of fats, B_{12}, vitamin A, and lactase deficiency.

Lab: Stool antigens. Stool O&P for cysts 70% to 85% accurate. Duodenal aspirate or examination of swallowed string. Often presumptive treatment is the easiest option.

Rx: Metronidazole 2 grams orally once daily × 3 d (children 5–7.5 mg/ kg every 8 hr × 5–7 d).
    Tinidazole 2 grams orally once.

Quinacrine, furazolidone, paromomycin also used but not in WHO formulary.

Amebiasis

Cause: *Entamoeba histolytica.*

Epidem: Common, 50 million infections, and 70 000 deaths/yr. Fecal-oral, many cyst carriers.

Pathophys: Ingestion of cyst, which produces trophozoites. They invade colon mucosa and may spread throughout the body, especially the liver then brain, skin, less frequently other tissues.

Sx: 90% asymptomatic. Insidious onset usual with abdominal and back pain, diarrhea with mucus and blood. Tenesmus > 50%.

Si: Fever 40%, tenderness, occasional abdominal mass ameboma.

Crs: Worse in pregnancy, children, malnourished, and those on steroids. HIV+ no worse.

Cmplc: Liver abscess most common in adult males, only 30% with present or history of dysentery. Sudden onset upper abdominal pain with fever. Same as pyogenic abscess. Peritonitis, fistula, metastatic spread. Differential: bacterial dysentery, IBDs.

Lab: Antigen test on stool. Stool O&P must be fresh to see trophozoites with ingested red blood cells.
Sigmoidoscopy will show ulcers 3 to 5 mm with normal mucosa between. Look for amoeba in biopsy.
Liver aspirate will only occasionally show trophozoites. Best seen in the last aspirate. Alkaline phosphatase elevated 75% in liver abscesses, other enzymes up in 50%.

Xray: Elevated right hemidiaphragm. Sonographic search of liver for abscess, usually right lobe. May increase in size for several weeks despite correct Rx. Most gone by 6 months but occasionally (10%) persist > 1 yr.

Rx: Must treat trophozoites and kill cysts; for trophozoites:

Metronidazole 750 to 800 mg orally (10 mg/kg in children) 3×/d for 7 to 10 d, or

tinidazole 2 gm orally for 3 d, plus for cysts:

diloxanide furoate 500 mg orally 3 × daily for 10 d, or

tetracycline 500 mg orally 4×/d for 10 d.

Prev: Cysts viable for days in feces, soil, water, longer if chilled to 10°C.

Killed by 5% acetic acid, iodine 200 ppm, or heat. Not killed in chlorinated water, must filter out.

Drain abscesses:

- if suspect bacterial infection or superinfection
- if patient not improving clinically after 3–5 days
- if rupture seems likely or if in the left lobe of liver

Introduce needle at point of maximum tenderness; ultrasound guidance is helpful.

Repeated drainage over several days may be needed for abscesses > 250 ml.

If a pleural effusion is found, suggests past or incipient rupture into pleural space. Tap it also.

Operate for ruptured hepatic abscess or perforated colon.

Protozoa-caused Diarrheas

Cause: *Cryptosporidium parvum*, *C. hominis*, and others (J Infect Developing Countries 2007;1:242).

Epidem: Common cause of diarrhea in children (4–17%), travelers, and adults. Cows and dogs reservoir. Incubation 2 to 14 d. Often chronic in HIV+.

Sx/Si: Watery diarrhea, cramping, weight loss, increased mortality independent of HIV status, fever 12% to 57%, vomiting 48%.

Crs: Immunocompetent course 6 to 22 d, HIV+ intermittent to chronic diarrhea.

Lab: Acid-fast stains show oocysts, 4 to 6 microns, sensitivity greatest in diarrheal stool. PCR available.

Rx: Supportive.

Paromomycin 500 mg orally 3×/d for 2 wk then once daily may be marginally effective in AIDS.

Nitazoxanide (not WHO formulary) 100 mg (1–3 yr), 200 mg (4–11 yr), 500 mg (adult) all twice daily for 3 d in HIV negative. Also treats most roundworms, flatworms, flukes, and giardia.

Cause: *Cyclospora cayatenensis*.

Epidem: Worldwide, higher in rainy season. Incubation 1 to 7 d.

Sx: Watery, crampy diarrhea, nausea, vomiting, weight loss, gas, bloating. May persist for weeks.

Lab: AFB stain 8 to 10 micron cysts.

Rx: TMP/SMX 160/800 twice daily for 7 to 14 d; pediatric 5/25 mg/kg twice daily.

Microsporida

Cause: *Enterocytozoon bieneusi* and *Septata intestinalis* (*E. intestinalis*).

Epidem: Worldwide.

Sx: Diarrhea, anorexia, nausea, cramping.

Cmplc: Cholangitis, dissemination in AIDS, nephritis. Persistent diarrhea.

Lab: AFB stain of stool. Small bowel bx.

Rx: Albendazole 800 mg twice daily for 4 wk or metronidazole 400 mg 3×/d for 1 wk.

Cause: *Isospora belli*.

Epidem: Worldwide, especially AIDS patients.

Sx: Chronic watery diarrhea, crampy pain, malabsorption.

DIARRHEA

Lab: AFB stain or hot safranin stain, 10 to 40 micron cysts, eosinophilia.

Rx: TMP/SMX 160/800 twice daily for 7 to 14 d; pediatric as above.

15.5   Chronic Persistent Diarrhea

Cause: Dependent on local conditions and HIV status.

Epidem: Lasting ≥ 14 d with or without blood.

Si: Often malnutrition and vitamin/mineral deficiency.

Lab: Useful to guide therapy.

Rx: One algorithm:

   Bloody diarrhea: Treat for Shigella; if continues after 2 appropriate antibiotic courses, treat with metronidazole 7.5 to 10 mg/kg orally 3×/d for 5 d.

   Watery not bloody diarrhea: TMP/SMX, then metronidazole, then albendazole plus zinc and folic acid, vitamin A, iron, magnesium, and copper, nutritional support.

15.6   Dysentery

Cause: Shigellosis the most common, amebiasis dangerous, most other etiologies do not require treatment.

Sx: Cramping with visible bloody diarrhea.

Lab: Shigella antibiotic sensitivities helpful as is stool for trophozoites.

Rx: Nalidixic acid 15 mg/kg orally 4×/d (maximum 4 grams/d) for 5 d or ciprofloxacin, pivmecillinam, or other fluoroquinolone, plus or minus metronidazole.

15.7   Supportive Treatment of Diarrhea

(Hospital Care for Children, WHO, 2005)

The treatment of diarrhea in children and adults, HIV+ or negative, is centered on oral rehydration, zinc supplementation, and continued feeding. Antibiotic therapy may be indicated in a minority of patients, preferably targeted at a specific organism based on local knowledge and laboratory testing but sometimes empirically.

In the management of diarrhea, first obtain a history, record the vital signs and weight, and perform an examination. Based on this information categorize the patient:

- acute watery diarrhea
- dysentery
- persistent diarrhea
- abdominal condition requiring surgery
- recent antibiotic use
- HIV+
- malnutrition
- degree of dehydration: none, some, severe

Severe Dehydration

Cause: Cholera, rotavirus, many others.

Sx: Watery diarrhea, vomiting, lethargy, or unconscious.

Si: Sunken eyes, poor skin turgor. Capillary refill > 2 seconds.

Rx:

- Treat cholera if epidemic in area.
- Start IV or interosseous (IO) fluids (see Table 15.1).
- Reassess frequently and give additional IV bolus as needed.
- Use lactated ringers if available (Hartman's solution) or normal saline.
- Start ORS as soon as possible at 5 ml/kg/hr.

Table 15.1 IV Rates for Cholera

	< 1 yr	1–5 yr	> 5 yr
Initial	30 ml/kg in 1 hr	30 ml/kg in half hr	20 ml/kg in half hr
Then	70 ml/kg in 5 hr	70 ml/kg in 2½ hr	10–20 ml/kg per hr

- Use nasogastric ORS at 20 ml/kg/hr if IV or IO not available.
- Reassess in 6 hr and recategorize.
- Laboratory tests usually not needed.
- Give zinc supplement.

Moderate (Some) Dehydration

Causes: Various etiologies.

Si: 2 or more: restless or irritable, thirsty and drinks eagerly, sunken eyes, skin turgor decreased.

Rx:

- oral rehydration salts (ORS) in clinic (Table 15.2)

    Plus breast milk when available:
- Give in small amounts, 5 to 15 ml.
- Wait 10 min if vomits, then retry.
- Reassess frequently.
- Send home after 4 hr if improved or admit or repeat Rx.

Table 15.2 ORS in Clinic

In first 4 hr, give at least:

< 6 kg	200–400 ml
6–10 kg	400–700 ml
10–12 kg	700–900 ml
12–19 kg	900–1400 ml
20+ kg	kg × 75 ml

- Offer food before going home after 4 hr of ORS.
- Educate mother or patient to return if fever, blood in stool, worsens.
- Start zinc therapy.
- Role of probiotics in developing countries (J Infect Developing Countries 2007;1:81; Am J Trop Med Hyg 2008;78:214).

Diarrhea with no dehydration or recovered from severe or moderate dehydration:

- Educate as above.
- Send home with ORS.
- Instruct to give ORS for each loose stool < 2 yr, 50 to 100 ml; > 2 yr, 100 to 200 ml.
- Give zinc therapy.
- Continue feeding.

Zinc reduces the severity and duration of diarrhea and the risk of diarrhea over next several months. Up to 6 months: 10 mg/d for 10 to 14 d. Older than 6 months: 20 mg/d for 10 to 14 d.

DIARRHEA

Chapter 16

Parasitic Diseases

16.1 Schistosomiasis

Causes: *Schistosoma mansoni, japonicum, haematobium, intercalatum, mekongi.*

Epidem: Cercariae swimming in water penetrate human skin, lose their tails as they traverse subcutaneous tissue entering veins, migrating through lungs and heart and are distributed about the body until settling in the hepatic portal system where they pair, mate, and migrate to preferred egg-laying site (*S. mansoni, japonicum, mekongi,* and *intercalatum* the inferior and superior mesenteric veins are preferred, with *S. haematobium* the vesical plexus). Egg production begins in about a month; the eggs pass through the capillary walls and are excreted in the urine (*S. haematobium*) or stool (others). Eggs hatch, become swimming miracidium, which penetrate the fresh water snail, form sporocysts then cercariae. Snails that can serve as intermediate hosts are limited and generally dictate the range of schistosomiasis. They can survive outside of water for weeks and survive from one wet season to the next.

200 million infected worldwide, 85% in Africa.

S. mansoni in > 50 countries, especially Brazil, Surinam, Venezuela, some Caribbean Islands, Nile Valley, Sub-Saharan Africa, Madagascar, Arabian Peninsula, and Indian Ocean Islands.

S. *haematobium* in > 50 countries, especially Nile river drainage, Sub-Saharan Africa, Arabian Peninsula, and Euphrates river.

S. *japonicum* in China, Sulawesi, and Philippines.

S. *intercalatum* in Central and West Africa.

S. *mekongi* in Lao PDR and Cambodia.

Pathophys: Mating pairs of adults deposit 20 to 300 eggs per d, 3000 in S. *japonicum*. 70 μm in size, the eggs are encased in granulomas wherever they are deposited.

Sx: Cercariae dermatitis minutes: 3 d after skin entry, pruritus and papules. Katayama syndrome 1 to 16 wk after invasion: fever, myalgias, malaise, rigors, headache, slightly enlarged liver and spleen (1/3), anorexia, vomiting, diarrhea, cough.

Si: Eosinophilia, CNS spinal cord embolization.
Chronic infections with S. *haematobium*.

Sx: Painless hematuria.

Si: Bladder hyperemic mucosa with granulomas, ulceration, fibrosis, and calcification. Ureter obstruction, granulomas in perineum, rectosigmoid, and any organ.

Crs: Adult worms may live years.

Cmplc: Urinary obstruction in bladder and ureters. Bladder cancer and stones.
Chronic infections with S. *mansoni*, S. *japonicum*, others.

Sx: Blood in stool, tenesmus, chronic diarrhea.

Si: Anemia, weight loss, portal hypertension with edema, ascites, splenomegaly, distant granulomas, rarely spinal cord and brain.

Crs: Hepatic fibrosis, intestinal polyposis.

Cmplc: Cor pulmonale (S. *mansoni*). Gastroesophageal varices with bleeding. CNS signs. Coinfection with hepatitis B and C common.

Diff: Katayama syndrome (fever and eosinophilia): trichinosis, liver flukes

Lab: Stool for O&P, rectal, bladder, or granuloma biopsy. Microscopic examination of urine. Viable egg will hatch miracidia (1 mm length). Incubate in tap water, under light, for 20 min. Hematuria by reagent strip is presumptive dx of *S. haematobium*. Eosinophilia.

Xray: Ultrasound of liver diagnostic (Am J Trop Med Hyg 1992;46:403).

Bladder calcifications.

Rx: Praziquantel 20 mg/kg 3 doses over one d or 40 to 60 mg/kg single dose; higher dose in *S. japonicum*, *S. mekongi*, and heavy infections. Give with food. 80% cure rate but reinfection a problem.

Note: This dose of praziquantel also treats and cures intestinal, liver, and lung flukes, *H. nana* diphyllobothriasis, hymenolepiasis, intestinal taeniasis (not CNS or ocular where it may cause a reaction). Avoid in pregnancy and breast feeding for 72 hr.

Oxamniquine is still used for *S. mansoni* only. Dosage is based on local sensitivities 15 to 60 mg/kg total dose, divided so that no daily dose > 20 mg/kg. Care when used in patients with epilepsy, not in first trimester.

Prev: Animal reservoirs important in some instances:

S. japonicum: dog, cow, pig, water buffalo, rat

S. haematobium: none

S. mansoni: rats (Guadeloupe, Brazil)

S. mekongi: dogs

Avoid drinking, bathing, working in contaminated water through supply of safe water and community participation. Improve sanitation and water supply. Molluscicides have limited applications. Mass treatment programs (Clin Trop Med Commun Dis 1987;2:449).

PARASITIC DISEASES

16.2 Trematodes, Liver Flukes

Causes: *Clonorchis sinensis, Opisthorchis viverrini, O. felineus.*

Epidem: Adults live in bile ducts of raw fish-eating mammals. Eggs passed in feces, ingested by snails, form free-swimming cercariae, penetrate and encyst in fish as metacercaria, excyst in gut and migrate to intrahepatic bile ducts.

> *O. felineus* found in E Europe to Siberia.
> *O. viverrini* in SE Asia.
> *C. sinensis* from Vietnam to Korea.

Pathophys: Adults live years, causing ductal fibrosis.

Sx: Hepatomegaly, diarrhea, anorexia.

> *O. felineus* may cause acute hepatosplenomegaly with chills, fever, high eosinophilia.

Si: Obstructive jaundice, weight loss, ascites.

Cmplc: Gallstones, cholangiocarcinoma.

Lab: Stool O&P, differentiation difficult. If definitive diagnosis needed, purge with $MgSO_4$ 1 hr after praziquantel and examine adult worms (EID 2007;13:1828, for photos of adults).

Rx: Praziquantel 40 mg/kg orally once or 25 mg/kg 3 × daily for 2 d. See schistosomiasis above for contraindications.

Fascioliasis

Causes: *Fasciola hepatica, F. gigantica.*

Epidem: Life cycle similar to Clonorchis but metacercaria cysts on fresh water plants. Live in hepatic ducts of sheep (*F. hepatica*), cows and water buffalo (*F. gigantica*). In humans, excyst in duodenum, migrate through bowel wall and liver and into bile ducts.

> *F. hepatica*: sheep-raising areas in Europe, Middle East, Central and S America, Africa.

F. *gigantica*: S and SE Asia, Africa, > 2 million people infected.

Sx: Usually asymptomatic; when severe causes diarrhea, malaise, liver pain, fever, night sweats, cough.

Si: Urticaria, hepatosplenomegaly, anemia.

Cmplc: Cholangitis and cholestatic jaundice.

Lab: High eosinophilia, up to 80%.

Egg production begins 1 month after symptoms so O&P not useful in acute cases.

Eating infected animal liver gives false positives. Egg production often scanty; duodenal aspirate better yield.

Alkaline phosphate elevated, eosinophilia, immunodiagnosis.

Xray: Ultrasound of worms in bile ducts, liver calcifications.

Rx: Triclabendazole: only give in hospitalized after overnight fast with food; 10 mg/kg orally single dose.

Praziquantel not usually effective.

Artesunate 4 mg/kg daily for 10 d 76% effective (Am J Trop Med Hyg 2008;78:388).

Prev: Avoid uncooked wild watercress, "morning glory" in Asia, "kjosco" in Andes. Causes considerable mortality in animals in which they can be protected by immunization.

Intestinal Flukes

Causes: *Fasciolopsis buski*, *Echinostomia sp.*, and many others.

Epidem: *Fasciolopsis* life cycle similar to *Fasciola* except pigs and humans infected, and infection acquired through metacercaria on plant parts or drinking contaminated water; S and S. E. Asia.

Echinostomia sp. acquired by eating raw snails, fish, clams, tadpoles. Asia, Turkey to Siberia.

Sx/Si: *Fasciolopsis* attach to duodenum or jejunum and can cause local reaction, ulcers and with massive infestation obstruction, fever, anemia, malabsorption. Other intestinal flukes often asymptomatic except in severe infections.

Lab: Stool O&P usually positive, eosinophilia.

Rx: Praziquantel 25 mg/kg orally once.

Lung Flukes

Cause: *Paragonimus sp.*

Epidem: Lives in lungs of cats, dogs, primates. Eggs coughed up and pass via sputum or feces into fresh water, miracidia hatch, invade snail, multiply, and either released to enter second intermediate host (crab, crayfish) or snail eaten by crustacean. When raw or undercooked crustacean eaten, cercariae released, penetrate intestinal wall, pass through diaphragm to lungs. Mature in 2 months, live 20 yr. Acquired primarily from eating raw, pickled, or wine-soaked crabs, crayfish, or shrimp.

Africa, especially Nigeria and Cameroon, S. America, Peru, Guatemala, Ecuador, Asia, 10 million infected in China, Taiwan, Thailand.

Sx: Chest pain and cough.

Si: Hemoptysis, brown sputum, pleural effusion pneumothorax. Occasional ectopic infections in CNS with eosinophilic meningitis, seizures, or nodules in skin, abdomen, heart.

Diff: Resembles TB and bronchiectasis.

Lab: Eggs in stool or sputum (with eosinophils). Serological testing.

Xray: Cavitating lung lesions.

Rx: Praziquantel 25 mg/kg orally 3×/d for 2 to 3 d or
Triclabendazole 10 mg/kg orally twice; treat in hospital only in case of CNS involvement.

16.3   Filariasis

(Am J Trop Med Hyg 2004;71, issue on filariasis)

Causes: *Wuchereria bancrofti, Brugia malayi,* and *B. timori.*

Epidem: Mosquito vector transmits infected larvae, which migrate in
humans to the lymphatics where they develop into adults. Adults
mate, ova in female worm hatch and produce microfilarial larvae,
which can be found in blood in daily periodicity that maximizes
exposure to mosquito vector. Most peak around midnight; occasionally microfilaria can be found during the day (especially in
nightshift workers and long-term hospitalized patients).

   B. malayi: Malaysia, Indonesia, Sri Lanka, S China, central
India, Timor.

   B. timori: Timor, Sunda Island group.

   W. bancrofti: Polynesia, Micronesia (nonperiodic), West
Indies, S America, Tropical Africa, W and E Asia, Melanesia
(periodic night).

   Incubation period > 1 yr.

Pathophys: Many asymptomatic, but symptoms and signs due to lymphatic blockage by adult worms with inflammation and blockage.

Sx: Acute adenolymphangitis with fever, chills, malaise lasting 1 wk.

Si: Acute tender enlarged lymph nodes, especially in groin and limbs.
Epididymo-orchitis, leg, arm, breast swelling.

Crs: Multiple acute attacks or chronic infection lead to lymphedema.

Cmplc: Chronic lymphedema with secondary bacterial cellulitis =
elephantiasis.

   Hydrocele, chyluria.

   Tropical eosinophilia (cough, wheeze, hypereosinophilia).

Lab:

- Nighttime blood drawn, lyse cells, see microfilaria in counting chamber. Occasionally found in urine or hydrocele fluid.
   Worms measure 200 to 300 μm, or

- Diethylcarbamazine (DEC) 2 mg/kg administered to provoke microfilaria into circulation and draw blood 30 to 60 min later. Never try in areas where onchocerciasis is found.
- Milipore (Nuclepore) filters provide quantitative numbers.
- Numerous antigen tests are available and very sensitive and specific.
- Occasionally seen on thick smears for malaria or in CBC.

Xray: Ultrasound of scrotal lymphatics may show "dancing worms" (Am J Trop Med Hyg 1999;60:119).

Rx: Ivermectin 200 μg/kg orally once a yr for $\geq$ 5 yr with Albendazole 400 mg orally, or DEC numerous regimes:

6 mg/kg daily divided after meals for 12 d, children < 10 yr 3 mg/kg daily or

3–6 mg/kg once yearly, or

above dose once a wk for 6 wk, or

once a month × 6, or

add to table salt 0.1% for *W. bancrofti* or 0.3% for *B. malayi*. Rx 6 to 12 months

Note: Immunologic symptoms of headache, fever, myalgias, urticaria, asthma common with first treatment (Mazzotti reaction). Lymphangitis and lymphedema may occur. Best to start with lower doses and avoid in pregnancy.

Prev: Mosquito nets and repellants. Mosquito control with DDT shown effective.

WHO has Global Programme to Eliminate Lymphatic Filariasis.

Ideal program for community involvement using innovative methods (PNG Med J 2000;43: entire issue).

Onchocerciasis River Blindness

Cause: *Onchocerca volvulus* (Br Med J 2003;326:207).

Epidem: *Simulium* black fly transmits larvae by bite, migrate in skin, form nodules after 10 to 15 months; adults release microfilariae, which black fly consumes during blood meal; microfilariae develop in fly. Adults live years.

Central Africa, Guatemala, Mexico between 500 to 1500 m. Smaller foci in Venezuela, Columbia, Brazil, Ecuador, Yemen.

Pathophys: *Wolbachia sp.* bacteria symbionts live in worms and are important for their fertility and contribute to the body's inflammatory response.

Sx: Itching, papular rash, thickened skin and nodules later. Visual loss.

Si: Lizard (thickened) leopard (depigmented) skin, hanging skin. Painless, smooth mm-cm nodules usually mobile. Punctate keratitis in cornea, iridocyclitis.

Dx: Slit lamp exam shows live microfilariae in cornea. Bloodless skin snips (see lab chapter), worms 270 to 320 μm long. Antigen testing.

Rx: Ivermectin 150 μg/kg orally once a yr.

Avoid in pregnancy, first week of breast feeding, and children < 15 kg. Caution: may cause orthostatic hypotension.

Avoid DEC as may cause Mazzotti reaction (see Filariasis) with worsening eye symptoms.

Suramin is an option; use only if treating African trypanosomiasis primarily.

Loa Loa (Eyeworm)

Cause: *Loa loa.*

Epidem: *Chrysops* fly bites and introduces larva, which develop into adults in skin and produce microfilaria. Rainforest and swamps of West and Central Africa.

Sx: Pruritus, fatigue, arthralgias.

Si: Worm migrating under conjunctiva, Calabar swellings (painless, nonpitting swellings, usually on arms, lasting hr to several d).

Lab: 3 to 5 cm adult worms, 200 to 300 μm microfilaria.

Hypereosinophilia.

Microfilaria in blood (noontime best), > 50 000/ml = heavy infection.

Serological testing available.

Xray: Calcified worms in skin.

Rx: DEC 1 mg/kg orally on d 1; 2 mg/kg orally on d 2; 3 mg/kg d 3; then 2 to 3 mg/kg 3 × daily for 18 d.

Caution: Mazzotti reaction (see filariasis) and meningo-encephalitis in > 1% heavily infected patients, pretreat with corticosteroids and antihistamines first 2 to 3 d.

Prophylaxis: DEC 300 mg weekly.

Guinea Worm

(N Engl J Med 2007;356:2561)

Cause: Dracunculus medinensis

Epidem: Humans drink water fleas infected with larvae, which penetrate stomach and intestines, migrate to connective tissue, mate, move to skin, grow over 8 to 12 months, forms ulcer, which opens, and larvae released into fresh water over next 2 to 6 wk.

Primarily S Sudan, Nigeria.

Sx: Blister, which ruptures with protruding worm.

Si: Visible worm.

Cmplc: Inflammation about worm, worse if broken, secondary cellulitis, tetanus.

Xray: May show calcified worms.

Rx: Slow removal over days by winding worm up on small stick.

Prev: Clean water, monofilament nylon mesh will filter out water fleas.

Eradication expected by 2009.

16.4 Roundworms

Hookworms

(N Engl J Med 2004;351:799)

Cause: *Ancylostoma duodenale*, *Necator americanus*.

Epidem: Larvae penetrate skin and move into blood, penetrate pulmonary vessels, coughed up, swallowed, mature in small intestine with noninfective eggs in stool. Eggs hatch in soil, develop into larvae, mature into filariform larvae, which can penetrate skin. Larve may live 2 yr in damp soil, adults' lifespan 1 to 9 yr. A. *duodenale* are also infective by direct ingestion as well as skin penetration.

Sx: "Ground itch" at site of skin penetration; fever, asthma, and bronchitis (during migration). Epigastric pain.

Si: Iron deficient anemia, hypoproteinemia, vesicular rash at entry points.

Lab: Eggs in feces, stool allowed to set overnight may show larvae, which may be confused with *Strongyloides*. Eosinophilia, microscopic blood in stool.

Rx: Albendazole 400 mg orally once; children 1 to 2 yr, 200 mg.

Mebendazole 500 mg orally once for children 1 yr to adults.

Mebendazole-resistance reported (Am J Trop Med Hyg 2007;76:732). Use Rx for 3 consecutive d or albendazole.

Levamisole 2.5 mg/kg orally once.

Caution: Avoid all in first trimester pregnancy, never with cestode infection in pregnancy.

Pyrantel 10 mg/kg orally once; if severe give daily × 4. Avoid in pregnancy; reduce dose in liver disease.

Enterobiasis

Cause: *Enterobius vermicularis* (pinworm).

Epidem: No multiplication in body; spread by egg ingestion in feces, soiled linens, dust, or eggs hatch about anal mucosa and migrate back into bowel.

Pathophys: Adult worms live in terminal ileum and cecum causing ulcerations, secondary infections. Pruritus when gravid females migrate and lay eggs about anus. Occasionally, worms migrate into vagina or into abdominal cavity.

Sx: Pruritus insomnia, vulvitis.

Si: Rarely granulomas in abdominal organs.

Lab: Adult female 1 cm long.
   Eggs about anus (cellophane tape applied in morning), occasionally found in stool.

Rx: Albendazole 10 to 14 mg/kg orally once for children or 400 mg for adults.
   Mebendazole 100 mg orally once.
   Pyrantel pamoate 10 mg/kg orally once.
   Wash bed linens, clean up dust, treat entire family.

Whipworm

Cause: *Trichuris trichiura.*

Epidem: Fecal-oral spread. Eggs embryonate in moist soil 3 wk, ingested, hatch in small intestine, penetrate villi, develop for a week, and migrate to large bowel and rectum.

Pathophys: Cause dysentery-like syndrome in heavy infestation with blood and protein loss.

Sx: Epigastric and right lower quadrant (RLQ) pain, anorexia.

Si: Weight loss, anemia, rectal prolapse with visible worms, growth retardation.

Lab: Typical eggs with plug on each end.

   Eosinophilia unusual; when seen, suspect concomitant infections.

Rx: Albendazole or mebendazole in usual doses.

Prev: Associated with pigs (*T. suis*), which may infect man. Also frequent co-infections with *Ascaris* and *Toxocara* as they have similar epidemiology.

   Evaluate effectiveness of albendazole before starting mass treatment programs.

Ascaris (Roundworm)

Cause: *Ascaris lumbricoides*, *A. suum* (pig ascaris).

Epidem: Common worldwide. Eggs passed in stool, embryonate 3 wk to 4 months in soil, egg swallowed, hatch, penetrate bowel as larvae, and enter bloodstream to lungs, enter alveoli, coughed up, and swallowed (10–14 d), matures in small intestine, eggs passed in stool 2 months after initial infection.

Pathophys: Löfler's syndrome with fever, cough, asthma, and eosinophilia with lung passage.

Sx/Si: Usually asymptomatic but pulmonary symptoms and bowel obstruction. Occasionally, migrating larvae can appear anywhere. Passage of worms per anus, mouth.

Cmplc: Larvae: Pneumonitis, asthma

   Adults: Biliary obstruction with cholangitis, bile duct stones about eggs. Urticaria, malnutrition, vitamin A deficiency (Am J Clin Nutr 1998;68:623), liver abscesses, granulomas, neurological invasion, and seizures.

   Migration especially common with fever, bowel obstruction, and general anesthesia.

Lab: Adults 15 to 30 cm long.

   Eggs in stool, larvae in sputum.

   Eosinophilia with larvae migration

Xray: Seen in bowel with contrast.

Rx: Single dose albendazole, mebendazole, levamisole, or pyrantel are effective. Bowel obstruction: NG tube and IV fluids followed by anthelmintic Rx. If surgery undertaken, try to milk obstructing worms down bowel and avoid enterotomy.

Toxocariasis

Cause: *Toxocara canis* (dog ascaris), *T. cati*.

Epidem: Cause of visceral larva migrans. Transplacental infection of puppies and kittens, children ingest eggs, hatch in stomach, penetrate mucosa, and enter circulation and trapped in capillaries.

Sx/Si: Enlarged liver, fever, asthma.

Cmplc: Granuloma formation in eye with strabismus (resembles tumor), brain, lungs, liver.

Lab: Hypereosinophilia
Serology tests available.

Rx: DEC start 1 mg/kg orally twice daily and increase to 3 mg/kg twice daily. Total treatment 3 wk.
Cover with oral and topical steroids for eye lesions.
Thiabendazole 50 mg/kg orally for 4 wk is a second-line drug. Albendazole (10 mg/kg/d for 5 d) and mebendazole also effective.

Strongyloidiasis

Cause: *Strongyloides stercoralis*
Two life cycles, 1) a soil cycle and 2) a parasitic cycle where filariform larvae penetrate skin or mouth, migrate to lungs, coughed up and swallowed, mature in duodenum, lay eggs, which hatch in mucosa; larvae passed in stool or develop into adults, which penetrate bowel wall and enter circulation.

Sx/Si: Pruritic rash at entry point, 1 wk later cough, pneumonitis, right upper quadrant (RUQ) pain.

Cmplc: Urticaria about anus and buttocks from autoinfection. In immunosuppressed patients or those on steroids, a massive overwhelming infection with abdominal pain, diarrhea, fever, pulmonary eosinophilia, gram negative meningitis, may be fatal.

Lab: Larvae in stool or duodenal aspirate (best).
Eosinophilia (except in severe complicated disease)
Serological testing.

Rx: Ivermectin 200 μg/kg orally once, or
Albendazole 400 mg orally once or twice a day for 3 d (80% cure).
Mebendazole (2-wk course) and Thiabendazole are less effective.
S. *fülleboni* are found in East and Central Africa and Papua New Guinea. Sx and si are similar and treatment is the same as S. *stercoralis*.

16.5   Tapeworms

Cause: *Taenia saginata* (beef tapeworm).

Epidem: Cattle feed on contaminated human feces, form cysticercus in muscle, improperly cooked beef eaten, larvae released and attach to intestinal wall, proglottides passed stool. Highland Ethiopia, other areas. Other hosts: ox, camel.

Sx/Si: Often asymptomatic, GI upset, passing motile proglottides.

Lab: Eggs in stool, proglottid identification.

Rx: Praziquantel 10 mg/kg orally single dose > 4 yr to adult.
Niclosamide 1 gm orally after light breakfast, 1 gm 1 hr later, purgative 2 hr after last dose. Chew tablet, give antiemetic before first dose.

Cause: *Hymenolepis nana* (dwarf tapeworm).

Epidem: Oral-fecal; man is only host.

PARASITIC DISEASES

Sx/Si: Usually asymptomatic, abdominal pain.

Lab: Ova in stool, serology.

Rx: Praziquantel 20 mg/kg orally single dose > 4 yr to adults.
Niclosamide is less effective, 2 gm orally d 1, then 1 gram daily × 6. Children < 2 yr give 25% of dose; children 2 to 6 yr give 50%. Albendazole and mebendazole in usual single dose cure 50%.

Cause: *Diphyllobothrium latum* and *D. sp.* (fish tapeworm)

Epidem: Eggs passed in stool of human, cat, dog, others; hatches coracidium in water; eaten by crustacean, which are eaten by fish; forms cyst in muscle. Improperly prepared food (smoked, raw or partially cooked, frozen, caviar) is ingested by host and develops into adult. Common in fresh water lakes in Siberia, Africa, S. America.

Sx/Si: Usually none, B_{12} deficiency no longer seen.

Lab: Eggs in stool.

Rx: Praziquantel 10 to 25 mg/kg orally single dose.

Cysticercosis

(Am Fam Physician 2007;76:91)

Cause: *Taenia solium* (pig tapeworm).

Epidem: Eggs passed in stool, eaten by pigs, monkey, dog, or human. Oncosphere penetrates gut, travels in blood to muscles (especially heart), but occasionally elsewhere, and forms cysticerci (5–20 mm). Infected incompletely cooked meat eaten, and worm attaches to small intestine, matures, and releases proglottides with eggs.

Sx/Si: Usually none with adult worms.
Infection with cysticerci: subcutaneous cysts; CNS cysts with seizures (especially focal seizures in children), eye lesions, and commonly muscle pseudohypertrophy with weakness.

Cmplc: Auto infection by fecal-oral route common.

Lab: Biopsy of visible lesions.

Eggs in stool, serology, immunoblot.

Xray: Calcified cysts in muscle.

CT lesions usually < 2 cm, 4 types: low density without enhancement (alive), hypo or isodense with ring or nodular enhancement (dying), diffuse brain swelling with areas of nodular and ring enhancement, small granulomas or calcifications (dead).

Rx: Treatment for cysticerci requires consideration of side effects (brain edema) and should be undertaken in hospital with steroids and anticonvulsants available.

Albendazole 15 mg/kg/d in 2 divided doses (maximum 800 mg total) for 28 d, then 14 medicine-free d. Repeat for a total of 3 courses (Ann Intern Med 2006;145:43) is preferred to Praziquantel 50 mg/kg daily in 3 divided doses for 14 d plus oral steroids started 3 d before and continued through treatment.

Treatment of adult worm: Praziquantel to 5 to 10 mg/kg orally single dose.

Dexamethasone 2 to 4 mg 3×/d will decrease plasma levels of anticonvulsants and praziquantel.

Prev: Adequately cook pork. Treat pigs with oxfendazole 30 mg/kg orally once at 3 months of age and every 3 months (Am J Trop Med Hyg 2001;65:15).

Hydatid Disease

Cause: *Echinococcus granulosus* (cystic), *E. multilocularis* (alveolar), *E. vogeli* (polycystic).

Epidem: Parasite of dogs and canid family, primarily in sheep-raising areas, but many other mammals susceptible from camels to tree kangaroos. Ingest egg from dog feces, embryo penetrates duodenum into intestinal blood vessels to liver, lungs, elsewhere and develop into cysts. Dogs acquire from eating raw viscera of sheep or other animals.

Pathophys: Cysts primarily in liver 60%, lungs 20%, kidneys, heart, CNS, bone, etc. Symptoms from mass effect, cyst rupture with anaphylaxis and dissemination of protoscolices and formation of multiple cysts or secondary infections.

Sx/Si: Symptomatic early occasionally or after years as growth is 1 to 5 cm/yr. Then abdominal pain, jaundice, hepatomegaly, biliary colic (5–25%) and/or chest pain, cough, hemoptysis. Secondary infection with bacteria common (10%).

Cmplc: Some patients remain asymptomatic and self-cure. Biliary cirrhosis, metastatic disease, and cyst rupture are common problems.

Lab: Eosinophilia rare; serology for screening and confirmation available.

Xray: Water lily sign (cyst with wavy fluid at base).
Ultrasonography (useful for screening; EID 2008;14:260) and CT (differentiates active from dead cysts).

Rx:

- Surgery in skilled hands has a > 90% cure rate of accessible lesions with < 2% mortality.
- Medical therapy less successful, 40% to 100% cure. For cystic disease, same as cysticercosis; for alveolar disease, continue for months or years. Monitor WBC and transaminases twice a month. Not in pregnancy.
- Percutaneous puncture with instillation of ethanol.

Prev: Treat dogs to prevent/kill worms. Prevent dog access to animal offal. Wash hands after being with dogs.

16.6   Eosinophilic Meningitis

Cause: *Angiostrongylus cantonensis* (rat lung worm) occasionally *Gnathostoma spinigerum* (not covered).

Epidem: Third stage larvae in snails (or transport hosts or vegetables in contact with snail) eaten by rat, eggs hatch in lungs, and first stage larvae passed in rat feces, eaten by snail. Larvae molt twice and are infectious. Human accidental host. Found worldwide, especially SE Asia and Pacific Islands.

Pathophys: Larvae penetrate gut, spread by blood throughout body and to CNS.

Sx/Si: Headache, paresthesias, hyperesthesia, meningismus.

Cmplc: Blindness, seizures, occasionally death.

Lab: Eosinophils in CSF; occasionally worms seen.

Rx: Supportive; in massive infection mebendazole and steroids for brain edema (Am J Trop Med Hyg 2006;74:1122).

Prev: Avoid raw or marinated snails and unwashed vegetables.

16.7   Trypanosomiasis

Chagas' Disease

(Postgrad Med J 2006;82:788; J Infect Developing Countries 2007;1:99)

Cause: *Trypanosoma cruzi.*

Epidem: Mexico to Argentina (42°N to 42°S) where triatomine bugs found. Higher risk living in mud houses with dirt floors near palm trees. Triatoma bug feeds on blood; trypomastigotes passed in feces and enters through scratched skin, mucous membranes, or occasionally through food contaminated with insect feces. Trypomastigote enters cell, becomes an amastigote, multiplies, and is released as trypomastigotes, which invade other cells, especially muscle cells. Transmission also possible through blood transfusion, congenital (1–5%). All mammalian species may serve as reservoirs. 11 to 18 million infected; 200 000 new infections annually.

Pathophys: Local reaction at entry site 5 d after infection, then signs of disseminated invasion with inflammation, then fibrosis. Later chronic stage with persistent parasitemia and immune reaction with damage to myosites and ganglion cells.

Sx/Si: Local reaction with unilateral conjunctivitis and eyelid edema (Romana's sign) or edematous skin ulcer with regional adenopathy (chagoma).

Acute stage in 5% (95% asymptomatic), usually children with fever, myalgias, malaise, facial or generalized edema, headache, generalized lymphadenopathy with hepatosplenomegaly, GI symptoms. Rarely (5%) death from meningoencephalitis in children and HIV+.

Chronic phase asymptomatic in two-thirds, in others mostly (95%) cardiac: CHF, conduction system abnormalities especially right bundle branch block (RBBB), atrial fibrillation, blocks, bradycardia, premature beats, and sudden death (Am J Trop Med Hyg 2007;77:495). 5% have megaesophagus and megacolon with dysphagia and constipation. Less commonly, gastric emptying delayed and salivary gland hypertrophy.

In HIV+ with CD count < 200 acute meningoencephalitis (resembles *T. gondii*).

Lab: Acute and congenital: thick blood smears.

Chronic have low trypomastigote counts so use xenodiagnosis; bugs feed on patient then examined in 4 to 8 wk.

Serology, use 2 different tests.

Rx: Acute Benznidazole 5 to 10 mg/kg daily, divided into 2 doses for 30 to 60 d, or

Nifurtimox 8 to 10 mg/kg daily, divided into 3 doses, after meals for 30 to 120 d (child 15–20 mg/kg). Neither in first trimester of pregnancy.

Chronic < 15 yr of age or < 10 yr infected, as above.

HIV+ treatment advised, then use secondary prophylaxis with nifurtimox 5 mg/kg, 3×/wk.

A number of new drugs under development.

Prev: Residual insecticide spraying of mud hut walls; treated bed nets; screen blood donors; spray chicken houses where bugs multiply; plaster walls to block hiding spaces.

Tip: Seropositive blood can be made safe for transfusion by adding crystal violet (250 mg/L) and store at < 4°C for 24 hr.

African Trypanosomiasis

Cause: *Trypanosoma brucei-gambiense* and *rhodesiense*.

Epidem: *Glossina sp.* (tsetse) fly transmits infection from wild and domestic animals to humans. W African (Gambian) spread by *Glossina palpalis* group near water, common in Congo, Angola, S Sudan, N Uganda. East African (Rhodesian) spread by *G. morsitans* group in cleared bush and savannahs in SE Uganda and Tanzania.

Found in 36 countries in Sub-Saharan Africa in small pockets with about half million infected and > 50 000 deaths a yr. Unusual in tourists.

Pathophys: First stage with wide dissemination of parasites with second stage marked by CNS invasion. Gambian (chronic) and Rhodesian (acute and more severe) sufficiently different to be covered separately.

Sx/Si: Gambian: Nonspecific fever 2 to 3 wk after bite with 85% lymphadenopathy especially of posterior cervical chain (Winterbottom's sign), headache 70%, myalgias, malaise, and facial edema. Later anemia and amenorrhea. Second stage begins 4 to 12 months later with intractable headache, weakness,

Parkinson's-like symptoms, delirium, daytime somnolence, and indifference progressing to coma.

Crs: Slow progression, which is reversible with Rx.

Sx/Si: Rhodesian: Painful circumscribed red bite 2 to 5 cm (chancre), occasionally with cellulitis starts after 5 to 15 d and lasts 2 to 3 wk. Regional adenopathy, fever, occasionally eye inflammation. Second stage starts within weeks and progresses rapidly, one-third with cardiac involvement, all with CNS involvement with same symptoms as Gambian.

Lab: Gambian: Lymph node aspirate or blood on those with positive screening test—agglutination card. Do LP and check CSF if positive.

Rhodesian: Trypanosomes found in blood, chancre, bone marrow, lymph nodes, and CSF; wet preparations show motile parasites, but they lyse in 20 min. Many diagnostic lab variations available.

Rx: Follow country specific dosage regimes. Treatment of second stage uses toxic drugs (see package inserts).

- First stage Gambian with negative CSF, use pentamidine 4 mg/kg IM daily or on alternate days for 7 to 10 doses.
- Second stage Gambian, use pentamidine as above for days 1 and 2 plus Melarsoprol starting at 1.2 mg/kg slowly IV and increase to 3.4 mg/kg daily over 3 to 4 d, rest 7 to 10 d, then 2 more 3- to 4-d courses with 7 to 10 d rest. Reactive encephalopathy fatal in 3% to 8%. Maximum dose 5 ml. Instead of melarsoprol use less toxic eflornithine 100 mg/kg slowly IV every 6 hr for 14 d; 150 mg/kg in children. Give for only 7 d if used following melarsoprol failure (Lancet 1992;340:652).
- First stage Rhodesian use suramin slowly IV 5 mg/kg on d 1, 10 mg/kg on d 3, and 20 mg/kg on d 5, 11, 17, 23, and 30.
- Second stage Rhodesian use melarsoprol as above.

- LP for trypanosomes should be monitored using concentration method at 1 d post rx and every 6 months for 2 yr.

Prev: Yearly active case detection for Gambian disease in populations with prevalence > 1%. Tsetse fly traps. Control is complex.

16.8 Trichinosis

(Parasitologia 1997;39:77)

Cause: *Trichinella spiralis*, 3 subspecies.

Epidem: Infected improperly cooked meat eaten, cysts hatch, larvae invades small bowel, migrate, and encyst in muscles beginning 7 d after ingestion.

> In temperate climate: rat-pig cycle.
> In Africa: hyena, jackal, lion-bush pig cycle.
> In Arctic: walrus, seal-dog, bear, mink cycle.
> Usually asymptomatic, cluster of cases common.

Pathophys: Inflammatory reaction to larval invasion of small bowel (acute), lungs (2–11 d), muscles and CNS (weeks-months) with inflammation and fibrosis.

Sx: Gastroenteritis, pneumonitis (one-third), myalgias.

Si: Macular papular rash, fever, periorbital edema, conjunctivitis, splinter hemorrhages.

Crs: Resembles typhoid, Katayama fever.

Cmplc: Myocarditis with arrhythmias, pericarditis, and CHF.
> Meningoencephalitis 10% to 20%, focal signs, coma, seizures early and years later.

Lab: Eosinophilia after 2 wk up to 50%, muscle enzymes elevated, muscle biopsy after 1 wk shows larvae, serology tests.

Rx: Mebendazole 200 mg daily or
> Pyrantel 10 mg/kg daily for 5 d, or
> Albendazole 400 mg daily for 3 d.

Prednisone for severe symptoms.
Immunity acquired from untreated attack.

Prev: Cook meat thoroughly. Inspection at abattoir.
Prolonged freezing $< -15°$ C for > 3 wk.
Separate pigs from rats; cook pig feed.

16.9   Community Mass Treatment of Helminths

(Preventive Chemotherapy in Human Helminthiasis. Coordinated Use of Anthelminthic Drugs in Control Interventions. 2006. WHO. Free online access.)

Mass treatment of geohelminths is efficient and effective when combined with a program of community participation in health education and sanitation. Monitoring and evaluation should be considered at the onset with regular community feedback. School-based programs will not succeed without broad community-based primary healthcare initiative. In general:

- Children ≥ 2 yr age should be treated.
- Pregnant women should not be treated because of possible unrelated complications of pregnancy.
- If there is a rainy season, treat before and after the rains.
- Where transmission is perennial, treat every 6 months.
- Drug resistance should be considered.
- Mass treatment is appropriate if prevalence $> 50\%$.
- Ascaris and trichuris occur primarily in < 10 yr olds.
- Schistosomes in 10 to 20 yr olds.
- Hookworm in > 20 yr olds.
- Filaria in teens and above.
- Sanitation with appropriate Ventilation Improved Performance (VIP) toilets is crucial to success.
- Women are the key to modifying behavior.

- Albendazole > mebendazole > levamisole = pyrantel in terms of efficacy and coverage for *Ascaris*, *Trichuris*, hookworm, and *Strongyloides*.
- *Enterobius* is also covered as is *Trichostrongylus sp*.
- Capillariasis is not covered except by prolonged treatment or mebendazole 500 mg once.
- Albendazole also treats cutaneous larva migrans in a single dose.
- Iron sulfate treatment should be considered if anemia is prevalent.
- Breast feeding mothers with infants < 1 wk of age should probably be excluded.
- Mebendazole may cause ascaris migration per os (oral or nasal), and patients should be warned.
- Pyrantel and piperazine are antagonistic.
- Nitazoxanide may have a role in mass treatments because of its broad spectrum (Am J Trop Med Hyg 2003;68:382).

Although many worm infections are limited and therefore insignificant, mortality is estimated at Ascaris (60 000) and Trichuris (60 000) worldwide each yr.

Chapter 17
Bacterial Infections

17.1 Pneumonia/Acute Respiratory Infection (ARI)

Cause: Usually bacteria, even in HIV infected.

Epidem: Leading cause of death in children < 5 yr. More common in immunosuppressed, malnourished. WHO classification for children:

- very severe: central cyanosis, unable to drink, severe respiratory distress
- severe: chest indrawing
- mild-moderate: RR ≥ 60 infant < 2 months, RR ≥ 50 infant 2 to 11 months, RR ≥ 40 child 1 to 5 yr plus crackles on auscultation

   Infants < 2 months: Group B strep, gram negatives, listeria, *S. aureus*, RSV *Chlamydia trachomatis*, CMV.

   Children: *Strep. Pneumoniae* > *H. influenzae* > *Staph. aureus*, *Klebsiella*, *Escherichia coli*, *Salmonella*; RSV > influenza, measles, pertussis, TB, leptospirosis, PCP (especially < 6 months) nocardiosis, aspiration, lymphoid interstitial pneumonia (LIP).

   Adults: *Strep. Pneumoniae* > *H. influenzae*, *S. aureus*, gram negative, atypicals, *Legionella*, *Melioidosis* (SE Asia rice farmers), Paracoccidioidomycosis (S America), TB, Leptospirosis, PCP.

   Parasitic: *Ascaris*, hookworm, *Strongyloides*, schistosomiasis, lung fluke, malaria (5–15% pulmonary sx).

Sx: Cough, fever, chest pain, ± sputum.

Si: RR > 20 adults, rales, signs of consolidation.
Nasal flaring and grunting in infants.

Cmplc: Empyema, meningitis, heart failure.

Lab: Check for anemia; lymphocytosis in whooping cough; neutro-penia in HIV and disseminated TB, eosinophilia with parasites, blood cultures often positive with *S. pneumoniae*.
HIV test
AFB & gram stain sputum

Xray: Consider when severe disease, suspected empyema, uncertain diagnosis or persistent fever, or suspected TB. Not usually necessary.

Rx: Follow national or WHO guidelines when possible.

Infants and Children with Very Severe Pneumonia (VSP)

Ampicillin 50 mg/kg IM or IV every 6 hr plus
Gentamicin 7.5 mg/kg IM or IV daily.
Change to amoxicillin 15 mg/kg 3 × daily when able. Treat 10 d, or
Chloramphenicol 25 mg/kg IM or IV every 8 hr.
Change to same dose orally 4×/d when able, or
Ceftriaxone 80 mg/kg IM or IV once daily.

HIV+ with VSP

Ampicillin + gentamicin parentially for 10 d, but if not better in 48 hr, change to ceftriaxone as above, or
Gentamicin plus cloxacillin 50 mg/kg IM or IV every 6 hr.
Change to oral when better and continue for 3 wk.
Also, if HIV+ co-trimoxazole (8 mg/kg trimethoprim plus 40 mg/kg sulfamethoxazole, 8/40), IV or PO every 8 hr for 3 wk.

Infants and Children with Severe Pneumonia (SP)

Benzylpenicillin 50 000 units/kg IM or IV every 6 hr for at least 3 d. When better, switch to amoxicillin 25 mg/kg 2×/d. Total treatment 5 d, **but** if not improving, search for complications and switch to chloramphenicol (dose as above) and treat 10 d.

HIV+ with SP

Treat as VSP **except** co-trimoxazole routinely if 2 to 11 months of age. Co-trimoxazole only if CXR suggests PCP if 12 to 59 months of age.

Nonsevere (mild-moderate) Pneumonia

Amoxicillin 25 mg/kg 2×/d for 3 d or
Co-trimoxazole (4/20) 2×/d for 3 d **but** if HIV+, treat for 5 d.
Penicillin and gentamicin better than chloramphenicol. Amoxicillin and procaine penicillin better than co-trimoxazole (Cochrane Database Syst Rev 2006;3).

Adult Pneumonia, Outpatient Management

Amoxicillin 500–1000 mg orally 3×/d for 5 days, or
Doxycycline 100 mg twice a day for 7 to 10 d, or
Azithromycin 500 mg daily for 3 d or 2000 mg once.

Adult Pneumonia, Hospitalized

Ceftriaxone 1000 to 2000 mg IV daily, or
Cefotaxime 1000 mg IV every 8 hr, plus
Azithromycin 500 mg IV daily, or
Levoquine 750 mg IV daily, or
Moxifloxacin 400 mg IV daily, or
Gemifloxacin 320 mg orally. Not ciprofloxacin.

Adult Hospital Acquired

Imipenem 50 mg/kg/d divided into 3 to 4 doses, max 4 gm, plus
Gentamicin 3 to 5 mg/kg/d divided into 3 doses.

Tips:

- Staphylococcal pneumonia is suggested by rapid clinical worsening with lung abscess and pleural effusions. Sputum is frequently positive. Skin pustules support the diagnosis. Use a penicillinase-resistant penicillin (cloxacillin) plus gentamicin and treat 3 wk.
- Pleural effusions should be drained promptly when identified; AFB and gram stained and cultured. If purulent, think empyema. Also, obtain a CBC, protein, and glucose.
- Empyema may have a pleural rub, persistent fever, and CXR signs of pleural effusion. It must be drained. Treat with chloramphenicol for 4 wk or antistaph drug if identified. If no improvement or thick pus, insert chest tube. Consider TB.
- Lung abscess may follow bacterial or aspiration pneumonias, behind an obstructed bronchus or extension from a subphrenic abscess. Hemoptysis and foul-smelling sputum are usual, physical findings seldom positive and CXR makes the diagnosis—a cavity with an air-fluid level. Treatment is postural drainage and antibiotics such as clindamycin 600 mg IV every 8 hr or chloramphenicol. TB should be ruled out. Bronchoscopy if no improvement in 2 wk.
- Try to save floxins for treating resistant TB.

Pertussis-Whooping Cough

(N Engl J Med 2005;352:1215)

Cause: *Bordetella pertussis, B. parapertussis.*

Epidem: More common in unimmunized infants and children but vaccine only 60% to 80% effective and seen in adolescents and adults.

Pathophys: Incubation period 7 to 10 d. Coughing leads to dehydration, malnutrition, anoxia, and seizures.

Sx: Mild fever, cough, and rhinorrhea changing in second week to paroxysmal cough, vomiting.

Si: Prolonged coughing spell followed by whooping inspiration (not heard in infants who have apnea). Subconjunctival hemorrhages, cyanosis, seizures, ulceration frenulum, rectal prolapse, bradycardia.

Crs: 100-day cough.

Cmplc: Secondary pneumonia and atelectasis seizures, anoxia, brain damage, malnutrition.

Lab: CBC shows marked lymphocytosis in 2 to 5 wk. Culture difficult; Bordet Gengou medium, most positive in first week before cough; ELISA.

Rx: Erythromycin 12.5 mg/kg 4×/d for 10 d to reduce infectiveness or for prophylaxis.

Chloramphenicol 25 mg/kg 3×/d or co-trimoxazole (see non-severe pneumonia) alternatives. Azithromycin another option.

Oxygen by nasal cannula.

Turn on side during paroxysms to avoid aspiration.

Suction as needed.

No cough suppressants.

Treat seizures lasting > 2 min.

Prev: Immunize contacts and children in family (even if fully immunized).

Prophylactic antibiotics for infants < 6 months in family with URI symptoms.

Consider prophylactic antibiotics in other close contacts.

Lymphocytic Interstitial Pneumonitis (LIP)

Cause: Unknown.

Epidem: HIV related, in children > 2 yr.

Sx/Si: Often asymptomatic early, persistent cough, CHF with hepatomegaly and finger clubbing, dyspnea, parotid swelling, generalized painless lymphadenopathy.

Lab: HIV

Xray: CXR shows hilar lymphadenopathy and reticular infiltrates (looks like TB).

Crs: PCP, TB differential.

Rx: Prednisone or prednisolone 1 to 2 mg/kg/d (if O_2 sat < 90% or cyanosis) for 2 wk then decrease over 2 to 4 wk. It is usually prudent to treat for severe pneumonia and/or TB.

17.2 Melioidosis

Cause: *Burkholderia pseudomallei*, a gram negative bacillus.

Epidem: SE Asia and N Australia especially but worldwide (20° S to 20° N) distribution. Cause of 20% of community-acquired sepsis in NE Thailand. Associated with soil and rainy season. Usual inoculation via skin. May have latency period lasting years. More common in immune compromised, especially diabetes. Probably 80% asymptomatic or mild flu-like syndrome. Rare person-to-person spread.

Sx: Fever, sx of sepsis, pneumonia (50–80%), skin abscesses (10–25%).

Si: Shock, DIC, hepatorenal failure. Lung abscess resembling TB. Parotitis in children.

Crs: Dissemination to any organ; 50% mortality in symptomatic adults.

Lab: Culture of pus, sputum, urine, blood. Gram stain: bipolar "safety pin" appearance.

Xray: Typical pneumonia infiltrates to nodular-cavitating fibrotic TB-like changes on CXR.

Rx: Ceftazidime 50 mg/kg IV every 6 hr, max 8 gm a d. Imipenem another option ± co-trimoxazole (TMP 320 mg/SMX 1600 mg) IV twice a day plus folic acid 0.5 mg PO daily.

Treat for at least 14 d acutely, extend up to 8 wk, then continue eradication therapy for 3 to 6 months using co-trimoxazole orally (dose above). Less effective options include amoxicillin-clavulanate or oral quinolones.

17.3 Diphtheria

Cause: *Corynebacterium diphtheriae.*

Epidem: Man-only reservoir, airborne or direct contact spread, occasionally food, especially milk. Carriers common (3–5%) in endemic areas. Incubation period 2 to 4 d.

Pathophys: Mildly invasive in pharynx and skin. Exotoxin causes local necrosis or pseudomembrane and distant myocarditis, nephritis, and demyelination.

Sx: Pharyngitis, fever, malaise, dysphagia.

Si: Tonsillar membrane, dirty gray color, bleeds when removed. Bull neck, respiratory insufficiency. Myocarditis after 1 to 2 wk, heart blocks, ST-T changes and CHF. Neuropathy of cranial nerves in several days to peripheral neuritis 10 d to 3 months later. Primarily motor.

Cutaneous diphtheria presents as chronic nonhealing ulcers, often superinfected, rarely causes toxin-related symptoms but is important in dissemination.

Dx: Delayed treatment results in poor outcome. Presumptively treat tonsillitis with membrane especially with temperature < 103° and palatal paralysis. Cultures require special medium.

Rx: Diphtheria antitoxin ≥ 20 000 units IM or IV. See package insert.
Penicillin G or V for 14 d, or Erythromycin.
Immunize when recovered.

Prev: Vaccine
Prophylactic antibiotics for close contacts if immunizations are not up to date.

17.4 Bartonellosis

(Clin Infect Dis 2001;33:772)

Cause: *Bartonella bacilliformis*, a gram negative bacillus.

Epidem: Oroya or Guaytara fever, verruga peruana, N 5° to S 16° western slope of Andes of Columbia, Peru, Ecuador between 800 to 3000 m in narrow valleys suitable to the night biting *Lutzomyia* sand fly.

Pathophys: Live in RBCs and cause hemolysis and in reticuloendothelial cells causing hepatosplenomegaly, lymphadenopathy, and characteristic skin lesions of superficial lymphatic endothelium.

Sx/Si: Asymptomatic carriers common.

Incubation period 3 wk. Insidious onset of acute stage (Oroya fever) with malaise, fever (78%), anemia with jaundice (71%), headaches, and bone pain. Hepatosplenomegaly (82%, 29%) and lymphadenopathy (89%); all are tender. Meningoencephalitis (25%) with seizures (6%), coma (4%) and stroke. Death 10% to 40%.

Crs: Survivors pass into verruga stage, which may start during the acute stage or follow up to 2 months later. Fever and severe joint pains subside when eruption of vascular nodules appear on skin and mucous membranes including esophagus to intestines and vagina. They eventually shrink and drop off. Occasionally larger 5 to 7 cm nodules develop on the knees and elbows with severe bleeding.

Cmplc: *S. typhi* infections, toxoplasma reactivation, disseminated histoplasmosis and bacteria sepsis. CHF, pericarditis, tamponade, miscarriage. Differential: pyogenic granuloma, yaws, Kaposi's, secondary syphilis, angioma, bacillary angiomatosis, lymphoma.

Lab: Hemolytic anemia with bacilli in RBCs.

Rx: Chloramphenicol 1 gm 4 × daily or tetracycline, streptomycin, co-trimoxazole, quinolones. Response in 24 hr in acute stage.
Rifampin long term for verruga.

Prev: Insect repellent, household spraying, case detection important. Untreated bed nets not effective.

17.5 Leptospirosis (Weil's Disease)

Cause: *Leptospira interrogans* and others.

Epidem: Contact with warm water contaminated with animal urine, especially rats and cows. Survive a month in water. Entry through break in skin or mucous membranes. High risk in fresh water sports and workers, miners, animal husbandry, and sugar cane harvesters. Seroprevalence 15% to 20% in some areas. Incubation period 7 to 12 d.

Pathophys: Biphasic disease, bacteremic 4 to 7 d followed by immune reaction in various organs.

Sx/Si: Acute influenza-like illness with fever, sore throat, headache, myalgias, nausea, and vomiting. Cough and abdominal pain common, conjunctival redness, rash, occasionally purpura. Second stage may merge into first with meningeal and/or hepatorenal syndrome. Jaundice, hepatomegaly, bleeding into skin, lung, GI tract, oliguric renal failure (acute tubular necrosis; ATN), shock, myocarditis.

Crs: Mortality 2% to 5%.

Cmplc: Renal failure usual cause of death, but hemorrhagic stroke, adrenal failure, myocarditis common.
Differential: Suspect leptospirosis when severe myalgias, jaundice, conjunctival suffusion with meningeal signs and pretibial rash.

Lab: Elevated bilirubin with mildly elevated transaminases.
Urine normal early. Spirochetes can be found in urine later.

CSF lymphocytosis.

WBC in blood elevated with increased polys.

Creatine phosphokinase (CPK), BUN, creatine elevated.

Serological testing positive after a week.

Rx: Treatment must be started early to have any effect.

Tetracycline 1 gram every 6 hr, or

Doxycycline 100 mg 2×/d, or

Erythromycin 500 mg 4×/d, or

Penicillin.

Prev: Prophylaxis with doxycycline 100 mg twice a day for a wk effective. NNT = 24.

17.6   Brucellosis

Cause: *Brucella melitensis*, *abortus*, *suis*, rarely others.

Epidem: Close contact with bovines, goats, camels, sheep, or pigs or their milk products. Increased risk if no acid in stomach (PPI or H_2 blockers). Common in Andes, Mexico (3–4%), Iran, Iraq, Saudi Arabia (15% general population), Turkey (4.8%).

Pathophys: Intracellular pathogens result in granulomas.

Sx/Si: Incubation period 2 to 4 wk. Insidious onset with fever, night sweats, anorexia, and lethargy. Hepatosplenomegaly in one-quarter and lymphadenopathy. Osteomyelitis common, especially hip, knee, spine. Orchitis 7%, endocarditis, nephritis, rarely meningitis. May become chronic with undulant waxing and waning of symptoms.

Crs: Fatal in < 10%. Most resembles TB in presentation.

Cmplc: Abortion.

Lab: Blood culture takes weeks, < 50% positive, bone marrow culture has higher yields. Serology available. Erythrocyte sedimentation rate (ESR) elevated in 50%. Gram stain of joint fluid, gram negative cocco-rods.

Xray: Often 30% to 40% involves ≥ 2 vertebrae (TB 10–20%). Blastic lesions unlike TB.

Prev: Avoid unpasteurized goat cheese. Intra-family infection 50%. Iron deficiency increases susceptibility and severity.

Rx: Doxycycline 100 mg twice a day for 6 wk, plus
>Streptomycin 1 gram IM daily for 15 d (best), or
>Rifampin 10 to 15 mg/kg orally for 6 wk.
>Pregnant or children: Co-trimoxazole plus rifampin for 4 wk,

or
>Co-trimoxazole 4 wk plus streptomycin 15 d, or
>Rifampin for 4 wk plus streptomycin.
>Relapse up to 10%; consider rifampin and doxycycline

for 6 months with aminoglycoside for 1 wk (J Chemother 2003;15:466).

17.7 Anthrax

Cause: *Bacillus anthracis.*

Epidem: Gram-positive rod, which forms long-lived spores found in soil. Animals and rarely humans inoculated through break in skin, inhalation of spores, or consumption of contaminated meat. Common in Iran, Africa, S America, and Russia or imported on hides.

Pathophys: Exotoxin causes edema.

Sx/Si: Skin exposure incubation 2 to 3 d with papule on first day, surrounding vesicles on second day, then ulceration progressing to black eschar. Painless, edematous, lymphadenopathy, which resolves over 2 to 6 wk; usually not on hands but on arms, neck, and head; most self-cure. Intestinal from eating contaminated animals, which have often died of the disease; vomiting, diarrhea, fever, GI bleeding. Occasionally oral edema. Most survive. Pulmonary infection with fever, chills, pulmonary edema, and death.

Complc: Bacteremia.

Lab: Gram stain shows large brick-shaped rods, which are easily cultured.

Rx: Benzylpenicillin G 100 mg/kg IM daily divided into 4 doses (maximum 2.4 grams or 4 million units), or
> Amoxicillin orally.
> Doxycycline, ciprofloxacin, or erythromycin alternatives.
Not chloramphenicol.

Prev: Vaccinate animals.
> Human vaccine available for special situations (military).
> Avoid meat from ill or dead animals.

17.8   Meningitis

(Pocket Book of Hospital Care for Children. WHO 2005. Overview of diagnosis and management in the tropics.)

Causes: Age, immune competence, underlying illnesses, immunization status (*H. flu*, BCG, *S. pneumo*), and local epidemiological conditions are crucial in the diagnosis and management.
> Consider the following:

- age: under 2 months: Group B streptococcus, Listeria, coliforms, *Salmonella*, *Klebsiella* and vaginal flora, *Strep. pneumococcus*, and *Staphylococcus*
- children under 2 yr of age: *H. flu*, *S. pneumo*, *Neisseria meningitides*, Group B strep, Salmonella
- under 18 yr: *H. flu*, *S. pneumo*, *N. meningitides*
- adults: *S. pneumo*, *N. meningitidis*, *H. flu* (rare)
- elderly: *S. pneumo*, all others.

Epidem: Meningitis belt in Africa, 16° N to 4° N; *Neisseria meningitides* occurs in epidemics during dry seasons.

Also more likely to occur after influenza infection. Most commonly spread from nasal carriage.

Strep. pneumococcus often accompanies pneumonia or upper respiratory tract infections, occasionally by secondary extension.

Hemophillis influenza largely preventable with vaccine series.

All 3 more likely after surgical or auto-splenectomy (sickle cell disease).

Sx: Headache, fever, stiff neck, irritability, then lethargy progressing to coma.

Si: Nuchal rigidity in older children (rare in infants), bulging fontanelle (15–30%), high-pitched cry, poor feeding, seizures common, hypotension, petechial rash in *N. meningitidis* and occasionally *H. flu.*

Complc: CNS thrombophlebitis and damage with focal and global neurological deficits, hearing loss, communicating hydrocephalus, death.

Differential: Aseptic meningitis; herpes, enterovirus, HIV, adenovirus, and mumps.

Encephalitis and meningoencephalitis, malaria.

Spirochetes: syphilis, leptospirosis, borrelia (lymphocytic).

Chronic: TB, brucella, fungal, *T. gondii*, cysticerosis.

Lab: CBC not helpful usually (J Emerg Med 1988;6:33).

Blood cultures; malaria smears; HIV screen

CSF studies:

Cell count WBC > 10/mm^3 abnormal usually > 200 (cloudy CSF)

Predominately polys = bacteria

Predominately lymphs = viral, TB, others, early bacterial

Predominately eosinophils = parasitic: *Angiostrongylus cantonensis* (Pacific Health Dialog 2001;8:176) or *T. solium* (N Engl J Med 2002;346:668)

Glucose < 40 mg/dl, protein > 45 mg/dl

Gram stain on spun CSF useful for *H. flu, Strep. pneumococcus,*
rarely positive with *N. meningitidis.*

Culture if available.

Rx: Antibiotics: The etiological cause often remains uncertain, and
a repeat LP is useful. Broad spectrum antibiotics should be used
unless a specific agent is known or expected.

Premature infants: Ampicillin and gentamicin or penicillin
and gentamicin. See chapter 34.

Infants < 2 months: Ampicillin and gentamicin or cefotaxime or ceftriaxone, or chloramphenicol.

Older infants > 2 months, children, and adults: Ceftriaxone
or cefotaxime if available or ampicillin or benzylpenicillin plus
chloramphenicol or chloramphenicol in oil (meningococcal
epidemics) or guided specific therapy.

Elderly and immunosuppressed: Consider TB and opportunistic infections; treat as adults above.

Premature or low birth weight infants:

- Ampicillin (less 1 wk age) 50 mg/kg/12 hr IV or IM
- Gentamicin 3 mg/kg once daily IV or IM
- Chloramphenicol best avoided
- Ceftriaxone best avoided, biliary sludging
- Cefotaxime 50 mg/kg/12 hr IV
- Benzylpenicillin 50 000 units/kg/12 hr IV

Infants less than 2 months:

- Ampicillin (0–2 wk age) 50 mg/kg/12 hr; ≥ 2 wk 50 mg/kg/8 hr
  IV or IM
- Gentamicin (0–2 wk age) 5 mg/kg/once daily IV or IM; ≥ 2 wk
  7.5 mg/kg/once daily IV or IM
- Chloramphenicol 25 mg/kg/12 hr IV or IM
- Ceftriaxone 50 mg/kg/12 hr IV or 100 mg/kg/once daily IM
- Cefotaxime (0–2 wk age) 50 mg/kg/12 hr IV
  (≥ 2 wk age) 50 mg/kg/8 hr IV

- Benzylpenicillin (0–2 wk age) 50 000 units/kg/12 hr IV
  (≥ 2 weeks age) 50 000 units/kg/6 hr IV

  Older > 2 months old infants, children, adults:
- Cefotaxime 150 mg/kg/6 hr IV, maximum 2 gm/dose
- Ceftriaxone 100 mg/kg/12 hr IV, maximum 2 gm/d
- Ampicillin 50 mg/kg/8 hr IV or IM, maximum 12 gm/d plus
  Chloramphenicol 25 mg/kg/6 hr IV or IM
- Chloramphenicol in oil 100 mg/kg/once daily, maximum 3
  gm/d for 3 d for meningococcal disease
- Benzylpenicillin 100 000 units/kg/6 hr IV or IM, maximum
  dose 24×10^6 units/d

  Treatment tips:
- Duration of treatment ≥ 10 d. If not improved in 3 d, redo LP
  and reevaluate.
- Trial of TB drugs may be indicated.
- Look for cerebral malaria and treat, steroids contraindicated.
- Change to oral therapy can be considered after 5 d if stable and
  appropriate drugs available.
- Consider local antibiotic resistance if known and substitute/
  add drugs, ie, vancomycin 1 gm/12 hr for adults with suspected
  penicillin resistant S. pneumo.

  Nursing: oxygen if hypoxemia.

  Diazepam and phenobarbital for seizures.

  Watch for hypoglycemia, NG tube feed, regulate temperature, avoid fluid overload (inappropriate ADH secretion).

  Steroids: may be useful, especially in children with H. flu
  meningitis (N Engl J Med 1990;319:968); not advised by WHO
  as studies negative in tropics (Arch Dis Child 1996;75:482).
  Definitely useful in TB meningitis. Dexamethasone 0.6 mg/kg/d.
  One dose for H. flu and 2 to 3 wk for TB.

Prev: Immunization: H. flu, N. meningitides, S. pneumonia, BCG

Antibiotics are used for close day care and family contacts to prevent disease and clear nasal carriage.

For meningococcus: Ciprofloxacin 500 mg twice daily × 2 adult (resistance reported) or Rifampin 10 mg/kg twice a day × 2 d children

For *H. flu*: Ciprofloxacin 500 mg twice a day × 4, adult; or Rifampin 20 mg/kg twice a day × 4, children

Vaginal irrigation with chlorhexidine useful (BMJ 1997;315:216). Treatment of mothers in labor with known Group B streptococcal carriage or premature rupture of membranes (PROM).

Chapter 18

Insect-Borne Diseases and Hemorrhagic Fevers

18.1 Dengue Fever

Cause: A severe viral illness caused by RNA flavivirus. Antigenically related to YF, JE, and West Nile. Dengue has 4 serotypes.

Epidem: Spread by *Aedes* mosquitoes. Incubation period is 2 to 7 d. About 1 million cases are reported from over 60 countries annually.

Sx/Si: Children have nonspecific viral illness with fever, rash, and rarely shock. Older children and adults have mild to severe "break-bone fever" disease with myalgias, biphasic fever, severe headache, conjunctival infection, retrobulbar pain, and an early erythematous rash, which evolves in a few days to a scarlatiniform eruption beginning on the extremities. This rash accompanies the second fever, lymphadenopathy, and occasionally the shock of dengue hemorrhagic fever (DHF; see below). The second phase ends in 2 to 3 d when the fever breaks and the skin desquamates. Convalescence may be prolonged. The first attack is seldom fatal and immunity is type specific and long lasting.

Lab: Laboratory testing shows marked leukopenia. Diagnosis can be confirmed with a number of tests of IgM antibody. Muscle enzymes elevated (CK, lactate dehydrogenase [LDH], aspartate transferase [AST]) in severe disease and may be a marker for development of DHF (Am J Trop Med Hyg 2008;78:370).

Rx: Treatment is symptomatic. Aspirin should not be given due to its antiplatelet properties. Mosquito nets reduce transmission inside the hospital. *Aedes* mosquitoes are daytime biters. Mortality is less than 1%.

Cmplc: DHF/Dengue Shock Syndrome (DSS)
(N Engl J Med 2005;353:941)

This is a severe complication of a dengue fever virus infection, which occurs in a patient, most commonly a child, with immunity acquired at birth or through previous dengue infection with another type of virus. Pathogenesis is believed due to antibody-dependent enhancement of viral lode. Non-neutralizing antibodies enhance viral growth. The role of vaccine-induced immunity in DHF/DSS, if any, is unknown (Lancet 2002;360:1243).

On days 2 through 7 of a classic dengue attack, the patient suddenly worsens with shock, a positive tourniquet test with petechiae, ecchymosis, and hemorrhage. The liver may be enlarged and tender with elevated enzymes. Disseminated intravascular coagulation occurs. The platelet count is less than 100 000, and plasma leakage through capillaries leads to an increased hemoglobin and hematocrit (H&H).

WHO criteria for treatment are below:

- No hemorrhagic manifestations, well hydrated: home
- Hemorrhagic signs or borderline hydration: observe
- Bleeding or shock: admit
- Daily H&H and platelets
- Monitor fluids, BP, level of consciousness
- Antipyretics: no aspirin (ASA) or NSAIDs
- Fluids determined by serial H&H, intake and output (I&O), BP

- IV fluid for moderate dehydration use normal saline (NS)

Weight in kgs	ml/kg/d
< 7	220
7–11	165
12–18	132
19–40	88
> 40	twice maintenance: 2 (1500 + 20 [weight kg-20])

- Tourniquet test:
  - Determine blood pressure.
  - Inflate cuff to systolic + diastolic/2.
  - Wait 5 min, then deflate cuff.
  - Count petechiae in a 1-inch square area.
  - More than 20 petechiae is positive.

Prev: Control of *Aedes* mosquitoes reduces the prevalence of disease (see vector control). Research is ongoing with live attenuated vaccines but will be difficult. Personal protection with DEET.

Zika Virus

Cause: Transmitted by *Aedes* mosquitoes, a flavivirus.

Sx/Si: Symptoms similar to Chikungunya but milder. Characterized by a maculopapular rash, which starts on the face and spreads over the body, conjunctivitis, and arthralgias of the hands and feet. Other symptoms: fever, retro-orbital eye pain, headache, diarrhea, edema, and lymphadenopathy.

Epidem: Recently (2007) reported in Yap State, Federated States of Micronesia (Pacific Public Health Surveillance Network 6/22/07).

Crs: Lasts 2 to 4 d.

Cmplc: None.

Lab: Rapid laboratory tests for dengue may give false positive results.

Rx: None.

Chikungunya

Cause: Transmitted by *Aedes* and Culex mosquitoes, especially
A. *albopictus*, a member of the alphavirus genus.

Epidem: Ongoing epidemic began in 2005 and moving throughout
Asia with up to one-third of populations infected (New Engl J
Med 2007;356:769). Widespread in Africa. Incubation period 3
to 7 d (range 2–12). Monkeys are reservoir hosts.

Sx/Si: Abrupt onset with fever, severe joint pains, and prostration.
After 1 to 4 d, fever subsides for about 3 d then recurs, often with
a pruritic maculopapular rash on the trunk and extensor surfaces.
Nausea and vomiting may occur.

Crs: Recovery is 3 to 6 d later, but severe prolonged arthralgias with or
without effusions may continue for several months.

Cmplc: Severe infection is unusual (< 0.02%) and death is rare (Lancet Infect Dis 2007;7:319). Neonatal infection may occur.

Rx: Treatment is symptomatic. Aspirin should be avoided as the clinical disease may be confused with dengue. No vaccine is available.

Prev: Insect repellents and mosquito control are useful control
measures.

O'nyong-nyong

Emerg Infect Dis 2006;12:1249; Am J Trop Med Hyg 2005;73:32

Cause: An alpha virus closely related to Chikungunya.

Epidem: Transmitted by *Anopheline* and *Culicine* mosquitoes. Large
epidemics have occurred with over 70% of the population
affected; found in Sub-Saharan Africa.

Sx/Si: Self-limiting acute, febrile illness with lymphadenitis, epistaxis,
severe arthralgias, and conjunctivitis. A pruritic maculopapular

rash appears on the fourth day starting on the face and spreading to the trunk and limbs.

Crs: Recovery occurs in about a week, but arthralgias may persist.

18.2 Hemorrhagic Fevers

Yellow Fever

Cause: A severe flavivirus infection related to dengue fever spread by *Aedes* and *Haemagogus* (S America) mosquitoes.

Epidem: There is no direct transmission. Monkeys are the reservoir host. Most cases are acquired in forested rural areas (sylvatic) with the danger of spread to urban areas. About 300 cases per year occur in S America and perhaps 3000 in Sub-Saharan Africa.

Sx/Si: Symptoms are those of the viral hemorrhagic fevers ranging from an inapparent or mild disease to fulminant symptoms of fever, headache, myalgias, and bradycardia, accompanied by conjunctival infection, anorexia, nausea, and vomiting.

Crs: After about 3 d, there is a short period of remission lasting less than 24 hr followed by a recurrence of fever, upper GI symptoms, jaundice, and diffuse hemorrhaging. Renal and heart failure and shock follow. If the patient survives, this second stage lasts 3 to 5 d then recovery begins. Convalescence may be prolonged. Fatality rate is 20% to 50% in severe cases.

Lab: Neuropenia occurs early. DIC may occur. Liver chemistry and function tests are elevated (except alkaline phosphatase). Severe proteinuria is seen late in the course.

Rx: Treatment is symptomatic.

Prev: Yellow fever vaccine is effective. Adverse reactions are rare (MMWR 2001;50:343–5). Mosquito nets should be used by hospitalized patients.

INSECT-BORNE DISEASES AND HEMORRHAGIC FEVERS

Hemorrhagic Fever with Renal Syndrome (HFRS)

(J Infect Developing Countries 2008;2:3)

Cause: Transmitted by aerosolized rodent fecal, urine, or saliva excretions, this group includes the Hantaan (Far East), Dobrava (Balkans), and the milder Seoul (worldwide) and Puumala (Scandinavia-W Europe, Russia) hantaviruses and others. Sin Nombre (United States) and Andes (Argentina and Chile) cause a pulmonary syndrome (Emerg Infect Dis 1997;3:95–104).

Sx/Si: Patients with hemorrhagic fever (HF) with renal syndrome start with an influenza-like illness followed a few days later with petechiae and bleeding.

Crs: An oliguric period then ensues. Most deaths (mortality 1–15%) occur at this stage.

Lab: Laboratory findings include leukocytosis, thrombocytopenia, abnormal clotting studies, and proteinuria.

Rx: Treatment is symptomatic; ribavirin is effective.

Prev: Vaccines have been developed for Hantaan and Seoul viruses and are available in the affected areas. Avoid aerosol rodent feces and pretreatment of feces with a 10% household bleach solution prior to clean up.

Congo-Crimean Hemorrhagic Fever

Cause: A Hyalomma tick-borne illness.

Sx/Si: Characterized by fever, headache, myalgias, and dizziness with lymphadenopathy and tender hepatomegaly. Nausea and vomiting are common. Pharyngitis, conjunctivitis, and gingivitis occur.

Crs: Bleeding begins about d 4. Mortality is up to 50%.

Lab: Leukopenia, thrombocytopenia, and elevated transaminases and DIC may be detected in laboratory testing.

Rx: Ribavirin is useful.

Prev: Vaccines are available in some affected areas. Tick control measures and avoidance of body secretions of infected livestock or patients provide protection from transmission.

Omsk Hemorrhagic Fever

A tick-borne HF, also spread by direct contact with infected rodents, especially muskrats. Found in Western Siberia, the symptoms are typical of HFs. The disease usually has a biphasic nature with encephalitis occurring during the third wk. Mortality is 0.5% to 3%. Treatment is supportive; ribavirin is of some benefit.

Rift Valley Fever

Cause: One of the Bunyaviridae family of HFs, it is transmitted by a variety of mosquitoes and more frequently by direct contact with infected livestock in which it causes abortion.

Epidem: The disease is found throughout Sub-Saharan Africa, especially East Africa, Egypt, and the Arabian Peninsula (MMWR 2007;56:73–76). Outbreaks occur during wet seasons when mosquito numbers increase.

Sx/Si: Symptoms are usually that of a nonspecific viral fever, but retinitis, CNS symptoms, and HF may occur (< 8%). Mortality is < 1% generally but up to 30% in HF.

Rx: Ribavirin is effective treatment.

Prev: Animal vaccines are effective control measures along with mosquito avoidance. There is an inactivated human vaccine, but it is not commercially available.

Lassa Fever

A manual "Infections Control for Viral Hemorrhagic Fevers in the African Health Care Setting" is available online in English, Portuguese, and French through the CDC Special Pathogens Branch Web site (http://www.cdc.gov/ncidod/dvrd/spb/mnpages/vhfmanual.htm).

(A supplement to J Infect Dis 1999:179 is devoted to Ebola virus.)

Cause: Arenavirus spread by rodent (Mastomys) feces and direct contact with infected patient.

Epidem: West Africa: Guinea, Liberia, Nigeria, Sierra Leone, and probably other areas where rodent found. Estimated 100 000 to 300 000 infections/yr; 5000 deaths. Up to 10% to 16% hospital admissions in Sierra Leone and Liberia. Occasional epidemics.

Sx/Si: Exudative pharyngitis, fever, retrosternal pain, and proteinuria have a positive predictive value (PPV) of 80%. Abdominal tenderness.

Crs: 80% asymptomatic, 20% multisystem failure.

Cmplc: Hemorrhage, seizures, renal failure.

Lab: Elevated liver tests, leukopenia, thrombocytopenia.

Rx: Supportive.

Machupo (Bolivian HF), Junin (Argentinean HF), Sabia (Brazilian), and Guanarito (Venezuelan HF) all Arenavirus are spread by direct contact with rodent excreta and patient fomites.

Treatment is ribavirin and supportive care.

Filovirus HFs are Ebola and Marburg found in Sub-Saharan Africa.

Transmission is by contact with infected blood or secretions. Symptoms include headache, fever, myalgias, pharyngitis, abdominal pain, and diarrhea. Conjunctival infection and a maculopapular rash are present. Hemorrhage occurs later. CNS symptoms are common. Leukopenia, lymphopenia, and thrombocytopenia occur followed by a neurophil increase and large abnormal lymphocytes. AST and SGPT; alanine transferase (ALT) are increased; alkaline phosphatase and bilirubin levels are normal to slightly elevated.

Treatment is supportive. Barrier nursing care is essential. Fatality rate ranges from 25% to 90%.

Contact tracing is important to prevent dissemination as the incubation periods are up to 3 wk.

18.3 Japanese B. Encephalitis

Cause: Spread by the rice-paddy breeding mosquito *Culex tritaeniorhynchus* and other culucine mosquitoes. A flavivirus related to dengue and yellow fever.

Epidem: Found throughout South and Southeast Asia to Queensland, Australia (rare). Epidemics occur in the late summer with children frequently infected but seldom seriously ill.

Sx/Si: Fever, headaches, delirium, seizures, and focal neurological signs are presenting symptoms.

Crs: Incubation period is 6 to 16 d. Most cases are asymptomatic or with nonspecific symptoms. Encephalitis occurs in 1:300 but is devastating with high mortality (10–25%) and disability rates (25–50%). Neurological status may worsen until death or resolve through a slow recovery with residual symptoms.

Lab: Serological diagnosis is possible and helps to differentiate (along with geographic distribution) Japanese B. Encephalitis (JBE) from other types of encephalitis such as West Nile, Murray Valley, the equine encephalitides, and Rift Valley Fever. The CSF shows a mild to moderate lymphocytosis and increase in protein with a normal glucose.

Rx: Treatment is supportive. Steroids are helpful only if intracranial pressure is increased.

Prev: The disease is carried by birds, and the virus amplified in pigs. Vector control and repellents are useful. An inactivated vaccine is available, 3 injections at 0, 7, 28 d are required, but severe reactions may occur. Live vaccines are also available in other countries.

18.4   Leishmaniasis: Visceral, Mucosal, and Cutaneous

(Cutaneous: Am Fam Physician 2004;69:1455)
(Mucosal: Am J Trop Med Hyg 2007;77:266)

Cause: *Leishmania donovani* (visceral), *infantum* (visceral and diffuse cutaneous), *L. braziliensis*, *panamensis* (mucocutaneous) Brazil, Peru, Bolivia, *L. tropica*, *major*, and others.

   The spectrum of disease depends on the species and the patient's immunity.

Epidem: Most are zoonoses with mammalian reservoirs ranging from dogs and rodents to primates. Phlebotomus and lutzomyia sand flies are vectors. Geographic distribution ranges from 45° N to 32° S in isolated foci worldwide except Australia.

   Cutaneous and mucocutaneous disease affects 12 million people with 1 to 2 million new cases a year. Visceral has about half million annual cases. Outbreaks with 10% mortality have recently occurred (Ann Trop Med Parasitol 1992;86:481; Am J Trop Med Hyg 2007;77:275).

Pathophys: Sand fly bite introduces metacyclic promastigotes, phagocytosed by macrophages then develop to mastigotes, which may remain localized as a cutaneous or mucous membrane lesion(s) or spread throughout the body's macrophages.

Sx: Visceral (Kala-azar or Black Fever): Incubation period 2 to 6 months but wide range. Gradual or acute onset with fever, weight loss wasting, diarrhea, cough, and anemia with grayish color of skin.

Si: Cutaneous: Incubation 1 wk to several months; lesions on exposed (to sand fly bites) skin. Erythematous papule increases in size over weeks and ulcerates to a volcano-like lesion 0.5 to 10 cm in diameter. Often multiple lesions. Painless unless secondarily infected; occasionally satellite papules about larger ulcer or evidence of lymphatic spread.

Mucosal: Usually follows cutaneous lesion, which has cured, sometimes years earlier. Starts at nasal septum with mucosal invasion, stuffiness, epistaxis, ulceration, and septal destruction with collapse. Spreads to buccal mucosa and palate with granulomatous changes. Occasionally into laryngeal area with respiratory obstruction.

Visceral: Painless splenomegaly early, constant and massive later; hepatomegaly later with jaundice and ascites. Intestinal mucosa involvement causes diarrhea; other mucosal lesions cause menorrhagia and epistaxis. Usually normochromic/cytic anemia, leukopenia, thrombocytopenia. Death by secondary infections or hemorrhage.

Postvisceral dermal disease appears after apparent cure of Kala-azar. About 1 yr after treatment, depigmented macules develop into papules and nodules. Starts on face and fingers; may become widespread.

Crs: Kala-azar is fatal if untreated.

Mucosal and cutaneous lesions may self cure over a few months or years leaving a depressed scar; 10% reactivate later.

Differential diagnosis is aided by the history and geographic area but includes the following:

- cutaneous: discoid lupus, sarcoidosis, fungal infections; *Mycobacterium marinum*, *M. leprae*, TB, syphilis, and yaws
- mucocutaneous: fungal infections, rhinoscleroma, sarcoid, lethal midline granuloma, TB and leprosy, Wegener's, syphilis and yaws
- visceral: lymphoma, malaria, TB, schistosomiasis, typhoid, brucellosis.

Labs:

- Cutaneous scraping of margin and center of ulcer; multiple slides should be obtained; sensitivity 50% to 75%.

- Punch biopsy of edge of lesion; needle aspirate sent for staining.
- PCR available.
- Cultures allow species identification and drug sensitivity study.
- HIV test as it reactivates latent infections.
- Spleen puncture is used when platelet count adequate and clotting normal in Kala-azar.
- Bone marrow or lymph node aspirates positive.
- Peripheral blood may be positive in HIV+ patients.
- Leishmanin skin test similar to PPD test.

Rx: Cutaneous: self healing, especially *L. major* and *peruviana* or drug therapy for visceral, mucocutaneous, or cutaneous.

Pentavalent antimony 20 mg/kg IM or IV every other d for 30 d or daily for 20 d (28 d for mucosal).

Meglumine antimoniate 85 mg/ml, sodium stibogluconate 100 mg/ml; meglumine better cure rate, 88% vs. 51% (Am J Trop Med 2007;77:266). Primary resistance common in India. Requires 2 negative aspirate for test-of-cure.

Amphotericin B 0.5 mg/kg/d IV or 1.0 mg/kg/every other d IV for total dose 20 mg/kg.

Liposomal amphotericin B 2–4 mg/kg/d IV for a total of > 20 mg/kg over 7 to 10 d (expensive but most successful).

Pentamidine 2 mg/kg IM every other d, 7 injections. Total 2 to 4 gm. Cure rate 35% (Am J Trop Med 2005;72–133).

Paromomycin 11–15 mg/kg/d IM or IV for 21 d (N Engl J Med 2007;356:2571).

Fluconazole 200 mg/d for 6 wk for cutaneous (N Engl J Med 2002;346:891).

Miltefosine (N Engl J Med 2002;347:1739) 25 mg/kg/d (weight 8–20 kg); 50 mg/kg/d (weight 20–25 kg); 100 mg/kg/d (weight > 25 kg) for 28 d. Caution teratogenic; not in lactation.

Itraconazole 400 mg/wk × 6 (Arch Dermatol 1989;125:1540).

Topical paromomycin for *L. major* and *mexicana*.

Excision not advisable.

Allopurinol not effective; neither is aminosidine (Am J Trop Med Hyg 2007;76:1128).

Azithromycin cure rates for cutaneous < 25%.

Expect improvement in 7 to 10 d. Follow up at 3, 6, 12 months for sustained cure. HIV+ rarely cured.

Prev: Reduce sand fly vector contact:

- pyrethroid-impregnated ultra-fine bed nets
- pyrethroid-impregnated curtains (Br Med J 2002;325:810)
- deltamethrin-impregnated dog collars
- body covered with clothing
- insect repellents
- indoor residual spraying
- twilight and night feeders.

18.5   Typhus and Spotted Fevers

Epidemic Louse-borne Typhus

Cause: *Rickettsia prowazekii*.

Epidem: Transmitted by *Pediculus homanus*, body louse. Common in times of war and in refugee populations, especially in cool mountain regions.

Pathophys: Focal occlusive end-angiitis due to toxins from organisms on endothelial surface.

Sx: Headache, limb and shin pain, nausea, vomiting, delirium, dry cough.

Si: Fever, injected conjunctiva, rash begins on d 2 to 4 on trunk and proximal limbs, pink evolving to purple macules, and occasionally petechiae. Meningoencephalitis in 50%.

Cmplc: Peripheral gangrene, myocarditis, secondary infections. May cause hemolytic anemia in glucose 6 phosphate dehydrogenase (G6PD) deficiency with renal failure.

Differential typhoid (closely resembles) hemorrhagic fevers, cerebral malaria, louse-borne relapsing fever.

Lab: Usually not helpful. Felix-Weil test + OX-19 and OX-2.

Rx: Chloramphenicol 500 mg 4×/d for 7 d, or Tetracycline, doxycycline, quinolones. Steroids in severe cases. Rapid response within 48 hr confirms dx.

Prev: Wash patient, burn clothing.

1% malathion to sheets and hospital garments.

Prophylaxis of contacts with doxycycline 200 mg orally once.

Murine, Endemic Typhus

Cause: *R. typhi*.

Epidem: Transmitted by rat flea, *Xenopsylla cheopis*. Found worldwide.

Sx/Si: Milder than louse-born, headache, myalgias, rash.

Lab: Felix-Weil + OX-19, OX-2.

Rx: Same as *R. prowazekii*.

Tick-borne Spotted Fevers

(MMWR 2006;55(RR-4):3)

Causes: *R. rickettsii* (Rocky Mt-US, Columbia, Brazil), *R. conorii* (Boutonneuse Africa-India), *R. africae* (S African), *R. sharoni* (Israel), *R. sibirica* (Siberian), *R. japonica* (Japan), *R. australis* (SE Asia and Australia), and others. Various ticks and mammal hosts.

Sx/Si: Tick bite eschar variable. Fever, headache, myalgias, dry cough, rash appears 2 to 3 d later especially on feet, wrists, forearms. Rash initially macular becomes petechial then hemorrhagic.

Cmplc: Gangrene, meningoencephalitis, DIC, pneumonia, renal failure.

Lab: Serology.

Rx: Chloramphenicol, tetracycline, doxycycline in usual doses.

Scrub Typhus

Cause: *Orientia tsutsugamushi*.

Epidem: Pacific Russia to Queensland Australia and Micronesia to Pakistan. Often in pockets when larvae mites live in grasslands.

Sx/Si: Incubation 5 to 10 d. Fever, painful lymph nodes, bite eschar (10–92%), headache, myalgias, hepatosplenomegaly, nausea, vomiting, cough. Rash on arms, thighs, trunk. Eschar less common in India (Emerg Infect Dis 2006;12:1590).

Cmplc: Meningoencephalitis, myocarditis, uremia, respiratory distress.

Lab: Weil-Felix OX-19, OX-2, and OX-K positive ≥ 1:80. PCR available.

Rx: Doxycycline 200 mg orally once in adults, 100 mg once in children. May retreat if recurrence. Chloramphenicol in usual dose. Ciprofloxacin used in Thailand where resistance reported.

Chemoprophylaxis with doxycycline 200 mg weekly is effective.

Chapter 19

Typhoid Fever

(N Engl J Med 2002;347:1770)

Causes: *Salmonella typhi* and *paratyphi*, gram negative bacilli, which are easily grown in the laboratory.

Epidem: A common disease where sanitation is poor. There are 20 million cases and 600 000 deaths per year. Transmission is through food or water contaminated with feces or urine from a carrier or patient. Shellfish are important sources as are dairy products. The incubation period depends on the ingested dose and is usually 10 to 20 d for *S. typhi* and 1 to 10 d for *S. paratyphi*. Only humans are infected.

Sx: Onset is insidious, and patients often present after 1 to 2 wk of illness. Headache is most common symptom followed by abdominal pain, fever and rigors, myalgias, malaise, and cough. Constipation is more common than diarrhea; vomiting unusual except in children. Delirium may be present and mimics cerebral malaria or psychosis. Usually the patient seems apathetic, with a drawn haggard face—a key sign.

Si: On examination, signs of bronchitis are common with coarse crepitations and rhonchi. Splenomegaly occurs in about 1 in 4 but may be helpful as a diagnostic sign in nonmalarious areas. A slightly distended abdomen is frequent. Rose spots are not seen on dark skin but may be sought on the trunk of fair-skinned patients or on the conjunctiva. They are pale, pink, raised, and fade on pressure. Jaundice (1% adults, 5% children) and an enlarged tender liver may occur. Meningismus without meningi-

TYPHOID FEVER

tis (3%) is unusual as is frank pneumonia. Relative bradycardia occurs but is uncommon.

Crs: Convalescent carriers are common with positive stool cultures persisting for several months to over a year in 1% to 3% of patients. When possible patients should be kept in hospital until stool cultures are repeatedly (3–6) negative. Chronic carriers often have S. *typhi* in their gall bladders, and a cholecystectomy is sometimes curative. Urinary carriage is short lived except in those infected by *Schistosoma hematobium*. Retreatment with antibiotics may be helpful.

Cmplc: Complications occur in the third or fourth wk. Intestinal hemorrhage or perforation from typhoid ulcers in the lower ileum may be heralded by collapse, rise in pulse, fall in temperature, abdominal distension and pain. Perforation and hemorrhage require surgery, but the typhoid ulcers are friable and difficult to oversew. Segmental resection is quicker than multiple wedge resections (Am J Surg 2005;187:22). Mortality is about 20%. The ulcers are typically oval in the long axis of the bowl with marked mesenteric lymphadenopathy.

Less common complications include hemolytic anemia (2%), pneumonia (1–2%), renal disease (pyelonephritis, glomerulonephritis, renal failure), parotitis (lymphatic hypertrophy), osteomyelitis, and cholecystitis.

Differential diagnosis includes malaria. Typhoid is often misdiagnosed as cerebral malaria.

An experienced clinician knows the myriad presentation of typhoid, but the uninitiated are easily mislead. Typhoid can be diagnosed on clinical grounds about 80% of the time.

Lab: Laboratory findings are confirmatory. The bone marrow yields the highest (90%) culture rate. Use a large butterfly needle drilled into the sternum. Marrow/blood cultures are frequently ($> \frac{2}{3}$) positive from onset through the third wk. Urine and stool cultures may also be collected, the latter for proof of cure prior to hospital discharge.

A Widal test may be used if cultures are negative or unavailable; a 4-fold increase in 0 and H antigen titers is considered positive. It is not useful for diagnosing or following the carrier state. Dip antigen testing is sensitive after a week of fever.

Leukopenia is considered common or even a required finding but may not be helpful in children (S Afr Med J 1976;2:556).

Rx: Treatment is determined by local antibiotic sensitivities. Chloramphenicol was the drug of choice, but like ampicillin and co-trimoxazole, resistance is common (South East Asia Journal Tropical Medicine and Public Health 2006;37:1170). But when these older drugs have not been in use for a number of years, it appears that resistance will decline over time (J Infect Chemother 2006;12:402). Chloramphenicol dosage is 500 mg q 4 hr until defervescence then q 6 h for 14 d. The oral route is preferred. Amoxicillin and co-trimoxazole are given for 14 d. If possible, the lab should screen for nalidixic acid resistance. If resistance is reported, ciprofloxacin and ofloxacin are likely to fail despite the organism being reported as "sensitive." If sensitive to nalidixic acid, fluoroquinolones are preferred. One option is levaquin 500 mg/d for 7 d (SEAJTMPH 2006;37:126). Other antibiotics are ceftriaxone 2 to 3 gm/d IM or IV for 7 to 14 d, cefixime 20 to 30 mg/kg/d orally for 7 to 14 d, or azithromycin 1 gm/d for 5 d. The quinolones have a lower relapse rate. High dose steroids (dexamethasone: 3 mg/kg loading and 1 mg/kg/6 hr for 2 d or hydrocortisone 200 mg IV followed by prednisone 40 mg/d) reduces mortality in severely toxic patients. It should be avoided in the third week of illness as it masks the signs and symptoms of ileal perforation. Relapses may occur in up to 20% of patients usually a week after stopping antibiotics.

Prev: Prevention is through adequate sanitation and vaccination. See Chapter 5.4.

Other Salmonella Infections

There are a number of other salmonella species that infect humans and animals. Transmission is fecal-oral, usually through contaminated food. Asymptomatic carriers also play a role.

Incubation period is short, 12 to 48 hr. Symptoms begin with nausea, vomiting, headache, fever, and malaise. Crampy diarrhea is at first watery but later becomes bloody with signs of colitis. Bacteremia occurs in 5% to 10%, usually in children or immune-suppressed individuals. Meningitis in children, osteomyelitis in those with sickle cell disease, and vascular infections in adults with atherosclerosis may result. Reactive arthritis 1 to 2 wk after infection usually affects the knees and ankles of patients with the HLA-B27 antigen. Carrier states are common, lasting 1 to 2 months; chronic carriage is rare.

Treatment is reserved for the very ill, the young, elderly, and immunosuppressed. Antibiotics do not shorten the illness in healthy adults and may prolong the carrier stage. Antibiotic choice is the same as for typhoid fever.

Chapter 20

Viral Exanthems

20.1 Measles (Rubeola)

Cause: RNA paramyxovirus.

Epidem: Probably the leading cause of vaccine preventable death in infants and children; measles is also seen in adults who were inadequately protected by immunization. Atypical measles may occur in the partially immunized. Over 345 000 deaths in 2005 (WHO) down to 242 000 in 2006 due to immunization coverage of 80%. Very contagious by aerosol with over 75% to 90% of contacts becoming infected; it is rarely subclinical. Incubation period is 10 to 14 d. Epidemics are common.

Sx: The prodromal stage presents as a low-grade fever, cough, conjunctivitis, and coryza.

Si: After 2 to 3 d, pathognomonic Koplik spots occur—effervescent white sand-like spots on a reddened mucosa of the palate and buccal mucosa. The temperature rises suddenly about the fifth d of illness; the rash follows, starting on the head and extending downward to the feet over the next 2 to 3 d. It is usually maculopapular but may be confluent and even hemorrhagic. In dark-skinned patients, it may be easier to palpate than see. The rash may be less severe in those with HIV infection. Lymphadenopathy is present along with mild splenomegaly.

Crs: Otitis media, pneumonia, and diarrhea are common complications in younger children (20%); liver inflammation is more common in adults.

Lab: A low white count with relative lymphocytosis is seen. CSF shows a mild increase in lymphocytes.

Cmplc: The measles virus may cause an interstitial pneumonia or predispose to a secondary bacterial pneumonia (1/20). Latent tuberculosis may be activated, and a tuberculin skin test is unreliable. Encephalitis occurs in 1–2/1000 patients, usually several days after the rash appears. The leading cause of blindness in African children is due to measles-precipitated vitamin A deficiency resulting in corneal scarring. Mortality may be 10% to 25%. Many die of complications. Infants with malnutrition do the worst. Immunity from disease is lifelong. Subacute sclerosing panencephalitis (SSPE) is a late complication of measles occurring months to years later. The rate is probably 10:1 000 000 (J Infect Dis 2005;192:1686).

Rx: Treatment is largely symptomatic. Vitamin A (400 000 IU) reduces mortality (N Engl J Med 1990;323:160). Immunity is present in newborns and decreases after 6 months.

Prev: The live vaccine is effective and recommendations for age of first immunizations varies by country policy. One option is to immunize at 9 to 12 months of age and again at age 4 to 6 yr. During an epidemic, immunize after 6 months but do not count this as a first immunization (MMWR 1998;47:1–57). Immunize all previously unimmunized patients when admitting them to a hospital in case a measles patient is admitted. Respiratory precautions are indicated.

Vaccine-induced immunity is dependent on age of immunization (blockage by maternal antibodies), potency of vaccine (cold chain security and variety of virus), and second immunization. Under ideal circumstances, 1 dose is 98% protective. Deaths have fallen 60% from 1999 to 2005 due to vaccine.

20.2 Pox Viruses

Monkey Pox

(MMWR 1997;46:1168)

Cause: Orthopoxvirus.

Epidem: West and Central Sub-Saharan Africa (Congo Basin-Sudan). Transmission from monkeys or other animals (Emerg Infect Dis 2006;12:1827) to humans. Person-to-person spread has occurred but is unusual. Incubation period 5 to 17 d. Seroprevalence 1.7% (Am J Trop Med Hyg 2007;77:1150).

Sx/Si: Abrupt onset with fever for 2 to 3 d followed by single crop of papules over entire body, the face, soles of feet, and palms are involved. Papules evolve to pustules, which heal with scarring after 10 d. Lymphadenopathy is prominent (70–82%).

Cmplc: Death is unusual, usually in children.

Lab: Viral isolation possible, serology.

Rx: Supportive.

Prev: Small pox vaccine is effective.

Tanapox

Cause: Yabapox virus.

Epidem: Kenya, Zaire, other areas. Monkeys to man via mosquitoes.

Sx/Si: Mild, one to two 5 mm pox on exposed areas with cheesy contents; heal without scarring.

Chickenpox

Cause: *Varicella* virus.

Epidem: Worldwide, disease of children with zoster in adults and immunosuppressed, 14-day incubation period, infectious 2 d before and 6 d after appearance of rash. Spread by direct contact and airborne.

Sx: Centrifugal rash. Papule evolves to vesicle then to pustule (occasionally hemorrhagic), which opens, crusts over, and heals with scar. Several crops appear over 4 d.

Si: Fever < 39°C; occasionally headache and myalgias.

Cmplc: Systemic involvement common in older individuals and immunosuppressed. Pneumonia, encephalitis with cerebellar symptoms, DIC, renal, and hepatic involvement. Secondary infections. Embryopathy in pregnant women, especially between wk 8 to 20. Congenital infection if mother symptomatic around time of delivery. Neuropathic pain with zoster.

Rx: Acyclovir (Aciclovir) 10 mg/kg IV every 8 hr for 7 d for disseminated disease or eye involvement.

Oral treatment 20 mg/kg 4×/d for 5 d may shorten illness if started early.

Avoid aspirin as associated with Reye's syndrome.

Prev: Vaccine available.

VZ16 varicella-zoster immunoglobulin seldom available but useful in pregnant mothers, neonates, and immunosuppressed if given prior to symptoms.

Chapter 21
Cardiovascular Disease

21.1 Hypertension

Cause: Sodium chloride intake (Int J Cardiol 1997;59:185), low
  potassium, and low calcium diet. Renal disease common cause in
  developing countries. Rarely due to Cushing's or Conn's disease,
  coarctation, lead exposure, others.

Epidem: Urban migration increases blood pressure (BP; Br Med J
  1990;309:967) as does alcohol intake and obesity. Increased
  prevalence in Sub-Saharan Africans.

Sx/Si: None initially, targeted physical examination for retinopathy,
  cardiomegaly (left ventricular hypertrophy; LVH), large kidneys,
  pulses.

Crs: Left ventricular hypertrophy leading to heart failure, stroke.
     Coronary artery disease less common than in west.
     Renal failure, primary vs secondary difficult to sort out.

Lab: Urinalysis, H&H, renal function, electrolytes. Electrocardiogram
  (EKG) occasionally shows LVH (< 10%). Echocardiogram more
  sensitive.

Rx:

- "Western diet" and lifestyle should be avoided.
- Weight loss and exercise; limit alcohol and salt; stop tobacco.
- Drug treatment will depend on national policy and availability.
- Goal is 140/90 or less with diabetes mellitus.

- Compliance a problem, best treatment directed by local provider.
- NSAIDs should be avoided.
- Thiazides first line (Ann Intern Med 2004;141:39).
- Avoid hypokalemia with dietary changes.
- Beta-blockers safe and inexpensive.
- Angiotensin-converting enzyme inhibitors (ACEIs) good in renal disease, CHF, and diabetes mellitus. Less effective in Blacks. Never use in pregnancy, monitor renal function, accept up to 30% increase in creatinine (N Engl J Med 2002;347:1256).
- Other less expensive third-line drugs include the following:
  - Alpha methyl dopa: Safe in pregnancy. High doses may cause Coombs positive hemolytic anemia (1–5%).
  - Reserpine: Sedation and depression side effects; limit dose to ≤ 0.25 mg/d.
  - Alpha blockers especially helpful with prostatic hypertrophy.
  - Calcium channel blockers: Use long-acting types only, such as diltiazem.
  - Hydralazine use IV for preeclampsia.

Hypertensive Crisis

Management depends on the presenting symptoms and the drugs available. Preferred therapy is nitroprusside, IV beta blocker, and furosemide. Nifedipine sublingually not advised (JAMA 1996;276:1328).

21.2   Infective Endocarditis

Cause: Underlying valvular disease, especially rheumatic heart disease (RHD) and congenital anomalies. Pathogens similar to those in developed countries: *Strep viridans*, staph, enterococcus, group

D strep. Occasionally fungal, anaerobes, brucella (normal aortic valve).

Epidem: Diagnosis difficult with basic laboratory facilities. About 5% of all cardiac hospital admissions, < 5% right sided (IV drug users).

Sx: Fever > 90%; weight loss.

Si: Murmur (99%), cardiomegaly (75%), petechiae (75%), anemia (60%), splenomegaly (50%), clubbing, splinter hemorrhages, Osler's nodes less common.

Cmplc: Valve rupture, CHF, peripheral arterial emboli with mycotic aneurysms and rupture: stroke, meningitis, abscesses. Differential broad: rheumatic fever, TB, brucellosis, borreliosis, abscess, osteomyelitis.

Lab: Sedimentation rate elevated > 90%.
Blood cultures × 3 (< 30% + in basic laboratories) 10 cc each tube. Urinalysis 95% microscopic hematuria with multiple tests; H&H for anemia.

Studies: Echocardiogram + in > 80%.

Rx: Streptococcus or empiric therapy: Penicillin G, 10 million units IV divided doses plus aminoglycoside (gentamicin or streptomycin) for 4 to 6 wk; staphylococcus: nafcillin or oxacillin or cefazolin or vancomycin ± aminoglycoside for 4 to 6 wk.

21.3 Pericarditis

(Am Fam Physician 2007;76:1509)

Cause: Idiopathic (90%), uremic, bacterial (local and systemic spread), TB (chronic), amoebic (extension from left liver abscess), viral (coxsackie), post MI, sarcoidosis, meningococcemia.

Epidem: Viral etiology most frequent, but confirmation of diagnosis difficult.

Pathophys: Restriction of ventricular filling leads to CHF.

Sx: Dyspnea, cough, pleuritic chest pain better when sitting.

Si: Intractable CHF, tamponade and shock, ascites. No point of maximum impulse (PMI), decreased heart sounds, tachycardia, small pulse volume, friction rub. Pulsus paradoxus: > 10 mm Hg drop in systolic BP with inspiration.

Cmplc: Tamponade.

Lab: Sedimentation rate elevated in many, as opposed to low ESR in CHF.

      EKG: ST elevation and/or PR depression, low voltage electrical alternans-QRS alternate size

      Echo: excess pericardial fluid

Xray: Large heart, pleural effusions L > R, calcifications in chronic. High left diaphragm with liver abscess.

Rx: Aspirin or NSAIDs; watch fluid overload.

      Colchicine 0.5 to 1.0 mg/d reduces symptoms and recurrences (Circulation 2005;112:2012).

      Steroids plus TB Rx.

      Diagnosis: if purulence suspected or therapeutic tap required, do a pericardiocentesis.

- Have patient sitting.
- Attach EKG V1 lead to 20-gauge spinal needle with 3-way stopcock and 50 cc syringe or use Echo guidance.
- Prep skin with antiseptic.
- Enter below xyphoid aiming toward left clavicle.
- Advance until fluid encountered, aspirate, and send to laboratory.
- Withdraw needle if EKG pattern of injury (ST elevation) appears—indicates myocardial stick.

- Drain slowly but completely.
- May need to repeat daily.
- Suspect amebiasis if green-brown or chocolate-colored exudate; TB if protein high (> 40 gm/L), bloodstained (80%), and many lymphocytes.
- Avoid tapping for suspected viral or with concurrent meningococcal disease unless symptomatic.
- Make a pericardial window if constriction occurs.
- Drain amoebic liver abscess when present.

21.4 Atherosclerotic Heart Disease and Myocardial Infarction

Cause: Elevated lipids, diet, HT, tobacco use, diabetes mellitus, chronic inflammation with elevated C-reactive protein (N Engl J Med 2002;347:1557), arterial spasm, emboli, aortic valvular disease, hypercoagulable states.

Epidem: Western lifestyle disease. Increased risk worldwide if waist-hip ratio high (WHR; Lancet 2005;366:1640). WHR female > 0.83, odds ratio 1.90; male > 0.9, odds ratio 1.73, increases as ratio increases.

 Decreased risk with exercise, fish intake, moderate alcohol, control of HT, blood glucose, lipids, and aspirin intake.

Pathophys: Hemorrhage into lipid-rich plaque with platelet aggregation ~90%.

Sx: Angina, diaphoresis, dyspnea, GI complaints. Many with no symptoms.

Si: Signs of atherosclerosis: vascular bruits, decreased/absent peripheral pulses; S_4 gallop, S_2 paradoxically split, low-grade fever, shock, CHF. At d ≥ 2, occasional pericardial rub.

Crs: Heart failure. Prognosis same for Q-wave and non–Q-wave infarcts. Angina, mitral regurgitation.

Cmplc: Left ventricle (LV) aneurysm with CHF, emboli. Arrhythmias, especially ventricular tachycardia (Vtach) and premature ventricular contractions (PVC), heart block, cardiac rupture with tamponade, shock, stroke, pericarditis (Dressler's syndrome).

Lab: CPK peaks at 2 d, up in 12 hr, lasts 4 d.
SGOT (AST) peaks at 2 to 4 d, up in 24 hr, lasts 7 d.
LDH last to elevate 5 d.
Cholesterol.
EKG ST elevations (50% sensitivity).
In right ventricle (RV), infarct ST elevation in V_1 or right-sided leads
New right bundle branch block (RBBB) or left bundle branch block (LBBB).

Rx: ASA 325 mg dissolve in mouth (N Engl J Med 1997;336:847), then daily.
Beta-blockers IV or orally and continue indefinitely.
ACEIs within 24 hr.
Statins.
Heparin (JAMA 2005;293:427).
Nitroglycerine for pain, CHF, anterior MI. Care with RV and inferior MIs.
Angioplasty, thrombolysis, clopidogrel, pressors, pacers, surgery usually not available but helpful.
Pericarditis: do not treat with indomethacin; use other NSAIDs (N Engl J Med 1981;305:1171).
Treatment often limited in developing countries especially in rural areas. ASA, oxygen, nitrates, beta blockers, morphine, and diuretics usually available. An ideal treatment would be a single pill with ASA, a beta-blocker, a statin and an ACE I.

Prevention:
(Bull WHO 2007;85:421)

- Restrict salt (5 gm = 1 tsp/d).
- Consume fruits and vegetables, 5 servings (400–500 gm/d)

- Limit fatty foods, cooking oils (30 ml/d); use olive, soya, corn, rape seed. Use chicken, wild game, fish.
- Limit alcohol: men 2 drinks: women 1 drink per d.
- Physical activity 30 min/d.
- Stop tobacco.
- Medicate as above.
- Control BP < 130/80.
- Control blood glucose.
- Reduce body mass index (BMI) to < 25.

21.5　Congestive Heart Failure

(Am Fam Physician 2004;70:2145)

Cause: A broader differential should be considered in developing countries because treatment of the underlying illness may resolve the cardiac symptoms. HT, cardiomyopathies (idiopathic, infectious, toxic, peripartum, genetic, amyloid, ischemic, hypothyroidism, collagen-vascular), valvular, renal disease, high output (hyperthyroid, beriberi, severe anemia, atrial-ventricular [AV] malformation, hydatidiform mole, Paget's disease), arrhythmias, high altitude, neurogenic, preeclampsia, snake bite.

Epidem: More common in children in developing countries especially: congenital, acute and chronic rheumatic fever, myocarditis, endocarditis, suppurative pericarditis, acute glomerular nephritis, severe anemia, severe pneumonia and malnutrition. Five-year survival is poor unless reversible cause.

Sx: Respiratory distress with dyspnea, orthopnea, cough, abdominal fullness, nocturia, anxiety, fatigue.

Si: Tachycardia, S_3 gallop, basal crackles in lungs, occasionally wheezing, enlarged tender liver, cardiomegaly, pleural effusions R > L, edema, ascites, signs of increased right atrial pressure (jugular venous distension [4 cm above sternal angle at 45° elevation] and hepato-jugular reflux), weight gain.

Lab: Hb to rule out anemia

Urinalysis to detect glomerulonephritis (GLN).

ESR low except with infectious causes.

EKG may show LVH with outflow obstruction and hypertension or other changes suggestive of underlying disease.

Xray: Occasionally useful when in doubt. Shows upper lobe redistribution and perihilar fullness, cardiac enlargement.

Rx: Acute

- Give oxygen 2–3 l/min.
- Give furosemide 1 mg/kg IV; may double if no response.
- Reduce any fever with acetaminophen.
- Avoid IV fluids, unless shock.
- Give morphine to help with hypertensive etiology and anxiety.
- Nitrates 0.4 mg sublingual.
- Elevate head of bed 45°.
- Give dopamine for shock (not in high output failure): start 2 to 5 μg/kg/min, max 20 to 50 μg/kg/min. Dobutamine preferred if available.
- Treat underlying cause and/or begin chronic therapy.

Chronic

- Salt restriction 2 gm NaCl/d.
- Digoxin: Children 15 μg/kg orally once then 5 μg/kg/twice a d. Maximum 250 μg per dose. Adult 500 μg once, then 250 μg every 6 hr × 2, then 125 to 250 μg per d, lower with renal disease and elderly. Keep pulse > 50 in adults. Avoid digoxin in hypokalemia, Wolff-Parkinson-White syndrome (WPW), second degree and complete heart block.
- Diuretics for symptom control, furosemide, and/or thiazide. Caution: Will cause hypokalemia and precipitate digoxin toxicity unless addressed by additional therapy below.
- ACEIs. Enalapril start at 2.5 mg/d and increase (watch BP!) to maximum 20 mg. Not in pregnancy. Reduces mortality (JAMA 1995;273:1450).

- Spironolactone 25 mg orally daily. Reduces mortality (N Engl J Med 1999;341:709).
- Amiloride HC1 5 to 20 mg orally daily, spares K.
- Beta-blockers (metoprolol, bisoprolol and carvedilol) reduce mortality but are usually not available.
- Isosorbide dinitrate 30 to 120 mg/d in divided doses (insure 12-hr treatment-free interval to avoid tolerance) plus hydralazine 25 to 50 mg twice a day for refractory CHF.

Caution: Hyper- and hypokalemia are real dangers with the use of ACE I, spironolactone, amiloride, and diuretics, especially when digoxin is being used. If you cannot monitor potassium in your laboratory, you will need to make an educated guess keeping patient compliance and renal function and drug availability in mind. An EKG may occasionally be helpful showing peaked T waves (hyper) or U waves (hypokalemia).

21.6   Rheumatic Fever

(Am Fam Physician 1992;45:613; Lancet 2005;366:155)

Cause: *Streptococcus pyogenes* Group A, various M protein types. Some genetic susceptibility.

Epidem: About half million new cases per yr (N Engl J Med 2007;357:439) with 15 million people with RHD and a quarter million deaths. Predominately low income countries, up to 2% to 3% of children 5 to 14 yr have RHD (N Engl J Med 2007;357:470). Unusual under age 4 yr.

Pathophys: Shared antigens between streptococcus and human antigens in heart, brain, and joints but still not clear.

Sx/Si: Insidious onset with fever, malaise, and weight loss. History of sore throat only 20%. Diagnosis by Jones criteria with WHO modifications (see Table 21.1).

Table 21.1 Revised Jones Criteria for the Diagnosis of Rheumatic Fever

Major Manifestations*	Minor Manifestations*
Carditis	**_Clinical_**
Polyarthritis	Fever
Chorea	Arthralgias
Erythema marginatum	Previous acute rheumatic fever
Subcutaneous nodules	or evidence of preexisting
	rheumatic heart disease

	Laboratory
	Acute phase reaction:
	Leukocytosis
	Elevated erythrocyte
	sedimentation rate
	Abnormal C-reactive protein
	Prolonged PR interval or other
	electrocardiographic changes

Plus

Supporting evidence of a preceding streptococcal infection (eg, elevated or
increasing antistreptolysin-O or other streptococcal antibodies, positive throat
culture for group A streptococcus, recent scarlet fever).

*Two major manifestations or one major and two minor manifestations are required
to make the diagnosis.

WHO additions

The diagnosis of acute rheumatic fever (ARF) can be accepted
in the absence of the Jones criteria in the 3 categories of patients
described below. In the first 2 categories, evidence of a prior
streptococcal infection is not necessary.

1. Pure chorea
2. Insidious or late-onset carditis
3. Rheumatic recurrence

- Carditis is a new or changed murmur, especially mitral or aortic incompetence, a friction rub, pericardial effusion, and cardiac enlargement.
- Arthritis is usually migratory, polyarticular, and involves the larger joints.
- Sydenham's chorea is more common in adolescent females and starts as clumsiness, weakness, involuntary movements, and ataxia. Often confused with psychiatric disease as it frequently occurs alone.
- Rash occurs in severe cases; erythema marginatum is transient, migratory, nonpuritic, macular, and worse with elevated temperature. Easily missed on dark skin.
- Subcutaneous nodules are rare, occur over extensor surfaces, and occiput and over spine. Often symmetrical, painless and mobile, 2 to 10 mm in size.
- Fever is universal except in pure chorea and late onset carditis. Responds to aspirin.
- Arthralgia is a minor criteria that cannot be counted toward diagnosis if arthritis is present.
- Recent streptococcal infection is by culture or serological testing.
- EKG changes include prolonged PR interval or Wenckebach phenomenon (2° type 1 block).
- Other common symptoms include epistaxis, weight loss, mild anemia, renal (> 50%) and liver (> 60%) involvement.

Crs: Usually < 3 months.

Cmplc: Chronic RHD, CHF with repeated attacks common. Echocardiogram-screening finds 10 × more patients with RHD than auscultation (N Engl J Med 2007;357:470). Not included in Jones criteria.

Lab: Elevated ESR, antistreptococcal tests 80% sensitivity, mild anemia, leukocytosis, and EKG changes.

Rx:

- Primary prevention and treatment of AFR: 10 d penicillin or erythromycin or 5 d azithromycin.
- Aspirin 100 mg/kg d divided doses maximum 6000 to 8000 mg. Therapeutic level is 25 to 30 mg/dL or until tinnitus and then reduce slightly.
- Prednisone for severe carditis 1 mg/kg d. Once improved, taper off 2 to 3 wk.
- Bed rest in hospital, especially carditis.
- Chorea mild tranquilizers.

Prev: Secondary prophylaxis (Table 21.2) should be instituted on any patient with AFR and those with suspected or proven RHD.

Table 21.2   Secondary Prophylaxis of Acute Rheumatic Fever

Drug	Dose	Frequency
Benzathine penicillin G	> 27 kg patient: 1 200 000 units IM	Every 3 to 4 wk
	< 27 kg patient: 600 000 units IM	Every 3 to 4 wk
Phenoxymethyl penicillin	125 to 250 mg orally	Twice daily
Sulfadiazine*	> 27 kg patient: 1000 mg orally < 27 kg patient: 500 mg orally	Once daily
Erythromycin†	250 mg orally	Twice daily

IM = intramuscular

*Not to be given in the third trimester of pregnancy. Other sulfa drugs have not been studied and their effectiveness in rheumatic fever is unknown.

†Only in individuals allergic to both penicillin and sulfadiazine.

- Continue prophylaxis for at least 5 yr after last attack or through puberty until early 20s, depending on country protocol.
- Give preprocedural antibiotics prior to dental work or certain surgeries; for those with RHD: 2 gm amoxicillin orally.

Control:

- Echocardiographic screening may have a role in case finding.
- All patients should be registered in a case file, which is used to ensure regular secondary prophylaxis.
- Primary prevention is preferable; a 10-day course of penicillin is necessary (JAMA 1981;246:1790).

Chapter 22

Endocrinology

22.1 Diabetes Mellitus

(Int J Diabetes Developing Countries online; Talabi Centre for Diabetes Studies online treatment guide)

Type 1

Cause: Hypoinsulinemia due to viral-induced autoimmune destruction of islet cells; occasionally pancreatic disease.

Epidem: Highest prevalence in Caucasians; much lower in tropics but varies greatly by ethnic groups. Rate depends on genetic makeup and environmental exposures. Migrants assume risks of host countries (Br Med J 1987;295:479).

Sx/Si: Polyuria, polidypsia, polyphagia, with weight loss, fatigue, and dehydration. Blurry vision.

Lab: Glycosuria, elevated glucose, often ketosis.

Rx: Management is frustrating in tropics as regular insulin dosage based on blood or urine sugar is difficult. Regular monitoring requires availability of health services. It is best that the patient moves near to a health center. Giving them employment at the hospital facilitates their care. One solution is to base insulin dosage on second voided urines:

- Hospitalize the patient for education if possible.
- Determine the spill point of glucose in the urine. At what blood glucose level does the patient first have glycosuria?

- Do this by having the patient empty their bladder and discard that urine. A half hour later have them void and test that urine and the blood sugar simultaneously.
- Find the point where glucose first appears in the urine. Typically:

Blood Glucose	Urine Glucose Test Strip
< 200	negative
250	≥ 1+
300	≥ 3+

- Taste the urine or place urine near an ant hill and return later if urine glucose test strips are unavailable.
- Use this information to adjust daily long-acting basal insulin, and if possible, test urine before meals to arrive at a dosage of short-acting (soluble, regular) insulin.
- Check urine ketones if glucose consistently ≥ 3+.

    Note: Urine glucoses are unreliable in pregnancy.

Type 2

Cause: Insulin resistance due to obesity (90%).

Epidem: As overweight and obesity increase, so does diabetes mellitus (DM; increased 3 × in 20 yr; N Engl J Med 2007;356:213). Greatest problem in Middle East, South, Southeast, and East Asia and Pacific Islands. In Tonga, uses 60% of health budget; in Nauru, 50% adult prevalence. Substantial genetic predisposition with increased risk with Western diet. Thrifty genotype hypothesis (Am J Hum Genet 1962;14:353) proposes a selective advantage in those predisposed to DM; they are better adapted to surviving famine.

Cmplc: Diabetic nephropathy most common cause of end-stage renal disease in Asia; over 30% in China.

    Retinopathy: after 15 yr 2% blind, 10% usually impaired. Neuropathy with limb amputations.

Cardiovascular disease rate is doubled.

Increased infection risk.

Obstetrical macrosomia, congenital malformations.

Lab: Fasting whole blood glucose ≥ 120 mg/d (6.7 mmol/L). Fasting plasma glucose ≥ 140 mg/d (7.8 mmol/L).

Random whole blood glucose (capillary) > 200 (11.1).

Random plasma blood glucose (venous) > 200 (11.1).

HgbA$_1$C not a diagnostic test, lower in iron deficiency and sickle cell (SS) anemia. Keep < 8% or lower. Cholesterol keep < 200; LDL < 100 if possible.

Urine glucose and protein.

Rx:

- Diet and exercise first. Diet should be divided by calories: 25% to 35% from fat; 10% to 15% protein (0.8–1 g/kg ideal body weight); 50% to 60% carbohydrates. Traditional diets should be encouraged.
- Modify cardiac risk factors: smoking, lipids, HT.
- Add oral drug:

     Metformin, start 500 mg daily and increase weekly to maximum 2 gm in divided doses. Use care in renal, heart, hepatic failure. Stop in sepsis, shock, and before iodine-containing radiographic contrast media and surgery. Sulfonylureas, several available: Glibenclamide 2.5 to 5 mg daily to start, 15 mg daily maximum. Not with porphyria or breast feeding.
- Add long-acting insulin if control sub-optimal.
- Add ACEIs for HT or proteinuria.
- Control lipids by diet or drugs if available.

Prev: Encourage traditional lifestyle and diet for primary prevention. Monitor BMI. Secondary prevention more difficult, but aggressive treatment of HT, smoking cessation, prevention and monitoring for foot ulcers important. Community action programs are effective (Diabetes Care 2000;23:898; Med J Aust 1995;162:632).

Gestational Diabetes

Traditionally managed by diet, exercise, and insulin with goal of blood glucose < 140 mg/d (7.8 mmol/L). Can use sulfonylureas in second and third trimester (N Engl J Med 2000;343:1134). Metformin also safe.

22.2   Addison's Disease

Cause: Adrenal destruction due to TB, meningococcemia, AIDS, idiopathic, metastatic carcinoma.

Sx/Si: Fatigue, salt craving, weight loss, nausea, vomiting, hypotension, vitiligo, hair loss, increased pigmentation on buccal mucosa, and scars/creases.

Lab: Low sodium, high potassium.
   Cortisol levels diagnostic but seldom available.

Rx: Acute replacement:

Hydrocortisone: 100 to 500 mg IV slowly every 6 hr 4 times.
   Child < 1 yr 25 mg, 1 to 5 yr 50 mg, 6 to 12 yr 100 mg.

Chronic replacement:

Hydrocortisone: Adult 20 mg orally daily in am, 10 mg early evening; child 10 to 30 mg daily, divided as above, or
Prednisone 5 mg daily, divided, or
Dexamethasone 0.75 mg daily.
A mineral-corticoid such as fludrocortisone (100–300 micrograms daily) should be added to prednisone or dexamethasone.

22.3   Thyroid Disease

Hyperthyroidism

Cause: Autoimmune, thyroiditis, adenoma, elevated human chorionic gonadotropin (HCG) from molar pregnancy, others.

Pathophys: Graves' thyroid stimulation by immunoglobulin; HCG molecule resembles thyroid stimulating hormone (TSH).

Sx: Weight loss, palpitations, tremor, warm sweaty skin, amenorrhea; with Graves' goiter, proptosis, vitiligo.

Si: Tachycardia, onycholysis, lid lag.

Cmplc: Thyroid storm, especially with surgery.
Cardiac arrhythmias, especially AFib, myocarditis, and CHF. Osteoporosis long term.

Lab: TSH low. Alkaline phosphatase elevated 50%.

Rx: Acute treatment if required:
Propranolol 2 to 10 mg IV or 20 to 80 mg orally or other beta-blockers and
Potassium Iodide 60 mg orally (15 drops saturated solution) once then up to 3×/d (maximum 14 d), and
Dexamethasone 4 mg IV, IM, orally 3 × a d, and
Propylthiouracil 1 gm orally once then 300 to 600 mg orally daily until euthyroid, then 50 to 150 mg daily maintenance. Watch for aplastic anemia with CBC every 2 wk.
If rash develops use carbimazole. Propylthiouracil may cause neonatal goiter and hypothyroidism. Use lower dose in pregnancy or replace thyroid hormone in mother. Breast feeding okay.

Iodine Deficiency

Cause: Inadequate dietary intake, thiocyanate inhibits iodine transport (cassava, lima beans, sweet potatoes, cabbage family), lithium.

Epidem: 1.5 billion at risk. Goiter in 200 to 300 million; 20 million with brain damage from fetal iodine deficiency. Western Africa especially Guinea; African highlands: Atlas Mountains, Kenya, Tanzania, Rwanda, Cameroon, Burundi; Andes especially Ecuador, Peru, Bolivia; Asian highlands, Papua New Guinea highlands.

Sx/Si: Goiter is soft and nodular, tracheal pressure, hoarseness. Usually no hypothyroid symptoms.

Endemic cretinism with defects in hearing, speech, mental retardation, small stature, spasticity.

Cmplc: Increased fetal and perinatal mortality.

Lab: Low urinary iodine excretion < 100 μg/d.

TSH elevated, elevated cholesterol.

Rx: Thyroid replacement if symptoms.

Iodine in oil (IM or orally):

Adult < 45 yr 480 mg IM, then orally yearly.

Adult pregnant 480 mg IM or 200 mg orally once.

Adult > 45 yr 76 mg IM.

Infant < 1 yr 190 mg IM or 100 mg orally.

Children 1 to 5 yr 380 mg IM or 200 mg orally.

Dose once a year. Doses may vary by country guidelines. Given when goiter prevalence > 3%.

Prev: Iodine 150 μg per d orally as iodized salt, added to wells (Am J Pub Health 1993;83:540) or water, or iodine in oil as above.

Note: High doses of iodine may precipitate hyperthyroidism in elderly. Not to be given to breast feeding mothers.

Chapter 23

Gastrointestinal Disease

Endoscopy has revolutionized the diagnosis and management of gastroenterology, and a skilled technician and equipment is often available at larger hospitals. The clinician without endoscopic abilities will need to make do with more traditional diagnostic methods considering the wider range of diagnoses found in tropical areas.

23.1 Esophageal Disease

Dysphagia can be divided into oropharyngeal (neurologic, goiter, mechanical) and esophageal (infectious, trauma, tumor/mechanical, other). Careful examination for signs of the primary illness and observation of the patient's swallow may help in the diagnosis, as may a barium swallow.

Infections: Candidiasis, cytomegalovirus, herpes simplex (all common in HIV+ patients), Chagas' disease.

Trauma: Foreign body, stuck pill, corrosives, acid reflux.

Tumor: Carcinoma is common in East and Central Africa, N China, Iran.

Mechanical: Achalasia, strictures.

Esophageal Varices

Cause: Portal HT.

Epidem: Cirrhosis, portal vein thrombosis, Budd-Chiari syndrome. Etiology of about 25% of upper gastrointestinal (UGI) bleeds.

Sx/Si: Hematemesis, melena, evidence of cirrhosis.

Crs: If survive initial bleeding, then rebleeding common, hepatic encephalopathy.

Lab: Protime or whole blood clotting time.

Hemoglobin.

Type and cross whole blood or packed red blood cells (PRBCs) and clotting factors.

Xray: Seldom indicated, sensitivity 50%. Endoscopy for diagnosis and treatment.

Rx:

- Transfusions with clotting factors.
- Octreotide 50 μg IV bolus and 50 μg IV an hr for 5 d (seldom available).
- Vasopressin (pitressin) 0.1 to 0.5 units/min IV (not with coronary artery disease [CAD] or CHF).
- Sengstaken-Blakemore tube tamponade is effective. Confirm placement with an X-ray and deflate 30 min q 6 hr.
- Propranolol reduces primary bleeding and perhaps rebleeding.
- If possible, refer for endoscopy.

23.2   Peptic Ulcer Disease

(Am Fam Physician 2007;75:351)

Cause: *Helicobacter pylori*, NSAIDs, idiopathic.

Epidem: Male > female, genetic influence.

Sx: Epigastric pain, often relieved by food or antacids, worse postprandial. Bleeding, pyloric obstruction with vomiting, perforation.

Si: Tenderness, anemia.

Crs: Chronic, relapsing without therapy.

Cmplc: Perforation with pancreatitis. Heavy worm infestation may cause epigastric pain, anemia, and heme positive stools. Giardia, gastroesophageal reflux disease (GERD), cancer, lead poisoning.

Lab: H&H

Xray: Consider perforation. UGI may show ulcer or obstruction. Gastric ulcers (but not duodenal) require endoscopy.

Rx:

- Surgery necessary for obstruction, uncontrolled bleeding, perforation.
- Stop NSAIDs, ASA, alcohol, smoking.
- Treat for *H. pylori:*
  Omeprazole 40 mg orally daily plus
  Metronidazole 400 mg 3×/d plus
  Amoxicillin 500 mg 3×/d.
  All for 1 wk.

Prev: The adult dose above can be used for an eradication regimen. Presumptive treatment should be considered prior to long-term NSAID therapy. H_2 blocker therapy alone has a 70% relapse rate at 2 yr.

23.3   Tropical Sprue/Postinfective Malabsorption

(Gut 1997;40:428)

Cause: Postinfectious.

Epidem: Defined as chronic diarrhea and malabsorption with weight loss over 3 months duration. More common in tropical S America and S and SE Asia in long-term residents.

Pathophys: Persistent bacterial overgrowth with toxin production and villous atrophy.

Sx/Si: Diarrhea with pale, fatty copious stools.
Malabsorption with weight loss, megaloblastic anemia, glossitis.

Cmplc: Differential includes: celiac disease (0.5% in Caucasians), lymphoma, HIV/AIDs (60% at some point), tuberculosis, and many intestinal parasites, chronic pancreatitis.

Lab: CBC, stool fat, O&P, serum albumin low. Small bowel biopsy helpful.

Rx: Once infectious causes ruled out as completely as possible in non-HIV patient, try tetracycline 250 mg orally 3 × daily plus folic acid 5 mg 3 × daily for a month. For HIV+ patients, try TMP-SMX then metronidazole then albendazole.

23.4 Pancreatitis

Cause: Alcohol, gallstone (rare—usually heme pigment with underlying hemolytic anemia), *Ascaris lumbricoides* (common), clonorchis, opisthorchis, anisakis occasionally, drugs, mumps and other viral infections, trauma, scorpion bite, penetrating peptic ulcer, elevated triglycerides, post-endoscopic retrograde cholangiopancreatography (ERCP).

Epidem: Less common than developed countries but increasing with Western diet and alcohol.

Pathophys: Ascaris ascends into biliary system (Lancet 1990;335:1503).

Sx/Si: Epigastric pain radiates to back, often nausea, vomiting, fever, hypotension. Pleural effusions.

Crs: Adequate laboratory support often not available for calculation of Ranson, Glasgow, or APACHE-II scores.

Cmplc: Pulmonary, adult respiratory distress syndrome (ARDS), pleural effusions, atelectasis.
Infection with abscess requires surgery.
Fistulas, renal failure, pseudocysts.

Lab: Amylase (false-positive), lipase, CBC, renal and hepatic tests if available. Triglycerides, glucose, and calcium.

Xray: CT can help with prognosis.

Abdominal film may show calcifications from previous pancreatitis, obstruction, free air from peptic ulcer disease (PUD) perforation.

Ultrasound for biliary obstruction, pseudocysts.

Rx: Nothing by mouth; NG tube if vomiting; ileus.

Hydration aggressive.

Antibiotics if severe (necrotizing).

Imipenem with cilastatin IV or IM 50 mg/kg/d (max 4 gm) divided into 3 to 4 doses; child 60 mg/kg/d (max 2 gm).

Albendazole for ascaris.

23.5 Acute Liver Diseases

Hepatitis A

Cause: RNA virus.

Epidem: Disease of children in developing countries with > 90% infection. Oral-fecal spread, shed in feces 2 wk before sx. Incubation 28 d (15–50). Household spread 20% to 50%.

Sx: Mild or none in infants and children, diarrhea common, nonspecific URI sx, rarely jaundice. In adults, fever, malaise, anorexia followed by jaundice with dark-colored urine then symptoms subside.

Si: Jaundice, right upper quadrant (RUQ) pain with hepatomegaly.

Crs: Lasts 3 to 6 months total, jaundice 6 to 8 wk. Fatalities in older adults 1/1000. Relapse in 3% to 20%.

Lab: Bilirubin, liver enzymes elevated. Lymphocytosis. Bile in urine.

Rx: Supportive.

Prev: Hepatitis A vaccines available, prophylactic if close contact.
Enteric precautions. Food and water sanitation.
Food handlers high risk for spreading.

Hepatitis B

Cause: DNA virus with core (HBcAg and HBeAg) and surface (HbsAg), antigens.

Epidem: Transmission from carrier mother to newborn most important in developing countries, especially if mother HBeAg+. Also transmitted through blood, child-child, sexual contact, inadequately sterilized needles and surgical equipment, tattooing, ritual circumcisions, and in dialysis units. Leading cause of hepatoma. 5% of world population carriers; 25% will have liver damage. Incubation 40 to 160 d.

Pathophys: Chronic infection more likely in neonates. Symptoms appear only when body recognizes infection in hepatocytes, which are attacked and killed.

Sx: Usually subclinical, especially in infants and children.

Si: Anorexia, jaundice, tender hepatomegaly, fatigue, nausea, vomiting, fever.

Crs: 95% of infants develop chronic disease, 30% of children, 3% to 5% of adults. Others clear virus in 6 months; ≤ 1% of adults die.
Chronic disease is HBsAg+ over 6 months.
HBeAg+ means continuing viral replication.

Cmplc: Hepatitis D infection, hepatocellular carcinoma. 1 million deaths/yr due to hepatitis B complications.

Lab: Bilirubin and liver enzymes elevated. HBsAg and anti-HBc positive in acute disease; anti-HBs denotes recovery; HBsAg over 6 months is chronic infection.

Rx: No acute treatment available; chronic disease treatment available but not covered here.

Prev: Immunization of infants, children born to HBsAg positive mothers, other high risk groups.

Mutant viruses are not covered by the vaccine and a problem in some areas (Hepatology 1999;30:1312), which requires monitoring. May be missed by routine lab tests for blood transfusions.

Part of WHO Expanded Program on Immunisation (EPI) program; national immunization policy may vary.

Hepatitis C

Cause: RNA virus, flavivirus family, multiple genotypes and subtypes.

Epidem: More common in developing countries (6–28% prevalence). Primarily spread by blood; vertical (maternal transmission 5–10%); needle sticks important; 10% to 15% prevalence in Egypt attributed to schistosomiasis campaign with inadequately sterilized needles (http://allafrica.com/stories/2000702070355).

Pathophys: Immune response often fails to clear virus but damages liver.

Sx/Si: Mostly asymptomatic, 30% have nonspecific symptoms, a few have jaundice.

Crs: 50% to 85% develop chronic hepatitis (hepatitis C virus; HCV) RNA > 6 months. Cirrhosis develops 20 yr later in 5% to 15%, hepatoma in 1% to 5%.

Alcohol, HIV+, obesity increase risk of cirrhosis.

Lab: Liver tests occasionally elevated acutely. Anti-HCV antibodies diagnostic.

Rx: Avoid alcohol, immunize against hepatitis A & B if appropriate.

Antiviral therapy not covered here; depends on genotype.

Hepatitis D

Cause: RNA virus requires hepatitis B virus to replicate.

Epidem: About 5% of hepatitis B carriers have coinfection.

Two types: simultaneous infection with B & D, which is usually benign, and fulminant new infection of D on preexisting B infection.

Sx/Si: Liver enzyme changes.

Anti-Hep D antibodies in patients with Hep B infection.

Rx: Available, high dose interferon.

Prev: Hepatitis B vaccine protects.

Hepatitis E

Cause: Single-stranded RNA virus, calicivirus.

Epidem: Areas of poor sanitation; oral-fecal; often waterborne outbreaks especially S and SE Asia. Pig reservoir. 40-day (16–60) incubation period.

Sx/Si: Fever, jaundice, liver pain and swelling.

Crs: Self-limiting; occasionally fatal < 4%, except pregnant women (20% mortality).

Lab: Increased liver tests, Hep E ELISA available.

Rx: Supportive.

Prev: Vaccine, trial complete (N Engl J Med 2007;356:895).

Treatment of Chronic Liver Disease with Portal Hypertension

Cause: Cirrhosis due to hepatitis B and C, schistosomiasis, alcohol. Less commonly: hemosiderosis, veno-occlusive disease, hyper-reactive malarious splenomegaly (increased portal blood flow). Indian childhood cirrhosis, others (Gut 1988;29:101).

Sx/Si: Ascites, varices-esophageal and hemorrhoidal, encephalopathy, fluid retention, prolonged bleeding.

Cmplc: Hemorrhage from varices, ascites with respiratory compromise, encephalopathy (less common with schistosomiasis).

Diff: Rule out peritoneal TB, ovarian tumor, nephroses.

Lab: Serum protein, liver tests, urine protein.

Search for chronic Hepatitis B and C, stool/urine O&P.

Hemochromatosis (ferritin, iron/IBC).

Other causes rare and difficult to treat.

Sonography: Pipe-stem fibrosis seen with high sensitivity in schistosomiasis. Needle biopsy often helpful and easily done.

Rx:

- Schistosomiasis treatment, if present.
- Salt restriction < 5 gm NaCl/d.
- Bed rest to encourage diuresis.
- Furosemide 40 to 120 mg orally daily, and
- Spironolactone 100 mg orally daily.
- Avoid paracentesis except for diagnosis or respiratory compromise.

  Hepatic encephalopathy treatment:

- Lactulose 20 to 30 gm 3 × daily, or
- Lactose in lactase-deficient individuals.
- Neomycin 6 gm daily if available, or
- Metronidazole 10 mg/kg/d divided in 3 doses, or
- Rifaximin (expensive).

  Spontaneous bacterial peritonitis (SBP)

- Low protein (1 gm/dL) ascites benefits from SBP prophylaxis with ciprofloxacin 750 mg orally weekly (Hepatology 1995;22:1171).

Liver Biopsy

- Check blood clotting, if able, and hemoglobin.
- Prep area in mid-axillary line.
- Inject local anesthesia.
- Have patient inhale, exhale, then hold breath.

- Obtain biopsy using large bore needle.
- Have patient roll onto right side.
- Observe several hr, expect shoulder pain, and watch for bleeding.

Chapter 24

Renal Disease

This chapter presumes a renal biopsy is not available.

24.1   Acute Glomerulonephritis (AGN)

Cause: Infection induced: poststreptococcal, endocarditis, less commonly other bacteria such as typhoid, strep pneumonia, diphtheria, leprosy; viral infection as in varicella, adenovirus, measles, hepatitis B & C, enterovirus; and parasitic infections like malaria and schistosomiasis.

Epidem: Often in epidemics following *Streptococcus pyogenes* group A with impetigo or pharyngitis. In children nearly 100% of AGN are poststreptococcal, in adults < 50%.

Pathophys: Immune complex deposition in kidney basement membrane.

Sx/Si: Red-brown urine due to hematuria, oliguria, proteinuria, facial, and extremity edema; HT.

Crs: Renal failure < 2% in children with strep.

Lab: Red cell casts in fresh urine, proteinuria; ESR and ASO titer elevated.

Rx: Penicillin or erythromycin × 10 d for presumed strep infection. Treat fluid overload and HT, salt restriction. Trial of prednisone warranted if no improvement with penicillin.

24.2 Nephrotic Syndrome

Cause: Minimal change nephropathy (5–75%, India highest; Arch Dis Child 1975;50:626). Chronic hepatitis B and C, chronic malaria especially *P. malariae*, schistosomiasis, IgA nephropathy (rare Africa), various forms of glomerulonephritis amyloid (chronic infections and HIV), snake bites, diabetes, other causes.

Epidem: Causes vary by region; etiology often unclear although attempt should be made to treat possible causative illnesses.

Pathophys: Often immune complex deposition in basement membrane.

Sx/Si: Edema, anasarca.

Cmplc: IgG loss may lead to infections.

Lab: Urine protein > 3 gm/d, often more.
Elevated cholesterol, low albumin, creatinine and BUN variable.

Rx: Diuretics and antihypertensive drugs.
Treat underlying cause.
Prednisone 1 to 2 mg/kg/d trial for uncertain etiology.
ACEI if able to follow renal function and electrolytes.
Penicillin prophylaxis in children to prevent infection due to loss of gamma globulin in urine.

24.3 Acute Renal Failure

A difficult problem to manage with basic facilities and laboratory tests. A number of treatable causes need to be considered. The list here is to remind the clinician that different etiologies are found in the tropics.
Prerenal:

- shock and ATN
- sepsis

- obstetrical disasters, septic abortion (AB), eclampsia
- trauma with rhabdomyolysis
- G6PD deficiency and hemolysis

  Renal:
- ATN
- snakebite
- GN
- common infections: pyelonephritis, leptospirosis
- nephrotoxins: paraquat, drugs
- hemolytic-uremic syndrome
- amyloid

  Postrenal:
- prostatic hypertrophy
- ureteral stricture and blockage
- stones
- schistosomiasis
- pelvic carcinoma and bladder cancer

24.4   Pyelonephritis

Cause: Gram negative rods in 95%.

Epidem: Increased in pregnancy, sickle cell, diabetes, obstruction.

Sx/Si: Fever, dysuria and frequency, flank pain.

Crs: Consider abscess if untreated or no improvement over 5 d.

Cmplc: Renal scarring, premature labor.

Lab: Urinalysis (UA), gram stain urine. Culture.

Rx: Ampicillin and gentamicin, or
   Fluoroquinolone, or
   TMP/SMX,
   all for 14 d.
   Consider TB or abscess if no improvement after 5 d.

Chapter 25

Neurology

25.1 Tetanus

(Ann Pharmacother 1997;31:1507)

Cause: *Clostridium tetani*, a spore-forming gram negative rod.

Epidem: Tetanus remains a significant cause of death in developing countries with poor immunization programs. Over 1 million cases and 300 000 deaths (200 000 neonatal) occur each yr. Tetanus is more common in hot, humid climates.

Pathophys: Once gaining entry to the body via a laceration or puncture wound, the spore changes to a vegetative state, which produces toxin that travels in a retrograde manner up the axons to bind irreversibly in the spinal cord and brain. This results in neural inhibition and muscle spasms or tetany along with an adrenal release of catecholamines with HT, tachycardia, and sweating. Puncture wounds with devitalized tissue, umbilical cord stumps, or burns are frequent antecedents. About 20% have no recent wound. Incubation period ranges from 1 to 2 d to perhaps several months.

Sx/Si: Diagnosis is clinical. Rigidity, dysphagia, backache, trismus, and risus sardonicus (sardonic smile) are early symptoms progressing to general muscle stiffness and occasionally opisthotonus.

The newborn feeds poorly with a stifled cry from a wrinkled face. The arms, hands, and legs flex and adduct past the midline. Onset of neonatal tetanus is usually at d 3 to 14 of life. The ability to cry is a good prognostic sign.

Crs: Spasms are paroxysms of rigidity. They may be spontaneous or set off by physical contact or a loud noise. Simultaneous contractions of antagonistic muscle groups are not seen in mild tetanus but begin about the second day in severe cases. After the first spasms, the period between them gradually shortens while the strength of inciting stimulus decreases. Respiratory distress, laryngeal spasms, cyanosis, and aspiration pneumonia are common. After 3 to 4 d of increasing frequency and severity, the illness plateaus and begins to improve by the tenth day. Recovery takes about a month.

Cmplc: Deaths are due to pneumonia, respiratory failure, and shock.

Rx: Treatment is human tetanus immunoglobulin, 500 units IV. Any wound should be debrided. Metronidazole (not penicillin) should be given for 10 d. Spasms may be controlled with drug-induced paralysis and mechanical ventilation. As treatment may take several weeks, a tracheostomy should be considered.

Conservation management (without ventilatory support) may be suitable for mild cases and is the only option in remote areas. Chlorpromazine and diazepam are suitable drugs. Phenobarbital or paraldehyde (0.2 ml/kg, up to 10 ml IM or twice the dose rectally every 6 hr) are substitutes. Use chlorpromazine 12.5 mg in neonates, up to 50 mg in adults, every 4 hr. Add diazepam 2.5 to 50 mg every 6 hr as needed. Titrate to control spasms and rigidity but not to suppress ventilatory effort. A tracheostomy facilitates suctioning of secretions. Morphine can be used to control autonomic instability. Short-acting beta blockers (esmolol) or magnesium sulfate 4 gm loading and 2 to 3 gm/hr IV (Crit Care Med 1987;15:987) may be helpful in HT and tachycardia, while inotropic agents and atropine will treat hypotension and bradycardia. Insensible fluid loss may be significant.

Prev: Vaccine and immunoglobulin if unvaccinated.

Debride wounds of dead tissue and foreign bodies.

25.2 Tropical Spastic Paraparesis

Cause: Human T-cell lymphotropic virus (HTLV-1).

Epidem: Hyperendemic: SW Japan (> 10%), Melanesia, Sub-Saharan Africa, Caribbean, Latin America. Transmission by sex, blood, breast milk.

Sx/Si: Progressive spastic paralysis, sphincter dysfunction, mild sensory loss, usually symmetrical. 20% disabled at 2 yr.

Crs: 1% to 4% lifetime risk of TSP if HTLV-1 positive.

Cmplc: Worsens course of HIV+. Associated with T-cell lymphoma. Immunosuppression with infection by Strongyloidiasis, scabies, TB.

Lab: Serology.

Prev: Screen blood prior to transfusion. Avoid breast feeding if HTLV-1 positive. Condoms.

25.3 Procedures

Lumbar Puncture

Patients with coma and fever, decreased level of consciousness or coma of uncertain etiology should have a lumbar puncture and cerebral spinal fluid examination whenever practical. A persistent headache may be another indication.

- Treat for meningitis if unable to do LP or LP delayed > 30 min.
- Rule out intracranial mass lesion by a funduscopic examination looking for sharp optic discs (particularly the nasal side) and venous pulsation (seen in about one-third of normals). Avoid if signs of increased intracranial pressure: unequal pupils, irregular breathing, focal paralysis, or generalized rigidity.

- Inability to do an adequate funduscopic exam or papilledema does not rule out doing an LP, but use the smallest gauge needle available and remove only a small amount of CSF.
- Obtain the patient's cooperation and have several experienced holders/assistants.
- Neither sterile gloves nor LP needle is necessary if unavailable. A small gauge butterfly needle works well for infants and children, a standard 1½-inch 22-gauge needle for adults.
- Identify the interspace you will use, pick one below the iliac crests. Mark an "x" with your fingernail.
- Wash with antiseptic solution.
- Give local anesthetic into skin.
- Insert the needle with the needle bevel turned to split the longitudinal fibers with patients sitting or on their side. Watch the airway!
- Advance the needle until you feel the "pop" of the dura.
- Put the patient in the lateral decubitus position and have your assistants relax their hold if opening and closing pressures are desired. Normal 6 to 14 cm, high > 20.
- Allow the appropriate amount of fluid to run out into clear containers (0.5–1 ml usually enough in each, allow 5 ml for TB culture).
- Obtain pressures by using the equipment in a prepared LP set or sterile IV tubing attached to the needle.
- Remove the needle, apply a bandage, and have the patient lie supine for several hr.
- Make a preliminary judgment on the fluid: clear (many etiologies including meningitis), cloudy (probably meningitis), very viscous or nonbloody clots (high protein—think TB), bloody or xanthochromic (old subarachnoid bleeding).
- Try the next interspace up if a traumatic tap is obtained (bloody fluid).
- Deliver the samples to the lab yourself.

Chapter 26

Hematology

26.1 Anemias

(Am J Trop Med Hyg 2007;77:44 for overview)

The diagnosis of anemia (Table 26.1) requires a look at the conjunctiva to raise suspicion, a careful physical exam, and ideally a microscope and simple laboratory to help differentiate the cause. Often a therapeutic trial supports the tentative diagnosis.

Table 26.1   Definition of Anemia

	Hb	Hct %
Newborn	< 13–14	< 40
Child < 6 yr	< 11	< 33
6–14 yr	< 12	< 36
Adult men	< 13	< 39
Adult women	< 12	< 36
Pregnant	< 11	< 33

- Blood loss
  Acute: bleeding
  Chronic: hookworm, schistosomiasis, whipworm, menstruation, childbirth, GI pathology
- Decreased red cell production
  Nutritional: iron, folate, B_{12}, protein, Cu, vitamins A, C, E, riboflavin, pyridoxine

HEMATOLOGY

325

Table 26.2　Etiology of Anemia by RBC Size

Microcytic	Normocytic	Macrocytic
Iron	Acute blood loss	Folate
Chronic disease	Cancer	B_{12}
Thalassemia	Hypothyroidism	Alcohol
Sideoblastic		Reticulocytosis

Infection: HIV, TB, SBE, osteomyelitis, other, renal and/or hepatic failure, cancer, aplastic, inflammation connective tissue, colitis

- *Hemolytic*
  Sickle-cell syndromes, thalassemias, G6PD, membrane abnormalities, immune complexes; nonimmune: malaria, venoms, burns, hypersplenism

The etiology of anemia can also be determined by RBC size (Table 26.2).

B_{12} Deficiency Anemia

Cause: Gastric resection and atrophy, dietary (India, Rastafarians), drugs (PAS), blind loop, giardia, distal ileal defect and tropical sprue.

Epidem: Breast fed infants of deficient mothers. Pernicious anemia common in S Africa and Zimbabwe.

Sx: Anemia, peripheral neuropathy, psychiatric (megaloblastic madness).

Si: Optic atrophy, melanin hyperpigmentation palms, soles, finger, and toe joints. In infants, hyperpigmentation, involuntary movements.

Cmplc: Anemia, thrombocytopenia, subacute combined degeneration cord (loss of position and vibratory sense and paresthesias), paraplegia, dementia.

Lab: Peripheral smear: macrocytes, hypersegmented polyps, low platelets. Bone marrow. Serum B_{12} level and anti-intrinsic factor Ab.

Rx: Hydroxocobalamin 1 mg IM 3×/wk for 2 wk. Modify diet. Infants 0.1 mg daily PO; treat mother also. If malabsorption, 1 mg IM every 3 months.

Folate Deficiency

Cause:

- high demands: pregnancy, lactation
- rapid growth: hemolysis, Burkitt's lymphoma, choriocarcinoma
- inadequate intake: prolonged cooking, food shortage, boiled cow's milk, goat's milk diet, alcoholism
- malabsorption: chronic diarrhea (giardia), ileocecal TB, inflammatory bowel disease.

Epidem: Especially common in pregnancy and premature infants.

Pathophys: Folates heat labile and water soluble. Stored in liver (3–6 month reserve). Good sources: liver, green vegetables, bananas, mangoes, peppers, eggs, cheese, yeast, sweet potatoes/yams. Poor sources: grains, cassava, nongreen vegetables.

Sx: Anemia, purpura due to thrombocytopenia, increased risk of infection.

Si: Glossitis, angular cheilosis.

Cmplc: Neurotube defects in infants of pregnant mothers.

Lab: Peripheral smear, macrocytes, macro-ovalocytes, neutropenia, hypersegmented polys. LDH and bilirubin elevated.

Rx: Folic acid 5 mg/d for 3 wk to replete stores. Prevention: premature infants 50 μg/d, pregnancy 400 μgm/d, chronic hemolytic anemias 5 mg/d. Therapeutic trial to differentiate B_{12} from folate deficiency: give folic acid 50 μg/d, check Hb or retic count in 1 wk. If no response, try B_{12} 1 μg/d and recheck in a wk.

Iron Deficient Anemia

Cause:

- Insufficient intake (breast milk 50% absorbed, meat 20–30%, plant < 5%, cooking utensils and dirt in food < 5%). Absorption enhanced by ascorbic and other acids and deficiency; decreased by plant ligands, tannin (tea), fiber, and clays in food.
- Increased physiological needs: pregnancy, prematurity
- Blood loss: parasites, GI bleeding, uterus
- Absorptive defects in duodenum: sprue.

Epidem: Estimated 1 billion people iron deficient. Most commonly due to inadequate intake.

Sx: Fatigue, impaired intellectual development in children, dysphagia.

Si: Palor, hyperdynamic circulation, angular stomatitis, koilonychia, glossitis, depigmentation.

Crs: With treatment, reticulocytes increase in about 1 wk and Hb 1 gm/wk.

Cmplc: Pregnancy: increased maternal and fetal morbidity and mortality, premature birth, low birth rate.

Lab: Ferritin elevated in tropics due to malaria and other illnesses. Not useful. Transferrin saturation: < 16% adults, < 14% children, < 12% infants. Peripheral smear: hypochromic, microcytic, ± target cells. To differentiate between: in β thalassemia MCV/#RBCs in millions < 14, in Fe deficiency > 14.

Rx: Oral iron: 200 mg ferrous sulfate contains 60 mg iron. Children 5 mg/kg/d, adults 60 to 120 mg/d. Give on empty stomach with vitamin C–containing food, not tea.

Parenteral iron: used for patients with malabsorption, poor compliance, or severe deficiency and rapid cure necessary (pregnancy).

One method is to use iron dextran 25 ml for adult < 60 kg, 30 ml for > 60 kg

- Start IV with 1 L NS.
- Give promethazine 12.5 mg IV.
- Put 5 ml of iron dextran in the liter of IV fluid.
- Run in 200 ml slowly.
- Add the remaining iron to the IV bag if not allergic (no hives, dyspnea, hypotension, etc).
- Run in over 4 hr.

Always give folic acid with iron in children, pregnant women, and severely anemic as deficiency may develop during iron therapy.

Identify and treat underlying causes. Transfuse if necessary.

Iron supplementation in those at risk:

- pregnancy 60 mg iron + folic acid 400 μgm bid
- preterm infants even if breast fed start at 1 to 2 months: 2 mg/kg/d maximum 15 mg/d
- bottle fed infants or cow's milk before 12 months

Iron fortification:

- of foods
- use iron cooking utensils

Dietary modification:

- Reduce tannins
- Ascorbic acid rich foods (destroyed by cooking).
- Increase animal protein

Control helminthic infections.

Other Deficiency Anemias

Pyridoxine-deficient anemia is hypochromic. Seen in INH, pyrazinamide, or cycloserine treatment of TB. Occasionally hereditary. Treat with pyridoxine 25 to 300 mg/d.

Vitamin A deficiency contributes to iron-deficient anemia as the addition of vitamin A increases the response to iron.

Riboflavin enhances the response to iron in riboflavin-deficient people.

Copper deficiency is seen in children with chronic diarrhea.

Anemia Due to Marrow Depression

Cause: Acute infection temporarily depresses bone marrow erythropoiesis, unnoticed except in those with high RBC turnover (sickle cell) or with concominant hemolysis (malaria, DIC). Parvovirus B19 causes aplastic crisis in those with severe hemolytic anemias and short RBC lifespan and hydrops in the fetus of an infected mother. Chronic infection (TB, HIV) and diseases cause anemia by depressing erythropoietin (N Engl J Med 2005;352:1011).

Rx: Treat the underlying cause when possible. Try pyridoxine high dose and folate. Erythropoietin works but expensive. Transfuse.

G6PD Hemolytic Anemia

Cause: Hereditary: Type 1 G6PD activity absent, chronic nonspherocytic hemolytic; type 2 < 10% G6PD activity, intermittent hemolysis triggered by oxidative stress; type 3 > 10% to < 60% activity, less severe hemolysis triggered by oxidative stress.

X-linked, more common in males 9:1. Heterozygous females have ~half RBCs susceptible. Expressed as % males susceptible. Protects against severe *P. falciparum* malaria.

Epidem: 400 million carry 1 or 2 genes for G6PD deficiency. 11% US African Americans, 62% Kurds, 32% Lake Victoria Luo,

> 50% Sardinians, Kurdish Jews, not in indigenous America or Australia.

Pathophys: G6PD reduces NADP to NADPH, which regenerates reduced glutathione, which restores sulfhydryl groups that prevents Hb oxidation and precipitation of Hb as Heinz bodies and cell membrane damage with hemolysis. In Caucasians, G6PD reduced in all RBCs; in Blacks only older cells (> 60 d).

Sx: Abdominal and flank pain.

Si: Newborn jaundice, acute hemolysis with anemia, jaundice, and splenomegaly.

Cmplc: Renal failure.

Lab: G6PD screening tests available, direct fluorescence or methylene blue reduction (blue to colorless). After hemolysis, centrifuge blood and test old cells at bottom of tube, or wait 6 wk. After hemolysis, peripheral smear shows fragmented, "bite" cells, and Heinz bodies (special stain required). Also elevated bilirubin.

Rx: Precipitants.

Antimalarials: primaquine, chloroquine*, quinine*, maloprim, fansidar, pamaquine, pentaquine

Antibiotics: all sulfa-containing drugs, dapsone, nitrofurantoin, nalidixic acid, chloramphenicol*, quinolones

Antiparasitics: niridazole (Ambilhar), betanaphthol, stibophen, nicidazole

Analgesics: high dose aspirin*, phenacetin

Others: methylene blue, henna dye, vitamin K analogs*, fava beans, naphthalene (moth balls)

Infections: severe viral and bacterial

*Not in type 3.

Treatment is supportive: transfusions, stop offending agent, prevent renal failure. With mild hemolysis, it may be possible to restart the drug cautiously, ie, dapsone, as only the older RBCs are lysed, and a steady state hemolytic anemia results.

HEMATOLOGY

Membrane Defects

Cause: Genetic: spherocytosis, Europeans; Ovalocytosis, SE Asia and Melanesia, up to 50% Sulawesi, 27% Coastal Papua New Guinea; elliptocytosis, W and N Africa, up to 2% Nigeria, Tunisia, Algeria, Morocco.

Sx: Spherocytosis: anemia, aplastic crisis
Ovalocytosis: none
Elliptocytosis: mild hemolytic anemia, jaundice, splenomegaly.

Lab: RBCs microcytic (spherocytosis) or oval-elliptoid.

Rx: Transfuse in spherocytosis. May protect against malaria.

26.2   Hemoglobinopathies

β-Thalassemia

Cause: Genetic, autosomal, homozygote = major, heterozygote = minor, various gene combinations = intermediate.

Epidem: Common throughout belt from Mediterranean to SE Asia and Melanesia. 3% of world's population are carriers. Confers partial resistance to severe *P. falciparum* malaria.

Pathophys: Block (homozygote) or decrease in hemoglobins β chain synthesis with increase in fetal Hb ($\alpha_2\gamma_2$) and Hb A$_2$ ($\alpha_2\delta_2$) and α chain precipitation.

Sx: Major: Failure to thrive, poor feeding.
Minor: None.

Si: Major: Splenomegaly, occasionally hypersplenism with thrombocytopenia, frontal skull bossing, recurrent fractures, osteoporosis, infections, and gout. If transfused, signs of iron overload.
Minor: Insignificant anemia.

Cmplc: Major: Need for transfusions and its complications. Death < 5 yr without transfusion, age 20 to 30 yr with transfusions and iron overload complications (diabetes, endocrine and hepatic failure, cardiac damage, CHF and arrhythmias).

Lab: Major: Anemia Hb 2–8 g/dL, microcytic (50–60 fl), anisocytosis (variable size), poikilocytosis (variable shape) and fragmented schistocytes, nucleated RBCs. Bilirubin increased as is Hb F.

Minor: Mild anemia Hb 9-11. Moderate RBC changes as in major with target cells Hb A_2 = 3.5% to 6%, Hb F ~3% in half of individuals. Testing may be available on laboratory spectrophotometer.

Rx: Genetic counseling in high risk populations.

Major: Complex problem involving transfusions to keep Hb ~10, iron chelation, folate, occasionally splenectomy.

Minor: Proper diagnosis prevents unnecessary treatment for iron deficiency.

Alpha Thalassemia

Cause: Genetic. (Table 26.3)

Table 26.3 Thalassemia Genotypes

Genotype	Smear	Hemoglobins
$\alpha\alpha/\alpha\alpha, \beta\beta$	Normal	Hb A $(\alpha_2\beta_2)$ > 95%
		Hb A2 $(\alpha_2\delta_2)\gamma$ < 3.5%
$\alpha-/\alpha\alpha, \beta\beta$	Silent carrier	Hb A
		Hb Barts (γ_4) 1–2%
—/$\alpha\alpha, \beta\beta$	Trait, mild	Hb A 90–95%
or	hypochromic anemia	Hb Barts 5–10%
$-\alpha/-\alpha, \beta\beta$		
—/$-\alpha, \beta\beta$	Moderate	Hb A remainder
	hypochromic	Hb Barts 5–30%
	anemia	Hb H 5–40%
—/—	Hydrops fetalis	Barts primarily

Note: a small amount of other Hbs are occasionally found.

Epidem: More common than β form, but homozygotes die in utero or infancy. All of Africa, Southern Europe, South Asia, and Melanesia. Protects against severe malaria.

Pathophys: Defect on chromosome 16, which contains 2 α genes: $\alpha_1\alpha_2$. Diploid cells contain 4 genes, 2 from each parent, $\alpha\alpha/\alpha\alpha$. Deletions or mutations with defective production are noted by "–".

Sx: Variable anemia.

Labs: Smear: hypochromic microcytosis, stippling siderocytes, targets, reticulocytosis. Same as β thalassemia.

Rx: Transfusions usually unnecessary, folate supplementation, rarely splenectomy.

Sickle Cell

Cause: Genetic.

Epidem: ~80 million carriers. Sub-Saharan Africa north of Zambesi River and migrants (US 7%). Also in Arabian Peninsula (> 30% some areas), central India, Turkey, and Western Black Sea.

Pathophys: Mutation in β chain of hemoglobin. Glu-Val amino acid substitution causes Hb S to polymerize at low oxygen tension resulting in sickle-shaped RBCs, which block microcirculation causing infarcts. Cells hemolyse easily. Chronic ischemia and infarcts cause complications. Most severe in Hb SS > Hb S β thalassemia (N Africa) > Hb SC > Hb SD (Punjab Sikhs) > Hb SB+ thalassemia (Liberia). Hb AS trait asymptomatic except under severe stress.

Sx: Symptoms develop after third month of life when Hb F falls. Often presents as hand-foot syndrome with digital infarcts, swelling, pain, and eventually digits of varying lengths. Polydipsia and polyuria due to medullary infarcts with enuresis.

Si: Initially poor growth and development with lumbar lordosis, bossing of frontal bones, skull, pallor, jaundice, enlarged liver, enlarged spleen in children until infarcts shrink, enlarged heart, delayed puberty.

Crs: Untreated 98% dead by age 4 yr. Treated > 50 yr of age (Lancet 2001;357:680).

Cmplc: Eventually growth may catch up and height exceeds others. Course punctuated by:

- Anemic crisis: Due to malaria, splenic sequestration, folate deficiency, acute infection especially parvovirus B19 and other stressors. Usually in infants 6 to 12 months but any age. Rapid decrease in Hb (> 2 gm) plus recticulocyte increase and enlarging spleen.
- Infarctive crisis: starts after 6 months. Bone pain (digits 6–24 months, long bones later). Sudden onset, pain, warmth, and swelling. Need to rule out osteomyelitis and infective arthritis.
- Acute chest syndrome, multiple causes. Need to rule out (r/o) pneumonia.
- Abdominal pain may be due to mesenteric infarcts, cholecystitis (common 10–30% patients) or usual causes of acute abdomen.
- CNS infarcts cause strokes, seizures, paralysis. Seen in two-thirds untreated children.
- Leg ulceration common in W Indies, usually above malleoli.
- Renal infarcts cause hematuria, papillary necrosis, and inability to concentrate urine. Priapism.
- Bacterial infections: especially with the encapsulated organisms, *S. pneumonia* and *H. influenzae*. Osteomyelitis with *S. typhi* (50%), *Staphlococcus* (25%), and others. Splenic infants decrease immunity.
- Chronic degenerative diseases: include avascular necrosis bone, retinopathy (blindness), and hepatic, renal, pulmonary failure.

- Pregnancy often complicated by cephalo-pelvic disproportion (CPD; mothers have small or malformed pelvis), sequestration crisis (25%), infarction bone, pseudoeclampsia (elevated BP and proteinuria), sepsis, and fetal growth retardation, preterm labor.

Lab: Hb usually 6 to 8 gm/dL. Smear shows, nucleated RBCs, anisocytosis, microcytosis and macrocytosis, target and sickle cells. Increased reticulocyte count 10% to 20%. Jaundice with elevated conjugated bilirubin. WBC count usually up with left shift and toxic granulations. Platelet count up with autosplenectomy. Hb electrophoresis Hb S and increased Hb F. The higher Hb F the better prognosis.

Xray: Bone infarcts, "hair on end" skull, vertebral fractures, and absorption digits.

Rx:

- Prophylaxis to prevent malaria.
- Daily folic acid.
- Prophylactic phenoxymethylpenicillin VK 125 mg twice a day throughout childhood < 6 yr, 250 mg twice a day 6 to 12 yr (JAMA 2003;290:1057).
- Immunize against *S. pneumonia*, *H. influenzae*, and Hepatitis B.
- Avoid precipitating factors: dehydration, chilling, hypoxia, infections, alcohol, and overwork.
- Limit transfusions or exchange transfusions to:
- Respiratory distress, CHF, Hb < 6 and falling in sequestration crisis, prior to delivery and Hb < 8, acute CNS involvement and prior to surgery.
- Hydroxyurea-Hydroxycarbamide (JAMA 2001;286:2099) for repeated crisis. Start 10 to 25 mg/kg/d and increase until poly (WBC) count depressed.
- Treat crisis with oral fluids or IV NS, pain management, antibiotics if judged necessary, bed rest.

- Patients with Hb S trait more prone to pyelonephritis, bacteriuria of pregnancy and painless hematuria. Partial protection against severe *P. falciparum*.

Other Hemoglobinopathies

Hemoglobin C disease, N Ghana incidence 16% to 28%. Homozygote mild anemia, splenomegaly, smear shows 100% target cells.

Hemoglobin D disease, Punjab, moderately severe anemia with splenomegaly and target cells.

Hemoglobin E disease, SE Asia, mild hypochromic hemolytic anemia with splenomegaly.

Chapter 27

Oncology

27.1 Overview

Infectious diseases and infant, child, and maternal mortality are significant problems in low and middle income countries. However, the number of deaths from noncommunicable diseases exceeds that of communicable and perinatal mortality in all regions except Africa. And, the number of deaths from chronic and noncommunicable diseases is expected to climb rapidly.

Cancer is the third (12%) leading cause of death worldwide, exceeded by cardiovascular (30%) and infectious-parasitic (19%). Some of these cancers are communicable (cervix-HPV) or secondary to preventable infections (hepatoma-hepatitis B&C, bladder-schistosomiasis), but most are lifestyle related (lung-tobacco, colon-diet). Prevention and early detection are often possible within the existing healthcare delivery systems (Table 27.1).

Healthcare providers in developing countries can educate the public and advocate for policies to promote the development and implementation of rational steps in cancer and chronic disease control.

The Institute of Medicine recommends the following:

- cancer control 5-year plans
- ratification of the Framework Convention on Tobacco Control (FCTC; WHO, 2003)

Table 27.1   Cancer Incidence by Region, 2000 (WHO)

	Africa	Americas	SE Asia	Western Pacific
1	cervix	lung	cervix	stomach
2	liver	breast	oral	lung
3	prostate	prostate	breast	liver
4	breast	colon	lung	colon
5	lymphoma	uterus	colon	esophagus
6	oral	lymphoma	lymphoma	breast
7	stomach	stomach	esophagus	leukemia
8	colon	leukemia	stomach	cervix
9	esophagus	skin	leukemia	oral
10	leukemia	cervix	liver	lymphoma
11	lung			

- hepatitis B vaccination and aflatoxin (mold found in maize, peas, millet, and peanuts) reduction
- cervical cancer prevention and detection programs
- development of standard treatment guidelines
- creation of government-supported cancer centers of excellence
- improved pain control
- enhanced cancer surveillance
- coordination-enhanced government involvement with NGOs

Tobacco Control

The FCTC is an international public health treaty written in 2003 and signed by 145 countries (United States had not ratified by 2008). It promotes the following:

- no smoking at indoor workplaces
- price and tax increases
- advertising bans
- packet warning labels

1.3 billion people smoke in the world; 70% of smoking-related illness will occur in low to middle income countries (N

Engl J Med 2007;356:1493). Lung cancer is the leading cause of cancer death (17.5%) in the world. It is up to healthcare workers to lead the way to change in their countries, which have most likely signed the FCTC.

27.2 Cervical Cancer

Comprehensive Cervical Cancer Control, WHO 2006; Planning and Implementing Cervical Cancer; Prevention and Control Programs Alliance, Cervical Cancer Prevention 2004.

Cause: Human papillomavirus (HPV) types 16, 18, 31, 33, 35, others.

Epidem: Seventh leading case of cancer-related deaths in developing countries with a lifetime risk of 2% to 4%. Cervical cancer affects 500 000 women annually with 270 000 deaths. Its slow progression of abnormal cytology to invasive cancer makes it ideal for screening and early intervention. A vaccine for primary prevention and several screening methods for secondary prevention are available (JAMA 2005;294:2173; Table 27.2).

- Pap smears
- visual screening with acetic acid or Lugol's iodine
- human papillomavirus testing

  Interventions for early disease include the following:

- cryotherapy, 85% curative

Table 27.2   Accuracy of Screening Methods

Test	Sensitivity	Specificity
Pap	31–78%	91–99%
HPV test	61–90%	62–94%
Visual acetic acid	50–96%	44–97%
Visual Lugol's	44–93%	75–85%

Source: International Agency for Research on Cancer (IARC).

- loop electrosurgical excision procedure (LEEP), 85% curative
- cone biopsy

Regular Pap smears with HPV testing is ideal but expensive and time consuming. Compliance becomes an issue. A single visit approach is appropriate in areas of limited resources and unreliable follow-up. At the visit, the following should be conducted:

- Discuss evaluation rationale and technique with the woman
- Conduct speculum exam and application 5% acetic acid (household vinegar).
- Offer treatment if acetowhite lesions seen.
- Refer suspicious lesions/cervical cancer for biopsy.
- Obtain consent.
- Consider pretreatment with NSAID and pregnancy test.
- Reinsert speculum and apply cryoprobe.
- Freeze 3 min or until cervix frozen.
- Thaw 5 min.
- Refreeze 3 min.

Complications are mild pain, cramping, occasional bleeding, passage of tissue, and discharge. Suggest 4 wk sexual abstinence followed by consistent condom use. This method, when used once or twice (age 35 and 40 years) a lifetime, reduces risk of cancer deaths by 25% to 40% (cost per year life saved (CPYLS) $500). It is the least expensive of all regimes. Do not treat pregnant women.

Note: Suspicious lesions, those with acetowhite > 70% cervix or into endocervical canal, require biopsy and close follow-up.

Primary prevention of cervical cancer is stopping transmission of HPV.

- condoms
- vaccines; 18 high-risk types; types 16 and 18 cause two-thirds of cancer

- male circumcision, 50% reduction (N Engl J Med 2002;346:1105)
- abstinence
- single sexual partner

27.3 Burkitt's Lymphoma

Cause: EBV; exposure to malaria

Epidem: Tropics about equator < 15° N and S below 1500 meters. Africa, PNG, rarely elsewhere. Ages 4 to 9 yr primarily. Most common pediatric cancer in Sub-Saharan Africa, incidence 1 to 7/100 000 children a yr.

Sx: Loose teeth, cranial nerve palsies, paraplegia.

Si: Jaw swelling maxilla > mandible (50–75%), abdominal swelling (60%), CNS (30%).

Crs: Fastest growing tumor, doubles every 3 d, 50% cure possible.

Cmplc: Differential neuroblastoma, Wilms' tumor, abdominal TB.

Lab: Biopsy is necessary; bone marrow should be obtained.

Rx: Aggressive debulking, cyclophosphamide, methotrexate, vincristine.

27.4 Pharyngeal Carcinoma

Nasopharyngeal Carcinoma

Cause: EBV, HPV, genetic factors

Epidem: Southern China and Chinese migrants especially; also Africa.

Sx: Recurrent otitis media, blocked nasal passage, bloody nasal discharge.

Si: Cervical adenopathy, cranial nerve palsies.

Crs: Rule out TB, lymphoma.

ONCOLOGY

Lab: Biopsy.

Rx: Radiotherapy, chemotherapy.

Oropharyngeal Carcinoma

Cause: Betel nut (*Piper betel*) chewing, tobacco, alcohol.

Epidem: S and SE Asia and Pacific Islands.

Sx: Pain.

Si: Leukoplakia.

Crs: Usually presents late.

Lab: Biopsy.

Rx: Radiotherapy.

27.5 Carcinoma Bladder

Cause: *Schistosoma hematobium*, smoking, chemical exposure, bladder stones, chronic infection.

Epidem: 20-year exposure to Schistosomal infection. Mean age 45 yr, M > F, squamous cell variety.

Sx: Painless hematuria, cystitis.

Si: Urinary obstruction.

Crs: Usually poor as invasive at diagnosis.

Lab: Cystoscopy, biopsy, urine cytology.

Xray: Calcified bladder.

Rx: Radical surgery may be curative.

27.6 Hepatocellular Carcinoma

Cause: Caused by chronic liver injury from persistent hepatitis B or C, hemochromatosis and aflatoxin (mold found in maize, peas, millet and peanuts).

Epidem: Common in tropical countries, incidence over 100/100 000 in some areas; seen in 20 to 40 yr age group, especially males.

Sx/Si: Presents as RUQ pain, mass (90%), wasting and ascites (50%), jaundice (25%), signs of cirrhosis and bone metastases.

Cmplc: Differential is amoebic liver abscess and oral contraceptive induced liver tumor (Ann Intern Med 1975;83:301), which regresses when oral contraceptive pills (OCPs) stopped (Ann Intern Med 1977;86:180).

Lab: Diagnosis is by percutaneous biopsy, elevated alkaline phosphatase (75%), and alpha-fetoprotein (60%).

Xray: Ultrasound will show the tumor.

Rx: Treatment is supportive. Chemotherapy has not been recommended in areas of poor medical services.

27.7   Cancer Tips

- When you diagnose a hydatidiform mole, look for metastases with a chest X-ray.
- Betel nut chewing, especially with tobacco use, causes oral cancer.
- Breast cancer rates in limited resource countries are probably increasing, and screening guidelines are under development (Breast J 2006;12:53).
- Squamous cell carcinoma often arises from areas of chronic inflammation such as tropical ulcers, draining sinus tracts of osteomyelitis, and in old burns.
- Malignant melanoma in dark-skinned people most often occurs on the soles of the foot or palms of the hand.

ONCOLOGY

Chapter 28

Dermatology

(J Am Acad Dermatol 2006;54; Tropical Dermatology [photos])

The variety of dermatological diseases seen in the tropics includes the usual problems common in temperate climates with a preponderance of infectious diseases that will be covered here. Heat and humidity, poor sanitation and hygiene, malnutrition, and HIV/AIDS may change the presentation and appearance of otherwise easily recognized diseases.

28.1 Hypopigmented Macules

Vitiligo

JAMA 2005;293:730

Cause: Genetic, idiopathic, autoimmune, pernicious anemia, Addison's disease

Si: Hair may or may not lose pigment.

Rx: Topical cosmetic cover-up with aniline dye.

Trimethylpsoralen 0.6 mg/kg/d orally followed 2 hr later by 15 min midday sun. Treat twice weekly for 3 to 6 months.

Postinflammatory Vitiligo

Cause: Often follows burns, ulcers

Tinea Versicolor

Cause: *Pityrosporum ovale*

Si: Nonpruritic scaly macules, occasionally patches.

Lab: Potassium hydroxide (KOH) prep shows hyphae and spores.

Rx: Selenium 2.5% apply 30 min × 7 d, repeat in 1 month or leave overnight on d 0, 3, 6.

> Miconazole cream bid × 4 wk.
> Sodium thiosulfate 15% bid × 4 wk.

Leprosy

See chapter 11.

Onchocercosis

See chapter 16.3.

Pinta

Cause: *Treponema carateum*

Epidem: Central and S America. Primarily children and adolescents.

Sx: Scaly papule evolves to scaly irregular plaque, < 1 to 20 cm, fades from blue-brown to depigmented hyperkeratotic lesions over months-years.

Lab: Positive syphilis test VDRL, RPR.

> Dark field exam of skin scrapings positive.

Rx: Benzathine penicillin 2.4×10^6 units IM once, children < 10, half dose.

> Treat family members.

28.2 Hyperpigmented Macules

Leprosy

See chapter 11.

Pellagra

Cause: Niacin deficiency

Epidem: Primarily corn (maize) diet.

Sx: Diarrhea, dermatitis, and dementia.

Si: Erythematous to vesiculation and crusting with hyperpigmentation and scale over sun-exposed skin. Casal's necklace, inflamed ulcerated mucus membranes.

Rx: Niacin.

Mongolian Spots

Cause: Usually present at birth.

Rx: Disappear spontaneously by age 5 yr.

28.3   Pruritic Papules

Scabies

Cause: *Sarcoptes scabiei* var. *hominis*

Epidem: Infants can be infected on the scalp; AIDS patients, lepromatous leprosy (Norwegian).

Pathophys: Characteristic burrows, 3 mm white thread-like, under skin.

Sx: Itching (except Norwegian).

Si: Finger webs, flexor creases, nipples, genitalia.

Cmplc: Impetigo frequent.

Lab: Burrows well outlined with India ink. Low power microscopic examination of skin scrapings shows mites and eggs.

Rx: Ivermectin 150 to 200 μgm/kg orally once (not in pregnancy or breast feeding if infant < 1 wk); 95% effective (Am J Trop Med Hyg 2007;76:392).

      Permethrin 5%, apply and leave on overnight.
      Hexachlorobenzene 1%, apply and leave on overnight.
      Hot sulfur baths in volcanic springs.
      DDT also effective.

Launder clothes and bedding and hang outside 24 hr.

Tip: Ivermectin 200 to 400 µgm/kg once, repeat in 7 to 10 d, cures head lice.

Flea Bites

Cause: *Pulex irritans*

Epidem: Common when pet dogs or cats in house or rat infestation.

Sx: Pruritic papules with central punctum. May have red or urticarial ring.

Rx: Often occurs when pet (preferred host) is removed from house; reintroduce pet. Residual DDT effective.

Tungiasis

Cause: *Tunga penetrans*, burrowing flea. Pigs natural host.

Pathophys: Female flea burrows into skin to lay eggs.

Sx: Usually feet, occasionally hands, buttocks, genitalia.

Si: Small papules with central black dot evolves in 3 wk to painful nodule with hemorrhagic punctum.

Lab: Remove with needle ~1 mm size.

Rx: Surgical removal, topical turpentine or chloroform.

Prev: Wear shoes.

Onchocerciasis

See chapter 16.3.

Myasis

Cause: Diptera (fly larvae)

Epidem: Central and S America and Africa.

Pathophys: Larva enters skin or mucous membranes and grows and develops over several wk.

Sx: Papule rapidly grows to furuncle or boil. Moving larvae occasionally seen.

Rx: Suffocate with petroleum jelly. Remove surgically.

Lichen Planus

Si: Polygonal, pruritic, purple flat topped 3 to 8 mm papules over flexor surfaces (especially wrist, mouth, and genitalia); whitish reticular pattern on surface; often linear; occasionally annular, atrophic, or ulcerative.

Cmplc: Healing lesions develop hyperpigmentation; differential secondary syphilis.

Rx: Topical or systemic steroids for 2 to 6 wk.

28.4 Nonpruritic Papules

Yaws

Cause: *Treponema pertenue*

Epidem: Tropical disease primarily of children 2 to 15 yr old. Spread by skin-to-skin contact.

Pathophys: Average 3 wk incubation period. Divided into early (< 2 yr), latent, and late (> 5 yr).

Sx/Si: Early primary yaws: first lesion (mother yaw) on skin begins as papule that grows to 2 to 5 cm, forms a papilloma, which may be pruritic, ulcerates, then heals over in 3 to 6 months. New lesions appear in a few wk to 2 yr with fever, malaise, and generalized lymphadenopathy; yellow-crusted raspberry-like granulomas, which may resemble condyloma lata of secondary syphilis or cause plantar hyperkeratosis (crab yaws). Bone involvement with osteitis, periostitis, dactylitis, limb swelling. Lesions heal with spontaneous cure or enter latency (10%) and then late stage manifestations with hyperkeratosis of palms and soles, gummatous osteitis, bursitis, ulceration of the oral pharynx and nose.

Lab: Dark-field examination of exudates show spirochetes; RPR/ VDRL positive.

Rx: Benzathine penicillin G, IM once: Children < 6 yr: 600 000 units; 6 to 15 yr old: 1.2 million units; adults: 2.4 million units or Erythromycin or tetracycline for 15 d.

Secondary Syphilis

See chapter 13.6.

Kaposi's Sarcoma

Cause: Herpes virus 8

Epidem: HIV+ patients who are immunosuppressed.

Sx: Violaceous vascular papules, nodules, and plaques.

Crs: Progressive.

Rx: Treat underlying AIDs.

Leprosy

See chapter 11.

28.5 Chronic Ulcers

Leishmaniasis, leprosy, tuberculosis, and syphilis (gumma) all cause chronic ulcers. See specific chapters. Patients with DM, SS disease, and chronic venous stasis often develop leg ulcers. Ulcerative lesions may have other causes:

- pyoderma
- spider bites, snake bites
- cutaneous diphtheria
- anthrax
- genital area (consider chancroid, LGV, syphilis)

- chagoma (chagas)
- African trypanosomiasis

Buruli Ulcer

Cause: *Mycobacterium ulcerans*

Epidem: Worldwide but especially Uganda and Zaire, mostly children. Probably mosquito spread (Emerg Infect Dis 2007;13:1653).

Pathophys: Toxin related.

Sx: After introduction under skin, proceeds from pruritic nodule to ulcer over 1 to 2 months; 85% on limbs.

Si: Undermined ulcer with necrotic base; limb edema, rare adenopathy; may invade bone.

Lab: AFB stain positive, sensitivity 40%, PCR sensitivity 98%.

Rx: May spontaneously heal over 2 to 3 yr or wide surgical excision (30% recurrence).

Rifampin 10 mg/kg/d, max 600 mg plus streptomycin

Streptomycin	
Weights (kg)	Dose (gm)
5–10	0.25
11–20	0.33
21–30	0.5
31–39	0.5
40–54	0.75
> 54	1

Amikacin 15 mg/kg/d, max 1 gm may be used if streptomycin contraindicated.

Nodule and ulcer < 5 cm: surgery + antibiotics (Abx) 1 hr before and for 4 wk.

Ulcerative plaques, edema, large ulcers > 5 cm, head and neck lesions: 4 wk Abx, surgery, 4 more wk Abx.

DERMATOLOGY

Bone and joint involvement: 1 wk Abx, surgery, 7 more wk Abx.

(Prov Guidance on the Role of Specific Antibiotics in the Management of Mycobacterium Ulcerans Disease, WHO;2004.)

Prev: BCG vaccine: some short-term protection; reportable disease in many areas. Soap, topical treatment of injuries is important.

Cancrum Oris (Noma)

Lancet 2006;368:147

Cause: Question *Treponema vincentii, Bacillus fusiformis, Fusobacterium necrophorum*

Epidem: Malnourished children, immune compromised.

Si: Unilateral rapidly progressive destructive mouth ulceration.

Sx: Painful, fetid odor.

Rx: Penicillin G, IV; debridement, treat malnutrition.

28.6   Vesicles

Consider these diseases depending on the history, physical findings, and distribution on the body:

- dermatitis herpetiformis
- discoid eczema
- contact dermatitis
- herpes simplex
- herpes zoster
- varicella (occasionally hemorrhagic in older age groups)
- monkey pox (see chapter 20.2)

28.7 Migratory Swellings

Consider parasitic infections:

- cutaneous larva migrans: slow moving
- strongyloidiasis: rapid, on buttocks
- *Loa Loa*
- gnathostomiasis
- fascioliasis
- sparganosis

Chapter 29
Ear, Nose, Throat

29.1   Ear Diseases

Otitis Media

Cause: *H. flu, S. pneumococcus, Moraxella catarrhalis*, others; viral.

Epidem: Common.

Sx/Si: Ear pain, fever, decreased hearing, red bulging drum; improved when tympanic membrane perforates. Chronic ear drainage.

Cmplc: Perforation, mastoiditis, meningitis, epidural abscess, lateral sinus thrombosis, middle ear destruction with vertigo, facial nerve paralysis, decrease or loss of hearing.

Rx: Amoxicillin 45 to 90 mg/kg/d divided into 3 doses for 5 d, or
Co-trimoxazole (TMP/SMX 4/20) mg/kg/d in 2 doses × 5 d.
Wick ear 3 to 4 × daily if pus. Use rolled up toilet paper, place in ear, leave 2 min, remove, and do again with dry paper. Continue until dry. This must be continued for a week. Chronic draining ear is managed with antibiotic ear drops once daily for 2 wk and ear wicking. Keep water out of ear.

Mastoiditis

Cause: Untreated bacterial infection of middle ear.

Sx/Si: Thick purulent discharge, low grade fever, ache behind ear. Pain with pressure over mastoid, loss of post-auricular skin crease, and protruding ear. Dull thickened ear drum.

Cmplc: As in otitis media.

Xray: Mastoid air cells cloudy with decalcification.

Rx: Myringotomy for drainage. Antibiotics for 4 to 6 wk.

29.2   Nose and Throat Diseases

Epiglottis

Cause: *H. influenza*, type B; rarely others

Epidem: Disease of children not immunized against *H. influenza*.

Pathophys: Upper airway obstruction by edematous infected epiglottis.

Sx/Si: Fever, sore throat, drooling, muffled voice, stridor. Child sits leaning forward.

Xray: Ill advised until airway secure, then directly visualize epiglottis.

Rx: Avoid exam of epiglottis until prepared for nasotracheal intubation or to undertake an emergency cricothyroid membrane puncture.

> Ceftriaxone IV or IM 20 to 50/kg once daily, or
> Ampicillin IV or IM 250 to 500 mg/kg q 4 to 6 hr, plus
> Chloramphenicol IV or IM or orally 25 mg/kg q 6 hr (reduce by 50% when improving) all for 10 d.

Prev: *H. influenza* vaccine.

Peritonsillar Abscess, Quinsy

> Am Fam Physician 2008;77:199

Cause: Streptococcal, other bacteria

Epidem: Complication of tonsillitis.

Sx/Si: Pain in throat, ear, neck. Fever, dysphagia, drooling, and lymphadenopathy; trismus and foul odor in mouth; unilateral swollen tonsil often past midline.

Rx: Begin antibiotics, penicillin, or chloramphenicol and do incision and drainage (I & D):

- Have patient sit, head forward.
- Apply local anesthetic spray, 2% lidocaine.
- Have an assistant hold the tongue in gauze and retract.
- Needle aspirate with 18- or 20-gauge needle into middle of abscess.
- Incise about 2 cm with scalpel to drain if pus found.
- Insert artery forceps and open to break up any loculations of pus.
- Aspirate with suction.
- Irrigate with saline.
- Have patient gargle with salt water for 5 to 7 d.

Chapter 30

Psychiatry

(Lancet 2007;370, series on global mental health)

There is not a book "Where There Is No Psychiatrist," although that is precisely the case in many developing countries. Mental illness is often treated and managed in the village by the family, community, traditional healers, or leaders. Aberrant behavior is tolerated, and the formal medical system is not frequently utilized; and when it is, patients and family prefer local health workers who speak the language and with whom they can relate more easily. The role of the expatriate is often to support the local staff with consultations and to assist in arriving at a diagnosis and treatment and, of course, to treat the local expatriate community who are frequently under considerable stress. Drugs available in developing countries are limited largely by cost.

Schizophrenia

Epidem: Acute or insidious onset from teens through thirties; worldwide prevalence about 1%.

Sx: Hallucinations (usually auditory or visual, delusions, loosening of associations); illogical, disconnected thoughts and statements, unusual mannerisms.

Rx:

- Chlorpromazine: Start at 25 mg orally or IM 3×/d and increase up to 100 to 400 mg each dose as necessary. Usual maintenance dose is 100 to 300 mg daily, less in the elderly. Avoid skin contact. Usually drug of first choice.

- Haloperidol: 1 to 5 mg orally or IM 2 to 3×/d up to 30 mg daily. Less in elderly.
- Fluphenazine depo preparation: Test dose 12.5 mg deep IM; if no adverse effect after 4 to 7 d, give 12.5 to 100 mg every 2 to 5 wk.
- Trihexyphenidyl: 1 mg orally twice a day, maximum 15 mg daily, is the usual anticholinergic drug available for treating side effects.
- Family counseling is important to explain drug therapy and to address psychosocial factors and stressors.
- It is important to rule out treatable delirium and dementia along with culturally related behavior.

Depression

Epidem: Onset at any age, first episode often in 20s.

Sx: Depressed mood, loss of interest or enjoyment in activities, fatigue, feelings of guilt, worthlessness, sleep and appetite disturbance, reduced concentration, ideas worthlessness, guilt, suicide. Often more somatic symptoms in non-Western societies, which may be attributed to spirits or spells.

Rx: Treatment effects are usually seen after 2 wk. If only a minimal response, reconsider diagnosis, consider hypothyroidism and consider combination therapy. Partial or good response, allow 6 wk total treatment; if not optimal, reconsider as above. For tricyclics, start treatment at a low dose and increase every 3 to 4 d over several wk. If the patient fails drug therapy or is an immediate suicide risk, consider electroconvulsive therapy (ECT). Always ask about suicide risks and posttraumatic stress disorder (PTSD).
   Tricyclic Drugs:

Amitriptyline: very anticholinergic, 150 to 300 mg daily.
Imipramine: less sedative, 150 to 300 mg daily.

Many others; most with orthostatic hypotension and anticholinergic side effects. Nortriptyline is an exception.

Selective Serotonin Reuptake Inhibitors (SSRIs):

Fluoxetine 20 to 80 mg daily.

Many others; GI and sleep problems, not anticholinergic.

Bipolar Disorder

Epidem: Prevalence about 1%, commonly a family history; onset usually 20s.

Sx: Gradual or acute onset of euphoria, pressured speech, distractibility, elevated activity energy with decreased sleep; may have hallucinations and delusions. Mania is punctuated by euthymic and depressive periods.

Rx: Acute mania is the same as schizophrenia using haloperidol or chlorpromazine. For acute episodes and prophylaxis against frequent recurrent episodes, use mood stabilizers:

Sodium valproate: 250 mg orally 3×/d, maximum 60 mg/kg/d; response in 2 to 4 d; first choice.

Carbamazepine: 100 mg orally 4×/d up to 1.6 gm/d; maintenance usually 400 mg daily; response in 7 to 10 d.

Lithium is too dangerous to use unless levels available.

Tip: Depression should be treated with a mood stabilizer.

Anxiety

Appears more common in expat population. In locals, frequently treated by local traditional healer. Somatization is a common presentation. Resolution of local conflicts and pressures should be first intervention. Panic attacks often respond to antidepressants. Long-term use of benzodiazepines is discouraged.

Acute transient psychotic episodes and dissociative states are common in stressed individuals. They provide a socially acceptable means of dealing with stress. Hospital admission and observation, judicious administration of a neuroleptic or benzodiazepine, if necessary, and a supportive hospital staff usually helps to resolve the symptoms and elicit a history. Underlying depression is common. Mass hysteria in school children is regularly reported (S Afr Med J 2003;93:10; Br J Psychol 1983;142:85).

Chapter 31

Things That Bite and Sting and Are Not to Be Eaten

William Alto & Chi Jokonya

31.1   Fish Poisoning

Ciguatera

Cause: Dinoflagellates concentrated in carnivorous fish.

Epidem: Worldwide.

Sx: Metallic taste, abdominal cramping, nausea, vomiting, diarrhea; paresthesia, pruritus feet and hands, temperature reversal.

Si: Pupil dilatation, weakness to paralysis, bradycardia, and hypotension.

Crs: Onset after 4 to 30 hr. GI symptoms resolve in a day; paresthesia may continue for months (Am J Trop Med Hyg 2007;77:1170).

Rx: Calcium gluconate IV for paresthesia; symptomatic treatment.

Scombroid Poisoning

Cause: Spoiled fish, usually tuna or mackerel.

Epidem: Worldwide.

Pathophys: Bacteria break down histidine in fish muscle releasing saurine (similar to histamine).

Sx: Fish has peppery taste. Histamine release-like reaction: headache, urticaria, angioedema, weakness, diarrhea.

Si: Hives, flushing.

Crs: Recovery < 24 hr.

Rx: Antihistamines.

31.2 Dangerous Sea Life

Stonefish

Cause: *Scorpaenidae* fish: stonefish, scorpion fish, and zebra fish.

Epidem: Pacific and Indian Oceans; stonefish are bottom dwellers, camouflaged, and often stepped on.

Pathophys: Venomous spines.

Sx: Immediate severe pain follows lymphadenitis, nausea, vomiting, diarrhea.

Si: Swelling, discoloration, necrosis around sting, seizures, occasional death.

Crs: Pain persists 1 to 2 d.

Complc: Gangrene, cardiorespiratory collapse.

Rx: 45°C hot water immersion; remove spine; antivenom available for stonefish and scorpion fish; supportive care.

Stingrays

Cause: Various species

Pathophys: Lacerations from barb plus venom.

Sx: Pain, swelling, necrosis.

Si: Shock, convulsions, GI symptoms.

Cmplc: Secondary infection common.

Rx: Remove spines and nonviable tissue; hot water neutralizes toxins; doxycycline prophylaxis.

Sea Urchins

Spines should be removed, or a secondary infection and granuloma formation may occur. Vinegar may dissolve with superficial punctures.

Jellyfish

Cause: Nematocysts of numerous types of jellyfish

Sx: Pain, burning.

Si: Whip-like pattern, swelling, vesiculation, erythema, seabather's itch in distribution of swimsuit.

Crs: Minor symptoms to respiratory arrest, DIC, convulsions.

Rx: Inactivate nematocysts with vinegar; antivenom for box jellyfish.

Cone Shells

Cause: Colorful shells of the Indo-Pacific area

Pathophys: Venom from radular tooth from pointed end of cone-shaped shell.

Sx: Paresthesia, numbness, respiratory and general paralysis.

Rx: Supportive.

31.3 Arthropods

Scorpion

Cause: Various types

Epidem: Fatal stings in S America, N Africa, Middle East, and S Asia; highest in children. Found worldwide in tropical and semitropical areas.

Sx: Pain, swelling.

Si: Systemic symptoms may be delayed up to 24 hr; autonomic excitation with catecholamine release; neurotoxic effects in some species, pancreatitis (black scorpion, Trinidad).

Rx:

- local anesthesia for pain relief
- delayed venom absorption with tourniquet and ice packs
- antivenom available
- alpha blockers for autonomic symptoms

Spider Bites

Am J Trop Med Hyg 2005;72:361

Lactrodectus

Cause: 3 important species: *L. mactans* (black widow, black button), *L. geometricus* (brown widow), *L. rhodesiensis*.

Epidem: Female 10 to 15 mm long, round body, colors and markings depend on species. Male 3 mm is no human threat. Black and brown widow: neurotoxic venom, severity of illness depends on amount of venom. Found worldwide.

Sx: Mild: Slight redness and swelling. 2 small fang marks like tiny red spots. Severe: May occur within 30 to 60 min with cramps and muscle spasms starting near bite and spreading, chills, nausea, vomiting, abdominal pain, anxiety, dizziness, sweating, excessive salivation, piloerection, pain in regional lymph nodes. Burning itching soles of feet, convulsions especially small children, and coma.

Si: Fever, hypothermia, bradycardia or tachycardia, very high BP, priapism.

Rx:

- Ice applied to bite site. Do not apply tourniquet.
- Too much movement should be avoided (may increase flow of venom to blood). Splint limb.

- Local anaesthetic around wound if pain severe and persistent.
- Calcium gluconate 10% for muscle spasm 0.2 ml/kg/dose slow IV.
- Dantrolene for muscle pain, 2.5 mg/kg IV then 0.5 mg every 6 hr for 12 to 24 hr for spasms.
- Dapsone 100 mg twice daily to reduce necrosis (JAMA 1983;250:648). Use for several weeks.
- TT if not received within 10 yr.
- Diazepam anxiolytic and muscle relaxant.
- Button spider antivenom (do not give if > 24 hr): antivenom 5 ml IM (need not be given close to the bite), observe for anaphylaxis. See package insert.

Loxosceles (Violin Spiders)

N Engl J Med 1998;339:379; 2005;352:700

Cause: Violin, brown recluse, fiddleback

Epidem: 6 to 10 mm long, dark brown violin shaped, long fragile legs, nocturnal, and most bite at night. Found in Americas.

Sx/Si: Painless swelling initially, later cytotoxic. Red skin followed by blister formation at bite site. Mild to severe pain and itching 2 to 8 hr after bite. Necrosis may occur, which may take months to heal. Systemic symptoms less common, fever and chills, skin rash, nausea and vomiting.

Rx:

- Immobilize and elevate.
- Antipruritic, local anesthetic.
- Dapsone.
- Early excision of the bite including all necrotic tissue is debated.
- Antivenom not available, steroids debatable, antibiotics if secondary infection.

Sicarius

Cause: Six-eyed sand spider, 10 mm long, body covered in bristles to which sand clings for camouflage, live in arid area, do not bite readily. May enter state of suspended animation, presumed dead, picked up, then bite.

Rx: As above for violin spider

Sac Spider

Epidem: 10 mm long, pale body, large black head found in gardens, southern Africa.

Sx/Si: Mostly bite at night; usually painless; may become inflamed, swollen, and necrotic; bite site looks greenish yellow due to venom. Local symptoms occur within 8 hr; systemic symptoms occur after 3 d, may mimic tick bite fever.

Rx: As above for violin spider.

Unidentified Spiders

Most are harmless.

Sx/Si: Local allergic reaction to bite that may not be venom; swollen, painful, itchy, cytotoxic apparent within 2 to 24 hr; anaphylaxis rare.

Rx: Give chlorpromazine or similar antihistamine

31.4 Snake Bites

Causes: *Crotalus sp.* (rattlesnakes: Americas); *Naja sp.* (cobras: Asia, Africa); *Vipera sp.* (vipers: Europe, Asia); and numerous others.

Epidem: Common cause of death in hunter-gatherers and agricultural workers. Identity of snake often unclear. Many bites have no venom injected. Annual incidence 200 to 650/100 000 in Sub-Saharan Africa.

Sx: Variable depending on toxins. Pain, vomiting, headache. Tender lymph nodes.

Si: Local necrosis and swelling that extends, rhabdomyolysis bleeding, shock, neurotoxicity, and paralysis. Redness of eye with cobra-spitting venom.

Crs: If envenomation occurs, often prolonged respiratory paralysis or local necrosis.

Cmplc: Limb necrosis, compartment syndrome. Internal bleeding, prolonged respiratory paralysis.

Lab: Monitor clotting if possible, blood in test tube, H&H, urine analysis for blood and myoglobin.

Rx:

- Splint limb. No tourniquet!
- Clean wound.
- Treat pain. Avoid IM injections if bleeding.
- Tetanus booster if appropriate.
- Identify snake if available.
- Give antivenom (specific or polyvalent) per package insert if envenomation symptoms. Children require the same dose or more than adults.
- Anticholinesterases may reverse neurological signs in certain species of snakes: cobras, death adders, mamba, kraits, coral snake. Tensilon test will identify.
- Fasciotomy or tracheostomy as needed.
- Surgical debridement, skin grafting later.
- Irrigate eyes for cobra venom spit; topical antibiotics, atropine, or epinephrine drops for pain.

31.5   Foods

Cassava Poisoning

Cause: *Manihot esculenta* (manioc, tapioca)

Epidem: Dietary staple in Asia, Africa and S America, principal source of calories for half billion people. Poisonous root must be processed properly to eat. Two roots can kill.

Pathophys: Cyanide in root released during processing as gas or after eating root. Cyanide processed in body to thiocyanate, which requires sulfur-containing amino acids that are reduced in malnutrition. Excess-free cyanide causes Konzo.

Sx/Si: Abrupt onset with severe weakness, tremor, cramps, hypertonicity and paraparesis; also optic neuropathy, deafness, and peripheral neuropathy.

Crs: Irreversible.

Rx: Usually not possible.

Prev: Proper preparation of root in ventilated area. Processing includes peeling, grating, soaking in warm water for several days to release cyanide gas, and then it is edible. Avoid bitter cassava (higher cyanide level).

Mushroom Poisoning

Cause: Over 100 species toxic, several deadly.

Sx/Si: Rapid (minutes to hours) muscarinic poisoning: lacrimation, salivation, diarrhea, sweating, miosis, shock, coma, convulsions. Delayed (6–24 hr) abdominal pain, vomiting, diarrhea lasts 1 d, then better; on d 3, hepatic failure and renal failure (ATN).

Pathophys: Renal and GI reabsorption of toxins.

Rx: Hemodialysis if available. If not, activated charcoal 1 gm/kg every 4 to 6 hr, forced diuresis, acetylcysteine.

Foods

Aspergillus flavus toxin present in moldy peanuts causes hepatoma. Best avoid eating peanuts.

Mango sap, leaves, and skin of unripe fruit; may cause irritant and allergic dermatitis.

Citrus skin may cause photodermatitis.

Jimson weed (*Datura stramonium*) seeds contain scopolamine and hyoscyamine. Treat as in atropine poisoning with activated charcoal and pilocarpine.

Trumpet flower (*Datura inoxia*) often prepared as tea; same as Datura.

Chapter 32

High Altitude Diseases

(Emerg Med Clin North Am 2004;22:329; N Engl J Med 2001;345:107)

Cause: Acute increase in altitude over 2000 m, 40% of individuals > 3000 m.

Epidem: Several syndromes:

- acute mountain sickness (AMS)
- high altitude cerebral edema (HACE)
- high altitude pulmonary edema (HAPE)
- high altitude retinal hemorrhage
- chronic mountain illness (CMS)
- high altitude pulmonary hypertension (HAPH)

Risk dependent on ascent rate, altitude, time at high elevation, exertion, temperature, elevation at sleep, barometric pressure (storms cause decreased pressure and increase relative altitude), preacclimatization, and individual factors including previous history of AMS, illness, medications, and age (children and teens more susceptible). Physical fitness is not preventive. Risks in Himalayan trekkers at 3000 to 5500 m (Br Med J 2003;326:915):

1 to 2 d: 49% AMS, 1.6% HAPE or HACE
10 to 13 d: 23% AMS, 0.5% HAPE or HACE
CMS usually residents of Andes or Himalayas.

Pathophys: Normal adaptations:

- 2,3-diphosphoglycerate (DPG) concentration increases, shifting Hb dissociation curve.

- Hyperventilation, carotid body stimulation.
- Respiratory alkalosis, 2° above, normalizes in 2 to 3 days.
- Polycythemia due to hemoconcentration initially then new RBC production.

Hypoxemia may result from relative hypoventilation causing pulmonary regional overperfusion/elevated hydrostatic pressure and capillary leakage. Both cause edema (N Engl J Med 2001;345:107).

Sx: AMS begins ≥ 1 hr (usually 6–10) after arrival > 2000 m. Headache (100%) and anorexia, nausea, vomiting, dizziness, fatigue, and difficulty sleeping. End-stage AMS is HACE with change of consciousness, truncal ataxia, lethargy progressing to coma.

HAPE: dyspnea at rest and moist cough.

CMS: breathlessness, palpitations, paresthesia, tinnitus, headache.

Si: Cheyne-Stokes respirations at night (normal), mental status changes, bizarre behavior, cyanosis, tachycardia. Asymptomatic retinal hemorrhages, > 4000 m. CMS: polycythemia, pulmonary HT, hypoxemia, cyanosis.

Crs: Spontaneous resolution of AMS in 1 to 2 d.

Lab: CMS: Hb ≥ 21 g/dL males, ≥ 19 g/dL females.

Xray: MRI white matter changes in HACE.

CXR will show interstitial fluid in HAPE.

Rx: Treatment AMS and HACE:

- Descent ≥ 500 m
- Oxygen 1 to 2 L/min or maintain SaO_2 ≥ 90%.
- Give dexamethasone 8 mg IV/IM/PO then 4 mg every 6 hr
- Consider acetazolamide (AMS) if unable to descend.

Treatment HAPE:

- Descent 500 to 1000 m.

- Oxygen 4 to 6 L/min initially then 2 to 4 L/min or maintain $SaO_2 \geq 90\%$.
- Provide portable hyperbaric therapy 2 to 4 psi.
- Give nifedipine 10 mg orally initially then 30 mg sustained release (SR) once or twice a day.
- Give albuterol/salmeterol 2 puffs q6h/q12h if no HACE (N Engl J Med 2002;346:1631).

Prev:

- Graded ascent 600 m/d.
- Rest day every 600 to 1200 m.
- Oxygen 1 to 2 L/min while asleep and for symptoms.
- Acetazolamide 125 to 250 mg bid, begin 24 hr before ascent and continue 2 d at maximum altitude. Pediatric dose 2.5 mg/kg bid. (Side effects: paresthesia, diuresis, sulfa allergy, alters taste carbonated beverages, pregnancy category C.)
- Adequate hydration.
- Dexamethasone 4 mg orally twice a day starting day of ascent; discontinue after 2 d at maximum altitude.

CMS and HAPH

Seen in residents at high altitude > 2500 m (High Alt Med Biol 2005;6:147).

- Migration to lower elevation. If unable:
  - Phlebotomy if Hb $\geq$ 21 g/dL males, $\geq$ 19 g/dL females.
  - Chronic oxygen therapy.
  - Medroxyprogesterone 20 to 60 mg/d for 10 wk.
  - Acetazolamide 125 mg twice a day for 3 wk.
  - *Rhodiola* (Tibetan herb)
  - Nifedipine SR 30 mg daily.

Chapter 33
Nutritional Diseases

Chi Jokonya & William Alto

33.1   Rickets (Children) and Osteomalacia (Adults)

Cause: Primarily caused by vitamin D deficiency and inadequate calcium intake (New Engl J Med 1999;341:563).

Epidem: Common in areas where women and children have limited sun exposure due to their clothing. Steatorrhea, postgastrectomy, and chronic seizure medications are other common causes.

Sx/Si: In children:

- More common in premature infants and those with low birth weight.
- Unusual with severe protein energy malnutrition, as stunting reduces bone growth requirements.
- Head sweating common, pale.
- Motor development delayed, poor tone.
- Tetany occurs.
- Bony lesions are frontal bossing, craniotabes (soft skull), delayed fontanel closure, delayed tooth eruption, rachitic rosary of ribs.
- X-ray findings of a widened and frayed epiphyseal plate (wrist best).

- Later bony abnormalities develop such as bow legs, knock knees, and pectus carinatum
- Increased risk of pneumonia.

  In adults:

- Painful walking due to kyphosis and limb deformities.
- Narrowing of the pelvis with subsequent obstructed labor.

Lab: Laboratory values will show an increase in alkaline phosphatase. Serum calcium will be low or normal.

Rx: Treatment is sunlight, vitamin D_3 2000 to 6000 IU/d, children; 50 000 to 100 000 IU/d adults for 3 months orally or 100 000 to 600 000 IU IV once.

Prev: Adequate calcium should be supplied 500 to 1200 mg/d. Breast fed infants at high risk (prolonged breast feeding, low birth weight, prematurity, mothers at risk for vitamin D or calcium deficiency) should receive vitamin D supplementation. Maize porridge, low in calcium and high in fiber, which inhibits calcium absorption, is commonly fed to children.

33.2   Vitamin A Deficiency

Cause: Diet low in vitamin A or malabsorption due to diarrhea.

Epidem: Vitamin A deficiency not only causes visual problems, but it increases mortality from ARIs (N Engl J Med 1990;323:929) and diarrheal illness in HIV infected infants (Am J Public Health 1995;85:1076). Measles infection precipitates symptoms.

Xerophthalmia is the leading cause of blindness in children. 250 million under 5 yr children have vitamin A deficiency; 3 million have xerophthalmia, and 10% of these are blind.

Sx/Si: Eye changes progress from mild disease with night blindness; often the child will bump into things in the evening or begin to wet the bed due to inability to walk to the toilet. Later, the cornea dries and Bitot's spots appear as foamy, white triangular areas on the temporal bulbar conjunctiva. The color and shape may vary (N Engl J Med 1994;330:994). The disease may rapidly progress to keratomalacia with corneal ulceration and perforation. Emergent treatment is indicated to save the less affected eye. Corneal scarring is the result.

Rx: Treatment of xerophthalmia (and children with measles):

At the time of diagnosis, the next day, and 2 wk later give orally (unless severe disease present)

- less than 6 months age   50 000 IU/d
- 6 to 12 months   100 000 IU/d
- 12 months and older   200 000 IU/d
- pregnant women   < 25 000 IU/d

Prev: Identification of one child with vitamin A deficiency usually indicates a family and often a community problem. Serious consideration should be given to high-dose universal distribution of vitamin A with intensive health education intervention.

Universal distribution every 3 to 6 months

- Less than 6 months age   50 000 IU
- 6 to 12 months   100 000 IU
- 12 months and older   200 000 IU
- mothers (after delivery)   200 000 IU

(If breast feeding mothers receive vitamin A, their infants < 6 months do not require treatment.)

Dietary prevention: Vitamin A is found in the following:

- breast milk (especially in treated mothers)
- mango, papaya
- carrots, green leafy vegetables, sweet potatoes, eggs, red palm oil, dairy products, animal and fish liver (oils)

33.3 Malnutrition

Kwashiorkor

Serious Childhood Problems in Countries with Limited Resources, WHO 2004; J Pediatr Gastroenterol Nutr 2007;44:487; Matern Child Nutr 2006;2:114.

Cause: Severe form of protein energy malnutrition (PEM) < 80% weight for height (edema may give false impression of better nutritional status) caused by inadequate protein intake in the presence of fair caloric intake.

Epidem: Undernutrition underlying cause of 53% deaths in children < 5 yr in developing countries. Most common 1 to 3 yr. Etiology is famine, limited food supply, illiteracy, war.

Sx: Lethargy, irritability, apathy, diarrhea, flaky paint dermatitis, edema, dementia, reddish pigment of hair.

Si: Decreased muscle mass, edema, large potbelly, skin changes, hepatomegaly, fatty liver, secondary immune deficiency, stunted linear growth, failure to thrive.

Crs: Treated early responds well; however, permanent mental and physical disabilities not uncommon; late shock and coma, death.

Cmplc: Lactose intolerance, dehydration, infection, diarrhea, decreased IQ, stunted growth, vitamin deficiencies (xerophthalmia due to vitamin A, beriberi due to vitamin B_1, pellagra due to niacin, scurvy due to vitamin C, rickets due to vitamin D).

Lab: CBC, urine, PPD

Xray: CXR

Rx: See Table 33.1: Treatment of Malnutrition
Phase 1: Length of time in phase 1 should be < 7 d as the diet does not allow for nutritional rehab. Use high energy milk (HEM; shown in Table 33.2) 1 kcal/ml; give 100 ml/kg/d.

Table 33.1   Treatment of Malnutrition

1st phase: 24-hour care	1–7 days
Rehydrate	Special formulation HEM (see below)
Start medical treatment	Systematic and prescribed for underlying diseases
Initiate nutritional treatment	8–10 feeds a d: 100 Kcals/kg/d up to 1.0–1.5 gm protein/kg/d

2nd phase: day care	± 14 days
Continuation medical treatment	Systematic and prescribed treatment
Nutritional rehabilitation	4–6 feeds/d: to > 200 Kcals/kg/d, 3–5 g protein/kg/d (10% Kcals from protein)
Transition to social environment	Maximum 300 Kcal/kg/d on demand
	Vary diet, psychosocial stimulation

- Review immunizations and give as needed.
- Treat any parasitic infestation with mebendazole 500 mg × 1 dose.
- Frequent small feeds: Day 1 to 2: 12 feeds of 8 ml/kg q 2 hr; Day 3–7: 8 feeds of 12 to 15 ml/kg q 3 hr.
- Indications for nasal gastric tube: severe dehydration or anorexia, too weak to drink, repeated vomiting
- 2 gm KCl/1000 ml HEM or supplement with bananas.

Phase 2 (shown in Table 33.3). Length of time in phase 2 depends on rate of recovery.

Table 33.2   Sample Composition of HEM for Therapeutic Feeding

	Grams per Liter	Protein (gm)	kcal
Dried skim milk	80	28.8	285
Vegetable oil	60		530
Sugar	50		200
Total	1 liter	28.8	1015

Table 33.3   Sample Meal Schedule for Phase 2

Time	Meal
0800	HEM + Banana
1000	HEM
1200	Porridge
1400	HEM
1600	Porridge
1700	Return home with package of biscuits

- Eventually replace porridge with local foods.
- Continue medical monitoring.
- Provide vitamins and minerals:
  - ferrous sulfate 100 mg/d from d 15 (do not start earlier due to risk of bacterial overgrowth)
  - folic acid 5 mg/d
  - multivitamins + vitamin C 125 mg/d (or fresh fruits and vegetables)
  - vitamin A: 6 to 12 months 100 000 IU orally every 3 to 6 months; 1 to 6 yr 200 000 IU orally every 3 to 6 months
- Provide psychosocial stimulation.
- Anticipate 10 to 20 g/kg/d weight gain during phase 2.
- Discharge to supplemental feeding program once 80% weight maintained for 2 wk with no edema and no medical issues.

  Some studies suggest antioxidants have increased survival and recovery benefit: reduced glutathione 600 mg twice a day, alpha lipoic acid 2 × 50 mg or N-acetylcysteine 2 × 100 mg/d (Redox Rep 2005;10:215), showed no benefit of antioxidants in prevention (Br Med J 2005;330:1095).

Marasmus

Cause: More severe PEM < 60% weight for height due to failure to take sufficient calories and protein.

Epidem: Usually occurs in first year of life, transition from breast feeding, poor foods in infancy. Acute gastrointestinal infections, chronic infections like TB and HIV exacerbate the problem.

Sx: Constipation or diarrhea, irritability, apathy, hungry, behavioral changes.

Si: Profound emaciation, dry skin, loose skin folds hanging over buttocks, dermatitis, failure to thrive.

Crs: Infection may stress a stable marasmus patient to develop kwashiorkor.

Complc: Decreased IQ.

Lab: CBC, urine.

Xray: CXR to rule out TB.

Rx: Slow feeding treatment protocol as for kwashiorkor.

Marasmic Kwashiorkor

Nutrition Guidelines; Medecins Sans Frontieres (MSF); Paris 1995

Cause: 60% to 80% weight for height: mixed type of undernutrition with edema, gross wasting, stunting, and mild hepatomegaly. Treat as noted above.

Chapter 34
Pediatrics

Chi Jokonya

34.1   Neonatal Resuscitation

Hospital Care for Children, WHO 2005; *Basic Newborn Resuscitation*, WHO 1997; *Management of the Sick Newborn*, Geneva, WHO, 1996 (Document WHO/FRH/MSM/96.12).

Anticipate Possible Asphyxia

Prepare for birth: 2 clean warm towels, a warm room, self-inflating bag and face mask, a clean delivery kit for cord care, a suction device, a radiant heater if available, a blanket, a clock. Have additional equipment in case of multiple births.

Dry baby with a clean cloth and place in warm environment or keep wrapped while assessing to prevent heat loss.

Assess:

- breathing, chest rising > 30/min or crying
- good muscle tone
- pink color

If yes, routine care

If no:

- Position baby's head so that it is slightly extended in the neutral position (a folded cloth under the shoulders may help)

- Clear the airway by suctioning first the mouth then the nose. (The baby may breathe from the stimulation provided by suction; if so no further action needed, give routine care.)
- Stimulate and reposition.
- Give oxygen as necessary.

If breathing and pink, routine care
   If not breathing, cyanosed:

- Select appropriate fitting mask (size 1 normal weight, size 0 small newborn).
- Make sure neck slightly extended and mask fits over mouth, nose, and chin, forming a seal.
- Give 5 slow ventilations with bag.

If breathing, observe closely
   If not breathing, chest not moving well:

- Check position and mask fit.
- Ensure airway is clear, suction.
- Ensure adequate ventilation pressure.
- Ventilate with bag and mask at 40–60 breaths/min.
- Make sure chest is moving with each compression

If breathing, observe closely
   Check the heart rate (HR):

HR > 60/Min	HR < 60/Min
• Continue to bag at 40–60 breaths/ min. • Make sure chest is moving with each compression. • Use oxygen if available. • Every 1–2 min stop to observe for adequacy of HR and breathing. • Stop bagging when respiratory rate (RR) > 30/min. • Continue oxygen until pink and active.	• Place thumbs just below line connecting nipples on the sternum. • Start chest compressions. • 90 compressions per 30 breaths/ min (3 compressions, 1 breath every 2 seconds). • Compress 1/3 AP diameter of the chest.

(If after 20 minutes resuscitation baby not breathing and no pulse, cease efforts. Explain to mother baby has died and allow to hold if she so wishes.)

Routine care after successful resuscitation:

- Leave the baby skin to skin with mother.
- Do a newborn exam.
- Encourage breast feeding within an hour, resuscitated babies at higher risk of developing hypoglycaemia, good suckling a sign of good recovery.
- If body temp < 36°C, baby has hypothermia; skin-to-skin contact and additional blanket; check body temperature hourly until normal.
- Difficulty breathing or other danger signs, arrange for transfer for special care.

Routine care of all newborns post delivery:

- Keep warm and dry, skin to skin.
- Encourage early, exclusive breast feeding, and feed on demand.
- Give vitamin K 1 mg/0.5 ml or 1 mg/ml IM once (do not use 10 mg/ml ampoule)
- Keep umbilical cord clean and dry.
- Give antibiotic eye drops to both eyes (tetracycline eye ointment) according to national guidelines.
- Give oral polio, hepatitis B, BCG per national guidelines.

34.2   Neonatal Seizures

Hospital Care for Children, WHO 2005

Epidem: Birth asphyxia, hypoxic ischemic encephalopathy, birth trauma, sepsis, hypoglycemia, hypocalcemia, neonatal tetanus, meningitis.

Sx/Si: Generalized or localized convulsions, irritability, lethargy, apneic episodes, high pitched cry, poor feeding, bulging fontanel, trismus, muscle spasms, fever, hypothermia, jaundice, pallor.

Cmplc: Status epilepticus with seizures persisting longer than 20 min during which time baby does not regain consciousness

Lab: Glucose, calcium, electrolytes if possible, LP (should not be done if signs of raised intracranial pressure, less likely in newborn with open fontanel).

Rx:

- Look for and treat the cause.
- Obtain IV access.
- Give oxygen if cyanosed or signs of respiratory distress.
- Keep warm and dry (cap, warm room, kangaroo care).
- Give IV glucose if glucose < 20 mg/dl; if 20 to 40 mg/dl, feed immediately and increase frequency of feeds.
- Try IO or give expressed breast milk (EBM) or glucose via nasogastric tube (NGT) if cannot gain IV access.
- Give phenobarbital 15 mg/kg × 1 dose, if convulsing; if convulsions continue, give further 10 mg/kg doses up to maximum of 40 mg/kg; if needed, continue maintenance of 5 mg/kg/d (watch for apnea).
- Start ampicillin and gentamicin if signs of sepsis, meningitis.

34.3 Recognizing the Sick Newborn

Lancet 2008;371:135–142; Integrated Management of Childhood Illnesses chart booklet, WHO; Pediatr Infect Dis J 2003;22: 711–717.

Adapted from the recent multicenter study: The Young Infants Clinical Signs Study Group. The above study has developed an algorithm of 7 signs and symptoms that are both sensitive and specific for the need for hospitalization in infants 0 to 6 days as well as 7 to 59 days. Integrated Management of Childhood Illnesses (IMCI) guidelines were not designed for the first week of life, and its use in this age group has resulted in wasted precious resources due to high sensitivity but low specificity.

Epidem: Of the 4 million babies dying annually, 75% die in the first week (WHO World Health Report 2005). Due to perinatal asphyxia, pneumonia, sepsis, meningitis, hypoglycemia, and hemolytic disease of the newborn.

Sx/Si: History of difficult feeding, movement only when stimulated, temperature < 35.5°C or > 37.5°C, respiratory rate > 60 breaths/min, severe chest indrawing, history of convulsion.

Lab: CBC, glucose, electrolytes, LP, consider CXR if available.

Rx: Oxygen, IV access, IV fluids or NGT feeding, keep warm, kangaroo care: caps, warm room, treat hypoglycemia/convulsions, treat sepsis with ampicillin and gentamicin.

34.4 Infections in Infants 1 Week to 2 Months

Pneumonia

Hospital Care for Children, WHO 2005, IMCI: WHO, UNICEF 2005; Lancet 2008;371:135.

Epidem: Clinically divided into very severe, severe, and nonsevere
H. influenza, S. pneumo, Group B streptococcus, gram negative bacilli, others.

Sx: Cough, dyspnea, fever.

Si: Alar flare, subcostal recessions, grunting, central cyanosis, coarse crackles on auscultation, bronchial breath sounds, pleural rub.

Dx: Very Severe Pneumonia:
Cough or dyspnea with ≥ 1 of the following:
- central cyanosis
- inability to feed/persistent vomiting
- convulsions, lethargy, or loss of consciousness
- severe respiratory distress.
- ± other clinical signs and symptoms of pneumonia

Severe Pneumonia

Cough or dyspnea with ≥ 1 of the following:

- subcostal recessions
- alar flare
- grunting
- ± other clinical signs and symptoms of pneumonia

Nonsevere Pneumonia

- Child has cough or dyspnea and tachypnea: 2–11 months ≥ 50 per min; 1 to 5 y ≥ 40.
- Rule out signs of severe or very severe.
- ± other clinical signs and symptoms of pneumonia.

Lab: CBC, blood culture

Xray: Consider CXR

Rx: Supportive:

- Clear secretions.
- O2 via nasal prongs or nasopharyngeal catheter (check prongs/ catheter every 3 hr for blockage).
- Pulse oximetry if available.
- Maintenance IVF, continue to encourage breast feeding and oral intake, NGT if too tachypneic or unable to take oral feeding.
- If temp > 39°C/ >102.2°F and causing discomfort, give paracetamol
- Antibiotics (see chapter 17.1).

Meningitis

See chapter 17.8.

Sepsis

Cause: Serious bacterial infection in a young infant (includes meningitis and pneumonia). S. pneumo, Meningococcus, gram negatives, Group B Strep, H. influenza.

Sx: Lethargy, poor feeding, vomiting, convulsions.

Si: Fever or hypothermia, pallor, cyanosis, jaundice, apneic spells, irregular breathing, grunting, shock.

Crs: Good prognosis with early diagnosis and antibiotics; however, illness may be fulminant and lead to death in a few hours or may be protracted.

Lab: Blood culture, electrolytes, urine.

Rx: Supportive therapy as for meningitis.

Give all sick neonates < 2 wk 1 mg IM vitamin K.

Ampicillin 50 mg/kg q 6 hr IM/IV, or

Benzylpenicillin 50 000 u/kg q 6 hr IM/IV, plus

Gentamicin 7.5 mg/kg (3 mg/kg low birth weight (LBW), 5 mg/kg normal birth weight (BW) ≤ wk old) IM/IV daily.

Continue treatment until stable/well for at least 4 d. If hospital acquired or concerns of possible staphylococcus, give cloxacillin 50 mg/kg q 6 hr instead of ampicillin plus gentamicin as above. If no response to treatment in 48 hr or condition deteriorates, add chloramphenicol 25 mg/kg q 8 to 12 hr (do not use in premature infants, LBW, avoid < 1 wk old).

If known pneumococcal resistance to penicillin, change to cefotaxime 50 mg/kg plus ampicillin 50 mg/kg both q 6 hr.

34.5 Emergency Drug Doses

Shown in Table 34.1.

Table 34.1 Emergency Drug Doses

Drug (Conc.) and indication	Dose	Administration/Remarks
Bicarbonate (0.5 mEq/ml) Documented metabolic acidosis	1–2 mEq/kg IV slowly	Not routinely given for resuscitation. Note: Use only 0.5 mEq/ml solution for infants

(continues)

Table 34.1 Continued

Drug (Conc.) and indication	Dose	Administration/Remarks
Epinephrine (1:10 000) Severe bradycardia and hypotension Heart rate should rise to ≥ 100 within 30 seconds After bolus infusion	0.1–0.3 ml/kg IV or intratracheal equal to 0.01–0.03 mg/kg/dose of 1:10 000 concentration For continuous infusion—start at 0.05 mcg/kg/min	Warning: Never use undiluted 1:1000 concentration Never inject into an artery IV push or IT followed by 1 ml normal saline Do not mix with bicarbonate If heart rate remains < 100, may repeat dose every 5 min as needed
Volume expanders Plasmanate, NS Hypotension or hypovolemia with evidence of acute blood loss or decreased effective plasma volume	10–15 ml/kg IV over at least 10 min but preferably over 30–60 min.	Consider if poor response to resuscitative efforts or weak pulses with a good heart rate
Glucose (D10W) Hypoglycemia	IV—2 ml/kg of D10W and/or constant infusion of D10W at rate of 100 ml/kg/d	(8 mg glucose/kg/min)
Naloxone (400 μgm/ml) Severe respiratory depression and maternal narcotic within the past 4 hr	10–100 μml/kg inject rapidly IM, IV, IT, SQ	Delivery room: 1 ml vial Never give to infant of opiate addicted mother (may cause seizures) May repeat in 5 min if no response during resuscitation Duration (1–4 hr) may be less than the narcotic, needing repeated doses
Dopamine To give 10 mcg/kg/min @ 1 ml/hr: weight (in kg) × 30 = mg of dopamine in 50 ml D5W/NS	Begin at 5 mcg/kg/min May increase in increments of 2.5–5 mcg/kg/min as needed up to 20 mcg/kg/min	Consider if poor peripheral perfusion, evidence of shock, or thready pulses after epinephrine and volume expansion (and bicarbonate)

Chapter 35

Obstetrics

35.1 Antenatal Care

Overview Safe Motherhood

Lancet 2007;370:1283–1371, issue devoted to maternal health; *Life Saving Skills, Essential Obstetrical Care*, Guidebook from TALCuk.org.

An estimated half million women die in childbirth each year, most in Africa and Asia. The lifetime risk of a pregnancy-related death is 1:16 in Sub-Saharan Africa (920/100 000 per pregnancy), 1:46 in South-Central Asia. Most mortality is from obstetrical hemorrhage, infection, eclampsia, obstructed labor, and unsafe abortion (N Engl J Med 2007:1365–1395).

One objective of the United Nations Millennium Development Goals is to reduce maternal mortality by 75% by 2015.

Reducing maternal morbidity and mortality requires careful regular prenatal care, skilled birth attendants with the ability to refer women to medical facilities with skilled surgical personnel (not necessarily a doctor), blood, and antibiotics.

The role of the antenatal clinic is as follows:

- Familiarize the woman with the maternity team and their methods.
- Integrate the MCH team into the community of women, their children, the baby's father, and the local midwives.
- Conduct a rapid assessment and management (RAM) of emergencies or urgent problems.

- Assess pregnancy status and prepare a birth plan.
- Share information.
- Respond to requests and illnesses.
- Deliver preventative services.
- Prepare and maintain prenatal records (antenatal cards).

Prenatal Visits

First: as early as possible in pregnancy	< 16 wk
Second: 6 months	24 to 28 wk
Third: 8 months	30 to 32 wk
Fourth: 9 months	36 to 38 wk

More frequent visits may be necessary per national policy or with problems in this or previous pregnancy.

Low-risk women should be encouraged to attend 4 clinic visits, high-risk women more. Where possible, local midwives (traditional birth attendants; TBAs) should be asked to bring their clients to the prenatal clinics in order to coordinate services.

This section provides a brief overview of ideal maternity services as presented in Pregnancy, Childbirth, Postpartum and Newborn Care: A Guide for Essential Practice: WHO, 2006. MCH staff will have their own routine, which should be respected and supported. One of the most important determinants of successful MCH clinics is consistency. The MCH team should arrive at their clinic site on time, in a reliable fashion, ready to deliver all services. All other health center and hospital tasks (except dire emergencies) should be second in priority to MCH clinics.

Preventive Measures

Institute these actions unless the national MCH guidelines dictate otherwise.

Tetanus Toxoid (TT):

Give 5 immunizations during the childbearing years. Dose is 0.5 ml IM.

TT1 at first antenatal visit.

TT2 at next antenatal visit (at least 4 wk later).

TT3 at least 6 months after TT2.

TT4 at least 1 yr after TT3 (often during next pregnancy).

TT5 at least 1 yr after TT4.

Iron/Folic Acid Tablets:

Give 1 tablet 60 mg/400 mg daily throughout pregnancy. Continue for 3 months postpartum or postabortion. Double the dose for anemic women. Take with vitamin C-containing fruits. Multivitamins may increase birth weight (N Engl J Med 2007;1423) and reduce early infant mortality (Lancet 2008;371:215).

Treat for Worms:

After the first trimester, mebendazole 500 mg or albendazole 400 mg once. For women with anemia, mebendazole 100 mg daily for 5 d.

Prevent Malaria:

Most countries have a national policy for preventative intermittent treatment of malaria. Advise women and children to sleep under a treated bed net. Give 3 tablets sulfadoxine 500 mg + pyrimethamine 25 mg at the beginning of the second and third trimesters for malaria prophylaxis. Treatment of acute malaria is different.

Increased Susceptibility to Infections:

Emerg Infect Dis 2006;12:1638

Pregnant women are more susceptible or have more severe clinical courses of these diseases:

- malaria: increased prevalence and parasite density
- measles: severity increased
- toxoplasmosis: twice as likely to seroconvert
- leprosy: increased relapse
- listeria: more common
- influenza: more severe

OBSTETRICS

- varicella: rate of pneumonia increased
- pneumocystis: increased infection and carriage

Laboratory Screening:

The extent of screening will depend on local resources and national policy. Recommended tests include:

- anemia: Hb and examination, iron, folate, worm, and malaria rx
- syphilis: RPR or VDRL and examination, antibiotics, check partner
- HIV: rapid HIV test and examination
- UTI: urine dipstick, history
- vaginal discharge: examination, microscopic examination, culture
- other tests that may be appropriate: blood type and Rh

Antenatal History:

If on antituberculosis medications, change streptomycin to another drug. If HIV+ and on ART, a change in medications may be necessary (see Table 14.9). Plan on PMTCT. Counsel on nutrition and food taboos, drugs, alcohol, tobacco, HIV and STIs and safer sex, take only prescribed medications, compliance with visits and medications, birth and emergency plan, family planning, breast feeding, and home vs hospital delivery.

Planning for a medically supervised delivery is best begun during the first visit. Based on the medical and obstetrical history and the physical exam, it is often possible to identify those at greatest risk. Ask the woman why she is seeking antenatal care. Encourage antenatal care and supervised delivery. Instill confidence in the woman for the local health center and staff. Try to keep maternity clinics relaxed and low pressured, with individualized attention. Develop a birth and an emergency plan. The greatest deterrents to supervised delivery are: no confidence in staff, distance, provision of care for the home and other children when away for delivery, and culturally unacceptable facilities or practices.

As a general rule the following women should deliver at a health facility:

- HIV+
- previous uterine scar or complicated delivery
- grand multiparity, ≥ 5
- severe medical illness: diabetes, heart disease, anemia
- malnutrition, protein, caloric, osteomalacia
- short stature (< 1.6 m has been used)
- very young (< 15 yr), very old (> 40 yr), first pregnancy and > 35 yr
- any danger signs, bleeding before labor, pre-eclampsia, etc
- malposition or multiple gestations suspected

Women should move near or into the hospital 3 wk prior to their due date. Suitable hospital-maintained local-style housing and gardens make this transition more acceptable. These "maternity villages" have reduced maternal mortality 10-fold and the stillbirth rate 6-fold (*Obstetrics and Gynaecology in the Tropics and Developing Countries*, Lawson and Stewart 1967).

35.2 Management of Labor

OBSTETRICS

Induction

Indicated for the following:
- preeclampsia with > 36 wk fetus
- severe preeclampsia or eclampsia at any gestation
- pregnancy ≥ 42 wk
- diabetic pregnancy ≥ 40 wk
- fetal death in utero after waiting 1 to 2 months
- placental abruption with DIC

Contraindications:

- grand multiparity ≥ 5 deliveries (relative)
- breech or transverse

- previous C-section
- maternal heart disease

These indications and contraindications may vary depending on the circumstances so read the appropriate section first.

Success will depend, in part, on the Bishop's score shown in Table 35.1.

You can ripen the cervix over time with a Pitocin drip (maximum 20 units in 1 L NS over 36 hr) or prostaglandin suppositories, misoprostol, or a Foley catheter placed through the cervix, inflated with 10 ml water, and hung over the bed with a 250 gm weight.

To begin an induction:

- Review the woman's last menstrual period (LMP) and estimated date of confinement (EDC) dates.
- Consider the urgency and ripen the cervix if possible.
- Rupture the membranes aseptically with an amino hook, long-toothed forceps, or a spinal needle if the presenting vertex is not engaged. Beware prolapse of cord!

Table 35.1 Bishop's Score for Induction of Labor

Finding	Score			
	0	1	2	3
Cervical dilatation	0 cm	1–2 cm	3–4 cm	> 4 cm
Cervical length	3 cm	2 cm	1 cm	0 cm
Cervical consistency	firm	medium	soft	—
Cervical position	posterior	midpoint	anterior	—
Fetal head (station) compared to ischial spine	–3 cm	–2 cm	–1 cm	≥ 0

Maximal score 13
Favorable ≥ 9
Unfavorable ≤ 8

- Prepare a Pitocin drip if no contractions at 1 hr.
- Use established guidelines or mix 4 IU Pitocin in 1 L NS (0.004 IU/ml).
- Start at 15 drops/min and increase 10 drops q 20 min.
- Aim for contractions every 3 min lasting 50 to 60 seconds. A skilled staff member must never leave the mother's side.
- If unsuccessful after 60 drops per min, double the strength of the Pitocin drip to 8 IU in 1 L NS.
- Adjust the rate of infusion to maintain good contractions.
- Stop momentarily if contractions are too close together or last longer than 90 seconds.

  Tips on using Pitocin:

- 1 drop = 1/15 ml. Read the IV set instructions; pediatric IV sets are 1 drop = 1/80 ml.
- Infusions greater than 0.03 micro units/min (36 ml/min) are the maximum (0.008 IU/ml).
- Pitocin works like antidiuretic hormone (ADH) and prolonged infusions will cause hyponatremia, water intoxication, and seizures. Never mix in D5W.
- Pitocin's half-life in the blood is < 3 min.
- Large doses of Pitocin (5–10 IU) given IV push may cause profound hypotension.
- Pitocin used unwisely will kill the mother and/or her fetus.

Using a Partograph: Induction

A *partograph* or *cervicograph* is an essential graphic aid in monitoring labor. All obstetrical staff should be trained to complete the chart in every labor. If examination gloves are in short supply, descent of the head is a substitute for cervical dilatation (Figure 35.1). The partograph is used for the following:

- to identify normal progression
- to detect dysfunctional labor and prompt early action
- to monitor cephalic or breech presentations

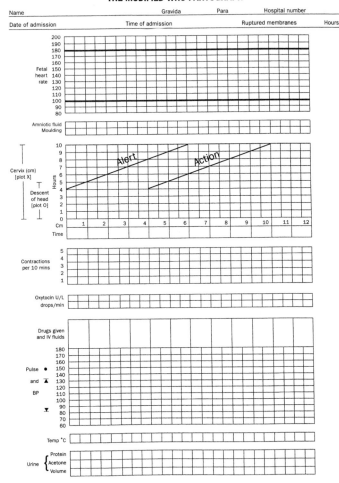

Figure 35.1 Partograph. (Reproduced with permission of WHO. *Pregnancy, Childbirth. Postpartum and Newborn Care: A Guide for Essential Practice*, WHO 2006.)

USING THE PARTOGRAPH

1 Record the following patient information:
   - Name
   - Gravida
   - Para
   - Hospital number
   - Date and time of admission
   - Time of ruptured membranes.

2 Assess cervical dilatation. If the cervix is at least 4 cm dilated, mark the dilatation on the Alert line. Use "X" to indicate cervical dilatation. Record the actual time on the X axis, corresponding to this point on the Alert line.

3 Record the following information on the partograph, starting from this point.

   Every 30 minutes, record:
   - Fetal heart rate
   - Contractions:
     - Palpate number of contractions in 10 minutes and shade the corresponding number of boxes
     - Use the following scheme to indicate the duration of contractions:

   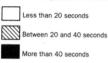

   - Oxytocin infusion: record the amount of oxytocin per volume IV fluids in drops per minute when used
   - Pulse rate

   Every 2 hours, record:
   - Temperature

   Every 4 hours, record:
   - Blood pressure

   At every vaginal examination, record:
   - Cervical dilatation: use "X"
   - Colour of amniotic fluid:
     - I = Membranes intact
     - C = Membranes ruptured, clear fluid
     - M = Meconium stained fluid
     - B = Blood stained fluid
   - Moulding:
     - 1 = Sutures apposed
     - 2 = Sutures overlapped but reducible
     - 3 = Sutures overlapped and not reducible
   - Descent of head by abdominal palpation: assess descent in fifths palpable above the pubic symphysis: record as "O"

   Drugs: record drugs given, each time they are given

   Urine volume, urine protein and acetone: record every time urine is passed

Figure 35.1   Continued

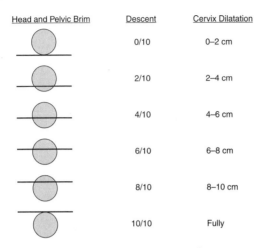

Head and Pelvic Brim	Descent	Cervix Dilatation
	0/10	0–2 cm
	2/10	2–4 cm
	4/10	4–6 cm
	6/10	6–8 cm
	8/10	8–10 cm
	10/10	Fully

Figure 35.2 Descent of the Head in Labor.

- when the cervix is ≥ 4 cm dilated
- when there are active, strong, frequent contractions

Plot the initial cervical dilatation at time zero (see Figure 35.1). The first diagonal line drawn at 2 hr is the alert line. The second diagonal line starting at 4 hr is the action line. As normal labor progresses with 1 cm of dilatation/hr, any delay will cross the alert line and prompt reassessment, possible intervention, or referral. If the action line is crossed, intervention or urgent referral to a facility where operative delivery is available is necessary.

If head descent is being used, divide the progressive movement of the head into 10 stations. Active labor is defined as the head 4/10 into the pelvis. Convert head descent into cm and plot on the cervicograph.

Obtain an APGAR score (Table 35.2) on every newborn at the time of delivery.

Table 35.2   APGAR Score

	0	1	2
Pulse	0	< 100	> 100
Respiratory effort	absent	slow irregular	crying, good
Muscle tone	floppy	some flexion	active
Reflexes	none	grimace	crying
Color	blue or pale	pink body blue extremities	completely pink

Do APGAR scores at 1 and 5 min. Repeat at 10 min if < 7 at 5 min.

35.3   Pregnancy Complications and Management

Antepartum Hemorrhage APH

Am Fam Physician 2007;75:1199

Vaginal bleeding before 20 wk gestation may be an abortion, an ectopic pregnancy, hydatidiform mole, implantation bleeding, or a number of other conditions. A speculum examination is indicated.

After 20 wk gestation, bleeding is defined as antepartum hemorrhage. The differential includes placenta previa, placental abruption, mole, or a cervical, vaginal, or labial lesion.

- Admit the patient or transfer when stable to the hospital.
- Determine the Hb, type and cross, and Rh factor (if appropriate).
- Resuscitate with IV normal saline and/or blood.
- Determine if this is placenta previa (painless bleeding, presenting part high), placental abruption, or partial abruption (painful hard uterus, frequent contractions).
- Obtain an ultrasound examination if possible.
- If uncertainty exists, vaginal examination should be done in the operating room already set up for an emergency

C-section if a placenta previa is identified and serious bleeding commences.

Molar Pregnancy

Suspect a molar pregnancy when:

- A "threatened" abortion continues to bleed after a week.
- The uterine size > dates.
- No fetal heart is heard after 12 wk with a fetoscope doppler or 20 wk with a stethoscope with no fetal movements.
- A pregnant woman presents with florid hyperthyroid-like symptoms (HCG resembles TSH and in high levels stimulates the thyroid.).

Diagnosis is confirmed by ultrasound examination or passage of typical grape-like vesicles in the uterine blood.

Treatment:

- Manage shock with fluid and blood.
- Start Pitocin 20 units in 1 L NS at 200 ml/hr.
- Perform a suction curettage when stable. Make a suction curette if need be out of firm suction tubing with holes cut in the side and the tip cut at a 45° angle. Follow with a sharp curette.
- Send samples to pathology.
- Give ergometrine (Methergine) l ampule after evacuation.
- Repeat curettage in 1 wk to insure the uterus is empty.

Follow-up:

- CXR to rule out metastasis
- Reliable contraception for 1 yr (Depo-provera)
- Follow-up every 2 months for clinical examination and pregnancy test. Do this for 1 year.

If the pregnancy test continues to be positive at the third month or turns negative and then positive, consider recurrent choriocarcinoma or a new pregnancy. Obtain an ultrasound.

Methotrexate may be curative for choriocarcinoma so follow the patient carefully.

Pre-eclampsia and Eclampsia

Pre-eclampsia:

- Elevated BP ≥ 140/90, which persists with the woman on her left side.
- Proteinuria > 2+, > 1/3 solid on boiling, or > 300 mg/24 hr.
- Generalized edema.
- Gestation > 20 wk, except in molar pregnancy.
- The diagnosis is supported by very active reflexes (clonus), headache, epigastric pain, changes in blood tests (see below).

Treatment:

- Admit the patient and nurse left side down.
- Keep a nurse in attendance.
- Place padded tongue blades between her teeth for seizures.
- Insert an IV, give NS or lactated Ringer's solution (LR) at 1 L/8 hr.
- Do not give diuretics for edema.
- Treat BP immediately if elevated BP persists over 6 hr or is dangerously high.
- Give 4 gm magnesium sulfate (20 ml of 20% solution) IV over 20 min, **and**
- Give 1 to 2 gm magnesium sulfate IV every hr, or
- Give 10 gm magnesium sulfate IM (5 gm 50% solution mixed with 1 ml (1% lidocaine) into each buttock with a long spinal needle).
- Check Hb, platelet count, kidney tests (BUN and creatinine), and liver tests if possible.
- Monitor urinary output and protein in urine.
- Wait 15 min after the last IV dose and give another 2 gm of magnesium sulfate for convulsions. If convulsions continue, give 10 mg diazepam slowly over 2 min.

Delivery is the best treatment for pre-eclampsia and eclampsia. If delivery is delayed:

- Give 5 to 10 gm of magnesium sulfate IM with 1 ml 1% lidocaine every 4 hr or continue at 1 to 2 gm IV/hr, or 5 gm IM q 4 hr.
- Ensure that the knee reflex is present, urine output is > 100 ml/4 hr, and respiratory rate is > 16 before giving magnesium sulfate.
- Do not give the next dose if all of these signs are not present. The antidote for magnesium sulfate overdose is calcium gluconate 1 gm IV (10 ml of a 10% solution) given over 10 minutes.
- Treat diastolic BP > 110 with hydralazine 10 IV or IM every 60 min until diastolic BP < 110. Or, use labetalol 5 to 10 mg IV every 60 min.
- Use furosemide 40 mg IV, oxygen, and stop IV fluids for pulmonary edema.

If magnesium sulfate is not available, use diazepam 10 mg IV; repeat if seizures recur. Give 40 mg in 500 ml NS or LR over 6 to 8 hr. Keep the woman sedated but arousable. Watch her breathing rate carefully and reduce the IV rate as necessary. Maximum diazepam is 100 mg/24 hr. Diazepam may be given rectally; start with 20 mg for the first dose. Do not give IM as absorption is slow.

- Do not rush to delivery until the mother is hemodynamically stable. A vaginal delivery is preferred.
- Expect a depressed infant if medications were given.
- Continue magnesium sulfate or diazepam for 24 hr after delivery.
- Do not give ergometrine (Methergine) postpartum as it increases BP. Use Pitocin (oxytocin) 10 units IM or an IV infusion 20 U/L NS.

HELLP syndrome (hemolysis, elevated liver tests, low platelets) may occur in severe pre-eclampsia. High mortality.

Prolapsed Cord

- Place the mother in a Trendelenberg (head down) position while supporting the presenting part with your hand.
- Administer a uterine relaxant if available: terbutaline 0.25 mg SQ, albuterol 4 mg orally, magnesium sulfate 4 gm IV slowly.
- Insert a Foley catheter; fill the bladder with about 1 L of saline and clamp. This will lift the presenting part out of the pelvis.
- Monitor the fetal heart carefully.
- Proceed to C-section.

    With twins, if the cord prolapses after the delivery of the first twin, do an internal version and a breech extraction. See twin delivery.

Symphysiotomy

A simple surgical procedure to divide the cartilage of the symphysis pubis and enlarge the birth canal.

Indications:

- A live fetus.
- Vertex presentation, not brow or mentum.
- Moderate cephalopelvic disproportionship with a failed attempt at vacuum extraction.
- C-section not indicated as woman unlikely to have supervised delivery in future and have significant risk of scar rupture.

Procedure:

- Have at least 2 assistants.
- Prepare the vacuum extraction set.
- Catheterize the bladder with a Foley and leave it in.
- Infiltrate 10 cc local anesthetic into the skin over and into the symphysis in the midline.
- Have the assistants hold the legs 80° apart. Do not allow the legs to fall apart!

OBSTETRICS

- Move the catheterized urethra to one side with your hand in the vagina.
- Make a stab wound through the skin and cut the fibers of the symphysis and arcuate ligament taking care not to cut through to the vagina.
- You will feel and hear the symphysis separate.
- Use vacuum if spontaneous delivery does not occur rapidly, pull downwards.
- Never use forceps.
- Compress the symphysis after delivery to control bleeding and suture the skin.

After care:

- Keep the catheter in 2 to 3 d or longer if necessary.
- Have the woman stay on her side to compress the symphysis.
- Ambulate after 1 to 2 d using a cane or walker.
- Wrap a bandage or bed sheet around the hips to stabilize the pelvis.
- Recovery takes 1 to 4 wk.

A symphysiotomy widens the pelvis and should facilitate subsequent deliveries. It cannot be repeated. If obstruction occurs with the next pregnancy, do a C-section.

Breech Delivery

There is a higher risk of fetal death or damage, especially if delivery is not carefully managed. Try external version first if conditions are met.

Management:

Obtain an ultrasound or X-ray (best unless there is an experienced sonographer) to determine frank (hips and knees extended), full or complete (hips extended and 1 or 2 knees flexed), or incomplete (one or both feet below the breech). Also, look for hydrocephalus (consider a destructive procedure) or hyperextension of the fetal head (do a C-section).

A C-section is usually advisable for the following:

- large fetus
- unfavorable pelvis
- not in labor with pre-eclampsia, prolonged rupture of membranes, previous C-section
- footling, full or complete presentation
- dysfunctional labor
- premature infant < 36 wk (prone to trapped head in undilated cervix)
- mother desires sterilization
- poor obstetrical history

Deliver with ≥ 2 assistants, 1 doctor for the baby, in the operating room if possible.

The first stage is managed using the partograph:

- Do not use Pitocin or artificially rupture the membranes.
- Check for a prolapsed cord when membranes do rupture.
- Do not allow the mother to push until full dilatation. If she continues to push, give morphine or meperidine (pethidine) to sedate her and ready nalorphine for the baby after delivery.

In the second stage:

- Empty the bladder.
- Have the mother in the lithotomy position.
- Allow 30 min of pushing; if undelivered, do a C-section.
- Anesthetize the perineum and cut a mediolateral episiotomy when the buttocks deliver.
- Have forceps with straight blades available.
- Deliver the leg by flexing one knee to the side of the trunk and pulling on an ankle. Repeat.
- Keep the baby's back up; wrap in a towel for support.
- Never pull; let the mother's efforts deliver the baby. If you pull, the baby's arms may extend trapping the head.
- Pull down, loop, and check the pulse once the cord appears.

- Delivery should occur in 5 min.
- Rotate the infant 90° to release the arm when the scapula appear, reaching into the vagina and sweeping the arm across the chest. Do the same for the other arm.
- Deliver the head by slow, controlled traction keeping it flexed. A finger in the mouth may be helpful as is suprapubic pressure. If this fails, allow the fetus to hang down over the perineum, its back towards you.
- Wait 1 to 2 min.
- Grasp the ankles, straighten the body and lift it up over the mother's body, swinging 180° while keeping the neck flexed once the suboccipital region is visible. Suprapubic pressure is applied.
- Suction the mouth and nose as the head appears.

Often a provider is called for a trapped head high in the pelvis. If the fetus is still alive:

- Cut a mediolateral episiotomy.
- Support the baby in your left supinated forearm, back up, your second and third fingers on its cheeks. Keep the head flexed.
- Put your right hand in over the baby's shoulders, 2 fingers on each shoulder, the middle finger on the occiput.
- Push down and back until the neck appears.
- Have an assistant provide suprapubic pressure.
- Apply forceps if necessary.
- Swing the baby up 180° as the head delivers.

Twin Delivery

Multiple Gestations

Women with twins or triplets are prone to more complications during pregnancy and delivery. Be certain the prenatal clinic staff consider the diagnosis when the following occurs:

- uterine size > gestational age
- uterine size > 40 cm

- uterine growth > 1 cm/wk
- term uterine size with small presenting part
- multiple fetal parts or > 2 poles on palpation
- persistent anemia
- family or personal history of twins
- polyhydramnios

All these women should be referred for imaging by ultrasound or X-ray. If multiple gestational confirmed:

- Admit to hospital or maternity village at 32 wk.
- Double iron/folic acid tablets.
- Follow Hb monthly.
- Monitor for complications.

Management of labor:

- Confirm fetal positions with X-ray, exclude multiple births (triplets), rule out locked or conjoint twins.
- Determine route of delivery based on X-ray.
- Start an IV with 1000 ml NS.
- Assemble adequate staff—at least 2 assistants.
- Clamp the cord with one clamp after delivery of the first twin. Check the position of second twin.
- Attempt an external version if transverse; hold the head in place and rupture the membranes. If this fails, rupture the membranes if needed; insert your hand into the uterus, bring down the legs and deliver.
- Clamp the cord of the second twin with two clamps.
- Check for a third baby.
- Add 20 units Pitocin to the IV and run at 200 ml/hr.
- Have Methergine available.
- Deliver the placenta(s).

If the mother arrives to you after delivery of the first infant with a dead, trapped second twin:

- If vertex or breech, start Pitocin to encourage uterine contractions and rupture the membranes.
- If transverse, sedate mother (ketamine is useful) and attempt a two-handed internal version. Pull the leg(s) down with one hand while pushing the arm and shoulder up with the other.
- If this is not possible, consider destructive delivery or a C-section.
- If indicated, give antibiotics.

Vacuum Extraction

Chalmers JA. *The Venthouse*. Yearbook Med Publishers, 1971 (classic text).

Indications:

- to avoid excessive maternal effort in certain medical conditions (heart disease, respiratory distress, eclampsia)
- fetal distress
- vertex (not brow or face)
- membranes ruptured
- head no more than one-fifth above pelvic brim (0 station)
- cervix fully dilated or nearly so
- bladder emptied
- adequate contractions
- mother who can push
- term infant ≥ 37 wk, ≥ 2000 gm
- second twin-vertex
- prolonged second stage

Technique:

There are several types of vacuum extractors available. Some have soft cups others have hard metal cups (Maelstrom). Use a 5 to 6 cm cup when available. First check the equipment and obtain an assistant.

- Confirm the fetal lie and engagement.
- Wash area with antiseptic solution.

- Place the mother in stirrups. Empty the bladder.
- Infiltrate the perineum with local anesthetic in case an epi-siotomy is necessary or use a pudendal block.
- Apply the cup over the posterior fontanel.
- Be sure the cervix or vagina is not included under the cup edge.
- Pump up the vacuum part way.
- Recheck and ensure there is an adequate leak-free seal.
- Pump up the vacuum to the maximum (100 mmHg).
- Pull with contractions in the direction of flexion of the head as the mother pushes. Keep the handle in line with the cup so the cup doesn't slide on the head. Cut an episiotomy if need be to obtain the correct angle of traction. The head should move with each pull.
- Release the vacuum as the head delivers.

Problems:

No progress after 3 pulls: C-section or symphysiotomy. If the baby is dead, perforate the skull.

Cup slips off—loss of suction.

- You may be pulling in the wrong axis.
- Air leak—check equipment.
- Pulling too hard; 40# is enough.
- Cup applied over caput; reposition the cup posterior to the caput.
- Loss of suction × 3 or cup applied for more than 30 min—quit.
- Fetal scalp trauma—stop.

Complc:

- vaginal abrasions 10%
- lacerations of scalp: cookie cutter like
- laceration of cervix 3%
- cephalohematoma 5% be sure the infant receives Vitamin K 1 mg IM
- subaponeurotic or subgaleal hemorrhage 2%

OBSTETRICS

- intracranial bleeding
- scalp necrosis (prolonged application)
- chignon: benign

The soft-cup vacuum extractor can also be used for delivery of the head during C-sections and for delivery of large ovarian cysts during laparotomy.

An option when neither forceps or a vacuum extractor is available is to have the mother hold on to a tied bed sheet and pull as the attendant pulls on the other end of the sheet lifting the mother partially out of the bed.

Cesarean Section

Surgery in Africa, May 2007

Helpful hints:

- Use other techniques if the fetus is dead or will die soon because of prematurity or malformations. C-sections are for live fetuses.
- Stabilize the mother first. Load with 500 to 1000 ml of NS or LR.
- Consider the risks: anesthesia problems, infection, bleeding, injury to bladder and ureter, and uterine rupture with subsequent deliveries.
- Always make a low segment horizontal incision in the uterus. Avoid classical or "T" incisions, which make the uterus prone to rupture with the next pregnancy. Classical incisions may be indicated for a live fetus in an obstructed transverse lie, a lower uterine segment with dense adhesions and inability to develop a bladder flap, constriction ring, anterior placenta previa with large vessels and no blood for transfusion. Try to do a tubal ligation (TL) if possible.
- Give antibiotics; for antibiotic prophylaxis, give a cephalosporin like cefazolin after the umbilical cord is cut. For

uterine and fetal infection, give 3 antibiotics: ampicillin, gentamicin, and metronidazole and start them before surgery.

- Find the foot and pull it out for a transverse lie. Deliver as a breech.
- Keep the uterus off the vena cava to maintain maternal venous return. Use a sand bag or IV fluid bag under the right buttock.
- Have an assistant correct any uterine rotation and hold it there before making a uterine incision.
- Consider the type of anesthesia carefully. A spinal can be deadly. If you are alone, use local and/or ketamine (see chapter 42).

Performing a C-section:

- Obtain consent for surgery and TL if necessary.
- Select anesthesia and prepare equipment and drugs.
- Consider antibiotics; if uterus infected, start now.
- Secure 2 units of blood.
- Have an assistant to care for the mother, another for the infant, and a third to assist you if possible.
- Position the mother on the operating table.
- Pass a Foley catheter.
- Prep the abdomen with soap then Betadine.
- Induce anesthesia.
- Open the abdomen.
- Identify the lower uterine segment, pick up the peritoneal reflection, and open it transversely.
- Develop a bladder flap and use a retractor to pull the bladder downward. If you were unable to empty the bladder because of difficulty passing a catheter, do it now with an 18-gauge needle attached to the suction.
- Open the uterus with a scalpel in the midline, have suction ready. Extend the uterine incision transversely with bandage scissors or traction.

OBSTETRICS

- Deliver the infant, clamp, and cut the cord. Obtain cord blood if necessary. Give one dose of prophylactic antibiotic now.
- Deliver the placenta and membranes.
- Start Pitocin 20 U/L of NS.
- Obtain culture if indicated.
- Clamp the lateral ends of the uterine incision and the upper and lower sides to control bleeding using ring forceps.
- Close the uterus with 1 or 2 layers of heavy absorbable suture such as 0 chromic. If the lower uterine segment is very thin, be sure it (but not the bladder) is included and the posterior wall of the uterus is not stitched into the wound.
- Inspect for bleeding, bladder injury, or other uterine tears.
- Do a TL if necessary.
- Irrigate the abdomen with saline.
- Leave the peritoneum unsutured.
- Close the fascia with a heavy nonabsorbable suture such as #2 Prolene.
- Pack the skin wound with antiseptic soaked gauze if the uterus was infected; otherwise, close the subcutaneous fat and skin.
- Consider retention sutures if the abdomen was grossly contaminated.
- Continue Pitocin 20 U/L NS or LR for 8 to 12 hr, 100 cc/hr.
- Monitor I & O and vital signs.
- Check the Hb the next day.
- Continue antibiotics for 7 d if the uterus was infected.

Cervical Tears

Always repair a torn cervix with good light and exposure. Use the OR (theatre). You will need an assistant. See Figure 35.3 Suturing of Cervical Tears.

Tears usually occur at 3 o'clock and 9 o'clock on the cervix. Anesthesia is unnecessary. Local anesthesia can be used for accompanying vagina or perineal repairs.

- Have the assistant push down on the uterus while using a retractor on the vaginal sidewall.
- Apply ring clamps to both sides of the tear and gently pull the tear into view.
- Start the stitch above the apex of the tear and sew towards you using a continuous locking O chromic suture.
- Place a ring clamp on the wound and leave it clamped for 4 hr if you cannot reach and suture the apex. After that time, loosen the clamp partially and leave it another 4 hr. If bleeding does not recur, remove the forceps 4 hr later.

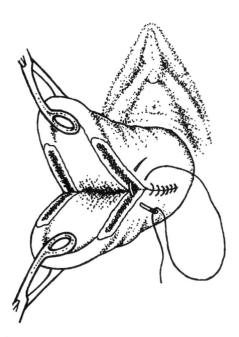

Figure 35.3 Suturing of Cervical Tears. (Reproduced with permission of WHO. *Surgical Care at the District Hospital*, WHO 2003.)

OBSTETRICS

- Do a laparotomy if the tear extends beyond the vagina and into the abdomen.

External Cephalic Version

Used to change singleton breech or transverse to vertex presentations. The technique is simple, usually safe, and successful in a majority of cases. Often the local midwives do the procedure themselves.

Conditions:

- presenting part not engaged
- ≥ 34 wk
- adequate amniotic fluid

Contraindications:

- antepartum hemorrhage
- previous C-section
- severe HT
- ruptured membranes
- twins

Technique:

- Confirm lie with X-ray or ultrasound if necessary.
- Monitor fetal heart.
- Flex the vertex toward the fetal chest while pushing the anterior thighs upward.
- Reverse directions if unsuccessful.

Often the uterus can be relaxed with 0.25 mg terbutaline SQ or albuterol 4 mg orally (give 1 hr before). If the mother is anxious, give diazepam 5 mg orally 1 hr prior. Excess force may separate the placenta.

Postpartum Hemorrhage

A blood loss greater than 500 ml, which occurs within the first 24 hr of delivery, is postpartum hemorrhage (PPH). Prevention is the best management. Anticipate PPH in high-risk women.

- history of PPH
- grand multiparity ≥ 5
- large uterus due to twins, polyhydramnios, large fetus
- long labor
- instrumented delivery
- extensive lacerations of the birth canal
- low lying placental attachment

A hospital delivery should be planned with an IV of normal saline started. Have Methergine (ergometrine) 0.5 mg available to give IV or IM unless BP is very high and/or Pitocin (oxytocin) 20 U/L of NS available.

At the time of delivery:

- Consider giving 10 U Pitocin IM or Methergine IM with delivery of the shoulder. Not with twins!
- Deliver the placenta promptly with controlled cord traction.
- Massage the uterus vigorously through the abdominal wall.
- Give uterotonics if needed. Pitocin may be run in as fast as possible then reduced to 200 ml/hr once bleeding is controlled. Methergine may be repeated hourly.

If bleeding persists:

Massage the uterus until firm, placing one hand in the vagina to support the uterus while the other hand massages through the abdominal wall. See Figure 35.4 Bimanual Uterine Compression.

- Call for help.
- Check that the placenta has delivered completely and no pieces or accessory lobes remain in the uterus if the uterus is firm but bleeding continues.
- Search for cervical or vaginal tears.
- Continue ergometrine and/or Pitocin.
- Draw blood for type and cross.
- Catheterize bladder.
- Remove placenta manually if it is retained.

OBSTETRICS

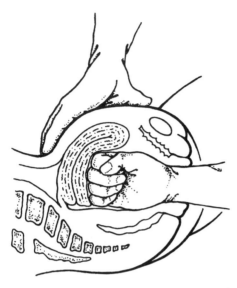

Figure 35.4 Bimanual Uterine Compression. (Reproduced with permission of WHO. *Surgical Care at the District Hospital*, WHO 2003.)

If the placenta has delivered and is intact and bleeding still persists:

- Check for DIC. Is her blood clotting? If not, see treatment of DIC (chapter 37.3).
- Take to the operating room.
- Place the patient in Trendelenberg position and, with an assistant's help, explore the vagina and look for tears.
- Consider hysterectomy or ligation of uterine arteries if the apex of a cervical tear extends above the vagina or bleeding still cannot be controlled.
- Have an assistant push down on the aorta to help control bleeding.

- Never rush to surgery with an unstable patient in shock or with untreated DIC.

Secondary PPH occurs more than 24 hr after delivery. Usual causes are retained products of conception with or without infection.

- Resuscitate the patient with IV NS or blood.
- Start a Pitocin infusion.
- Start antibiotics: chloramphenicol 1 gm or ampicillin 1 gm with metronidazole 500 mg IV.
- Do a uterine curettage with a large curette, or better still, a large suction curette.
- Secondary PPH following C-section is serious and requires laparotomy and perhaps a hysterectomy.

Women who have had a PPH will need iron and folic acid and reliable contraception. They should be told to seek prenatal care early and always deliver in a hospital.

Uterine Inversion

Postpartum inversion of the uterus is more common with fundal implantation of the placenta, placenta accreta, a relaxed uterine lower segment, and excessive cord traction. See Figure 35.5 Replacing Inverted Uterus.

Shock is usual and blood and fluid resuscitation should be immediately begun.

- Have an assistant give morphine sulfate and prepare for ketamine or general anesthesia (halothane works best).
- Wash the uterus with antiseptic solution; leave the placenta attached until all is prepared.
- Placing one hand on the abdomen, remove the placenta, and push the uterine fundus into the vagina, aiming for the umbilicus.
- Try hydrostatic correction if manual replacement fails.
- Place the woman in a deep head down (45°) position.

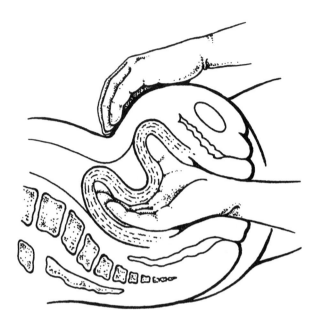

Figure 35.5 Replacing Inverted Uterus. (Reproduced with permission of WHO. *Surgical Care at the District Hospital*, WHO 2003.)

- Prepare 5 L warmed sterile saline or a disinfectant douche solution. Elevate the reservoir 2 m.
- Place a large catheter in the posterior fornix of the vagina.
- Seal the labia with your hands and fill the vagina with solution. As you fill the vagina with the douche, the uterus should gradually return into the abdomen.

If this fails, it is necessary to open the abdomen. Incise the lower peritoneum and protect the bladder as in C-section. The constricting cervical ring can be dilated with fingers while the uterine fundus is pulled up with a strong traction suture or tenaculum. An assistant should push from below. Cut the ring posteriorly if necessary to avoid bladder injury. Check for any other injuries, repair them, and close the abdomen. Once the uterus is replaced, start a Pitocin infusion of 40 U/L NS or LR and run at 100 ml/hr or faster if bleeding continues. Give Methergine or prostaglandins if necessary. Antibiotics are needed prophylactically (1 only) but use 3 if infection is present or develops.

Ruptured Uterus

The uterus may rupture due to obstructed labor, prolonged or injudicious use of Pitocin or prostaglandins to strengthen or induce contractions, or from operations used to relieve obstructed labor. The rupture is usually in the lower anterior segment; the tear is transverse or L-shaped and may extend into the bladder. Lateral tears may extend up into the fundus or down to the vagina and into the broad ligament and uterine artery. Posterior tears are usually transverse. Tears tend to follow lines of old uterine incisions. Ruptures are rare in the first pregnancy and increase with parity.

Dx: If the uterus ruptures along an old scar (C-section), there is dramatic sudden pain with cessation of labor. More commonly, there is a gradual onset of severe pain over the lower uterine segment. Blood may appear at the introitus and shock gradually develops. Generalized abdominal pain and guarding occur as blood and amniotic fluid spread throughout the abdomen. The contour of the uterus may change, and fetal parts become easier to palpate. Several signs in obstructed labor should cause the attendant to suspect ruptured uterus:

- Delivery of the placenta without delivery of the fetus.
- A gush of blood noted with a mobile presenting part.
- A prolonged postpartum bleed that does not respond to transfusion especially when the placenta is retained.
- Bright red blood in the urinary catheter.

The differential diagnosis includes placental abruption (not preceded by a prolonged labor), shock from any cause (usually sepsis), and a term extrauterine pregnancy.

Management is surgical and 6 or more units of blood should be obtained for transfusion and 3 antibiotics started immediately. Speed is essential. In brief:

- Remove the fetus and placenta.
- Control bleeding.
- Inspect the uterus for tears and close them with large bites of a running locking suture.
- Reflect the bladder off the anterior segment tears to avoid suturing it into the uterine wound.
- Identify the ureter prior to repairing lateral tears.
- Tie the fallopian tubes.
- Perform a simple supracervical hysterectomy if the lower segment is extensively damaged or badly infected.
- Repair the bladder in 2 layers. Be sure the systolic BP is greater than 100 mm to help identify all bleeders.
- Place a drain or two at the cervical stump and pass it through lateral stab wounds.
- Drain the bladder and leave the Foley catheter in for 14 d if the bladder was sutured.

Obstructed Labors with Dead Fetus

Destructive operations on the fetus are preferable to maternal surgery, but beware that you do not miss a ruptured uterus. If the baby is dead:

- Start an IV and give 2 antibiotics if there is evidence of prolonged labor. Gentamicin and ampicillin or chloramphenicol can be used.
- Empty the bladder and leave in a Foley catheter for 24 to 48 hr. If the bladder is empty, watch for a fistula.

- Vertex presentation with hydrocephalus: Perforate the head with a large needle or sharp straight scissors through a suture or fontanel. Smellies scissors are designed for this.
- Breech with hydrocephalus: Confirm by X-ray or ultrasound. Pull down on the legs and drain through the occiput.
- Vertex: Skull will be difficult to perforate. Drain the skull with scissors and use strong clamps to break up the bones carefully.
- Trapped breech with head retained: Sedate mother and tie 1 L bag of IV fluid (or similar weight) to fetal legs. If no delivery in 1 hr, perforate the head.
- Transverse lie: Have an assistant pull down on the arm and cut off the arm and head with a Blond-Heidler saw or strong scissors. A C-section may be needed.
- Always explore the uterus with your hand, feeling for rupture.

Repair of Vaginal, Perineal Tears and Episiotomy

Tears are classified as:

> First degree: vaginal mucosa plus connective tissue
> Second degree: plus muscle
> Third degree: plus complete anal sphincter
> Fourth degree: plus anal mucosa
> Repairs can usually be done with local or pudendal anesthesia. Use absorbable sutures.

- Check the rectum for mucosal or sphincter damage.
- Wash thoroughly.
- Close the rectal mucosa with 0.5 cm spaced 3-0 interrupted absorbable sutures placed through the muscularis and serosa, not the mucosa.
- Cover with the fascial layer; close with the same suture.
- Grasp the torn sphincter muscles with Allis clamps and repair with two or three 2-0 interrupted sutures. Include the muscle's fascial sheath for strength.

OBSTETRICS

- Check the repair by inserting a finger into the anus; check to be sure no sutures are through the rectal mucosa. Change gloves.
- Repair the vagina starting 1 cm above the apex of the wound using 2-0 or 3-0 running suture, stopping and tying at the opening.
- Close the perineal muscle and fascia with 1 or 2 layers of interrupted 2-0 or 3-0 sutures.
- Repair the skin with interrupted or a running subcuticular stitch.

Postprocedure Care

For a fourth degree tear, give a single dose of 2 antibiotics orally. Keep in hospital; give no enemas or rectal exams, and give stool softeners or a high fruit diet for 1 wk. Wash the perineum regularly and watch for foul drainage. If this occurs, remove sutures and dead tissue from any infected area.

Infected tears should be treated with 2 antibiotics. A secondary closure can be carried out several weeks later. Delayed primary closure is indicated for perineal tears that have been unattended for ≥ 12 hr. If it is a fourth degree tear, repair the rectal mucosa and the surrounding fascia as noted previously. Stop suturing here and keep the area clean and debrided with frequent antiseptic soaks. If the wound remains clean, resume the repair after about 6 d by suturing the torn sphincter muscles and continuing from there with a standard repair.

Retained Placenta

The placenta should always be delivered with controlled cord traction once it has separated. Separation is detected by a gush of blood and the cord lengthening 2 to 5 cm. Pitocin 10 units IM or Methergine 0.5 mg IM given with delivery of the shoulder may facilitate placental delivery. If the placenta does not deliver within 30 min of delivery of the infant, a retained placenta has occurred.

- Start an IV with normal saline.
- Have Methergine 0.5 mg or Pitocin 20 U/L of NS available.
- Check the vagina to be certain the placenta is not present or mostly out of the cervical os.
- Inject 20 units of Pitocin in 20 ml of NS into the maternal side of an umbilical vein as near to the vagina as possible and reclamp the cord.
- Wait 10 min and recheck the vagina.
- Pretreat the mother with ketamine 25 to 50 mg IV or morphine 5 to 10 mg IV or do a paracervical block (see chapter 42.2).
- Drain the bladder with a catheter.
- Enter the vagina and feel the cervical os using a clean gown and a new pair of sterile gloves.
- Place as many fingers as possible in the os and dilate it manually until the hand can be placed in the uterus. Stabilize the uterus by placing the other hand on the top of the fundus through the woman's abdominal wall.
- Develop the plane between the placenta and the uterine wall by sweeping the fingers around in a circle.
- Grasp the placenta in your hand and pull it out of the uterus in one piece once it is separated completely.
- Give an uterotonic drug.
- Inspect the placenta for completeness.
- Do a uterine curettage with a large dull curette if the placenta is not complete or retained products are suspected due to bleeding.

Antibiotics are not usually necessary unless the placenta has been retained for hours.

OBSTETRICS

If the mother arrives at the hospital late, but the placenta has been retained less than 72 hr, a similar procedure to above can be carried out but first:

- Start antibiotics IV (chloramphenicol 1 gm or ampicillin 1 gm and metronidazole 500 mg).
- Check the Hb.
- Type and cross match for 2 units of blood if Hb < 10 gm.
- Use ketamine or a paracervical block for better anesthesia.
- Give a uterotonic after delivery of the placenta.

If the placenta has been retained more than 72 hr, anemia and/or infection are probably present. Treat these first then proceed as above. If removal is impossible, abandon your efforts and cover the patient with IV antibiotics until the placenta discharges in fragments. Two weeks of observation and antibiotics may be necessary.

Women with a history of retained placenta should always deliver in the hospital as recurrence is common. Permanent sterilization may be lifesaving.

35.4   Antibiotics in Obstetrics and Surgery

This chapter bases its antibiotic regimes on those proposed by the WHO in *Pregnancy, Childbirth, Postpartum and Newborn Care: A Guide for Essential Practice*, second edition 2006. Exceptions may be necessary due to national policy, cost, and availability of medications. Dosages are for adults and should be adjusted for renal disease as appropriate.

One antibiotic:

- ampicillin 2 gm IV/IM then 1 gm q 6 hr, or
- chloramphenicol 1 gm IV/IM q 6 hr, or
- cefazolin 1 gm IV

Two antibiotics, add:

- metronidazole 500 mg IV q 8 hr, or
- tinidazole 1 gm orally q 12 hr

    Three antibiotics, add:

- gentamicin 80 mg IV or IM q 8 hr

    Allergic to penicillin (ampicillin):

- erythromycin 500 mg IV or IM q 6 hr

    Once the patient is free of fever for 48 hr, change to oral medications when possible. If malaria is suspected, treat appropriately (see malaria, chapter 10).

Chapter 36

Gynecology

36.1 Abortion (Miscarriage)

Abortion is considered a delivery of the fetus or embryo before 20 wk gestation or < 500 gm.

Threatened abortion: size of uterus equals dates, cervical os closed, usually little bleeding, and fetal heart may be heard by doppler or seen by ultrasound.

- Examine the os with a speculum to rule out other causes of bleeding.
- Treat cramping with oral acetaminophen (paracetamol) and observe.
- Obtain an ultrasound examination to rule out blighted ovum or hydatidiform mole.

Incomplete abortion: size of uterus often smaller than dates, cervical os opened ≥ 1 cm, heavy bleeding, fetal heart rarely heard, fetal tissue or membrane in os. A decidual cast (ectopic pregnancy), hyperplastic endometrium (dysfunctional uterine bleeding), or trophoblastic material of hydatidiform mole cannot always be distinguished by visual exam.

- Examine the os.
- Start an IV and treat shock if present.
- Give IV Pitocin infusion (20 U/L) or ergometrine 0.5 mg IM or IV.
- Remove tissue from the os with sponge forceps.
- Unless bleeding immediately stops, do a curettage.

- Use an ultrasound exam to confirm an empty uterus.
- Send any tissue for pathology examination if available.

Septic abortion may complicate an incomplete abortion or an induced abortion. The woman has a fever. The uterus and abdomen are tender, and shock may be present. Unsafe abortions: about 20 million/yr with an estimated 68 000 deaths.

- Start an IV and treat shock if necessary.
- Begin 2 IV antibiotics. Cover for aerobic and anaerobic bacteria.
- Perform a dilatation and curettage (D & C) once the patient is stable. Watch for perforation of the uterus. Occasionally a hysterectomy is indicated.
- Treat anemia.

Persistent fever may indicate septic thrombophlebitis, peritonitis, or pelvic/abdominal abscess.

Tip: Misoprostol 800 μgm vaginally may be used to complete first trimester, not septic, abortions. Vomiting and diarrhea are common side effects (Obstet Gynecol 1997;89:767).

36.2   Ectopic Pregnancy

Cause: More common in the first pregnancy, subfertility and history of PID or previous ectopic pregnancy; about 1% to 2% of pregnancies in Africa.

Sx/Si:

- abdominal pain (90–100%)
- anemia
- shock
- positive urine pregnancy test (> 90%)
- abdominal distention and tenderness
- 6 to 9 wk of amenorrhea (75–95%)
- mass on pelvic exam (< 50%), cervical tenderness
- vaginal bleeding, may be dark or bright red (50–80%)

Imaging: A pelvic ultrasound exam may be helpful or a culdocentesis. When in doubt, perform a laparotomy.

An unruptured ectopic pregnancy may occasionally be seen by transabdominal ultrasound (< 25% dependent on the quality of equipment and skill of the examiner). Transvaginal ultrasound improves diagnostic accuracy. If an intrauterine gestational sac is identified (> 5 wk), an ectopic pregnancy essentially is ruled out.

Rx: If quantitative HCG is available and the patient is stable, Methotrexate 50 mg/M^2 IM is an available treatment (N Engl J Med 1999;1974). Follow the levels down over about 5 wk or do a laparoscopy or laparotomy. Ninety-two percent success if HCG < 5000, 98% if < 1000. Pain is common 60%. Follow with ultrasound and Hb. Not if fetal heart or > 4 cm on ultrasound.

The treatment for an unstable patient is fluid resuscitation and laparotomy or laparoscopy.

- Open the abdomen.
- Set up an autotransfusion system if appropriate.
- Do a linear salpingostomy for ectopics < 4 cm. Make a linear incision over the ectopic, opposite the mesentery, remove with suction or pressure. No closure necessary.
- Do a salpingectomy for larger ectopics, those in the isthmus or uncontrolled bleeding.

36.3   Contraception

Family Planning: A Global Handbook for Providers 2007. WHO; available online at http://www.infoforhealth.org/globalhandbook.

How to Rule Out Pregnancy

Not being pregnant is important before starting many types of contraceptive methods. When pregnancy testing is unavailable or too expensive, ask the following:

GYNECOLOGY

- Do you have a baby less than 4 wk old?
- Do you have a baby less than 6 months old who is exclusively or almost exclusively breast fed?
- Did you have a miscarriage or abortion less than 1 wk ago?
- Was the beginning of your period less than 1 wk ago (or 12 d ago if starting an IUD)?
- Have you not had sex since your last period?
- Are you currently correctly using an effective contraceptive?

If any one question is answered "yes," the woman is probably not pregnant.

Family planning options in developing countries are often country specific. Programs are integrated into MCH teams for women while surgeons and medical officers do vasectomies. Condom use is part of the STI-HIV/AIDS division's health education efforts. The interested reader is referred to the publication listed above.

36.4 Infertility

Am Fam Physician 2007;75:849

A common problem that is difficult to investigate adequately at the district hospital, infertility is still important to undertake a preliminary investigation. In some cultures, a woman's ability to conceive may affect her marital status and security. Consider these issues:

- Intercourse with an individual wife may not be frequent enough to result in pregnancy in polygamous society.
- An older husband may be subfertile
- Anatomical problems
- Previous pregnancies by the man and in the woman
- Previous and chronic illnesses

A simple evaluation:

- Examination and sperm count on the male.

- Female pelvic examination to rule out fibroids, bifid uterus, infections especially pelvic TB (endometrial biopsy).
- Other testing may be indicated but is seldom available.

Never tell a couple they are infertile (depression, suicide, divorce). If a pregnancy subsequently occurs, infidelity may be suspected. Leave some hope.

36.5   Procedures

Culdocentesis/Colpotomy

Useful in the diagnosis of suspected ectopic pregnancy and drainage of collections of pus in the lower pelvis.

- Using a speculum blade and a tenaculum, elevate the cervix to visualize the posterior vagina.
- Wash the posterior fornix of the vagina with an antiseptic solution.
- Insert a spinal needle attached to a large syringe through the posterior vagina and into the pouch of Douglas.
- Aspirate:

    If nonclotting blood, consider ectopic pregnancy.

    If pus, take a long scalpel or clamp and perforate the posterior wall, put in your finger to break up any adhesions then push in a drain and suture it in place.

    If clotting blood (needle in vessel) or no fluid, try again several times. This may be normal, or see below.

- Clear or yellow fluid is found in normal women, in women with unruptured ectopics, or with ascites.

Dilatation and Curettage

Used for postabortion bleeding, menorrhagia unresponsive to medications, and diagnosis of postmenopausal bleeding, uterine polyps, hydatidiform moles, and suspected tuberculosis of the uterus. An endometrial biopsy using a suction cannula may be a better choice. Treat anemia and vaginal-uterine infections prior to a D & C.

Procedure:

- Obtain a pregnancy test if pregnancy is at all possible.
- Place patient in lithotomy position.
- Induce general anesthesia.
- Drain the bladder.
- Do a pelvic examination for uterine size, location, adnexal masses.
- Introduce a speculum.
- Grasp the anterior (upper) lip of the cervix with a tenaculum clamp and apply traction to straighten the uterus.
- Sound the uterus and record the measurement.
- Introduce progressively larger dilators. It is safer to hold a dilator with your thumb and index finger with the other fingers extended as you introduce the dilator into the uterus. This helps prevent a sudden uncontrolled forceful push of the dilator through the uterine wall.
- Introduce a sponge forceps to remove any polyps once the cervix is dilated.
- Curettage the uterus with a sharp curette or a suction curette, collecting the sample on a gauze pad placed in the vagina or in the suction bottle.
- Send samples for culture (TB in sterile NS) and pathology.

Pelvic Inflammatory Disease (PID)

Sexually Transmitted and Other Reproductive Tract Infections, WHO.

Cause: Usually polymicrobial, *N. gonorrhea*, *C. trachomatis*

Epidem: 75% in women < 25 yr. Exposure to infected or multiple partners. Increased risk in douching, new IUD, therapeutic or illegal abortions.

Pathophys: Inflammation of upper genital tract with scarring and tubal adhesions.

Sx/Si: Bilateral lower abdominal pain (90%), fever, rebound tenderness, cervical motion pain, adnexal mass; cervical discharge 75%.

Lab: WBC > 10 000 (50%), sedimentation rate > 15 (75%). Culture cervical discharge or culdocentesis.

Ultrasound: Occasional abscesses, free intraperitoneal fluid.

Rx:

Outpatient: Use treatment for GC + chlamydia and trichomonas as in chapter 13.2, continue for 14 d or use CDC recommendation: ofloxacin 400 mg twice a day plus metronidazole 500 mg twice a day or clindamycin 450 mg 4×/d; all for 14 d. Another option: cefoxitin 2 gm IM once plus 1 gm probenecid or ceftriaxone 250 mg once IM. Add doxycycline 100 mg twice a day to either for 14 d, or azithromycin 1 gm weekly ×2.

Hospitalized patient: 3 antibiotic regime (section 35.4), may substitute clindamycin 900 mg IV 3×/d for chloramphenicol, or second generation cephalosporin IV plus doxycycline IV or by mouth or WHO recommendations: Least expensive:

Ampicillin 2 gm IV or IM then 1 gm q 6 hr, plus
Gentamicin 80 mg IV or IM q 8 hr, plus
Metronidazole 500 mg IV q 8 hr (may give tablets PV).
Can substitute clindamycin 900 mg IV q 8 hr for ampicillin and metronidazole. Once better, continue for 2 d then stop and follow with doxycycline 100 mg twice a day or tetracycline 500 mg 4×/d for a total of 14 d of antibiotics.

Tip: Drainage of pelvic abscess(es) is often necessary. Consider culdocentesis. Severe PID may require laparotomy for drainage.

Prev: Hospitalization may facilitate the arrival of the sexual partner and his treatment, avoiding reinfection.

Chapter 37
General Surgery

Surgical Care at the District Hospital, WHO; *Surgery in Africa Monthly Review* online.

37.1 Introduction

Most medical providers will have had a minimum of surgical training and experience prior to an overseas posting. Even with some previous practice, they are unlikely to have seen such advanced illness or complicated trauma. If you are inexperienced in surgery, it is better to refer the patient than embark on a procedure beyond your capabilities. If transfer is impossible, at least try to speak with an experienced surgeon. This chapter will review some general principles and common surgical problems.

Wound Healing

Always (if possible):

- Place an incision along skin furrows (Langer's lines).
- Handle tissue gently; use nontooth forceps when possible.
- Keep tissue layers aligned and close dead space.
- Approximate, do not strangulate, skin edges.
- Remove devitalized tissue and foreign bodies.
- Use drains liberally and take advantage of gravity—put them at the lowest point. Advance (partially pull out) and then remove them when they quit draining.
- Protect the wound with splints.
- Consider circulation.

- Use delayed closure with contaminated wounds such as the skin incision with a ruptured appendix. Close the fascia. Pack the wound with gauze soaked in saline. Change dressing daily and debride as necessary.
- Prophylaxis against tetanus with tetanus immune globulin. Give a tetanus toxoid vaccine immunization if necessary.

Suture Material

Catgut: The degree of tissue reaction is directly proportional to the amount of suture material used. The tensile strength of chromic catgut exceeds that of plain catgut and both lose strength rapidly in infected wounds. Avoid running catgut sutures around drains where inflammation will weaken the suture; use interrupted sutures. As catgut is absorbable, use it for mucosal repair, uterine closure, the first layer of anastomosis of bowel repair, ligation of most blood vessels except the largest, and the first layer of deep wounds. Polyglycolic acid sutures have a greater and longer tensile strength than catgut and may be substituted.

Silk: Nonabsorbable, strong, and not prone to slip during knot tying, silk is readily available. Buried sutures should always be interrupted. Not suitable for vascular surgery. Used for the second layer of bowel anastomosis, skin closures, and in the mouth.

Cotton: Available in sewing kits, it can be used as a substitute for silk.

Plastic sutures: Nonabsorbable, they are ideal for vascular and tendon repairs and for facial and skin closures. Knots are prone to slip, and extra throws are necessary.

Various sutures: Vertical mattress sutures relieve wound tension and prevent wound edges from turning inward (see Figure 37.1).

Horizontal mattress sutures reinforce the wound and keep tension off the scar (see Figure 37.2).

Retention sutures pass through all abdominal layers and are used for debilitated patients, increased abdominal pressure, and

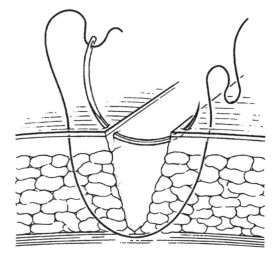

Figure 37.1 Vertical Mattress Suture. (Reproduced with permission of WHO. *Surgical Care at the District Hospital*, WHO 2003.)

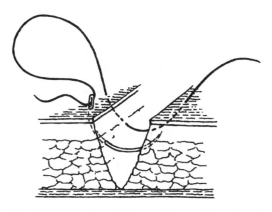

Figure 37.2 Horizontal Mattress Suture. (Reproduced with permission of WHO. *Surgical Care at the District Hospital*, WHO 2003.)

37.1 Introduction   **443**

suspected future wound infection to avoid or treat dehiscence (see Figures 37.3 and 37.4).

Sutures should be left in for an appropriate time to allow secure healing of the skin incisions, from 3 to 5 d on the face to 3 wk for incisions over joints on the limb.

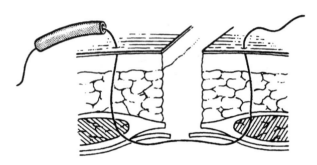

Figure 37.3   Retention Suture. (Reproduced with permission of WHO. *Surgical Care at the District Hospital*, WHO 2003.)

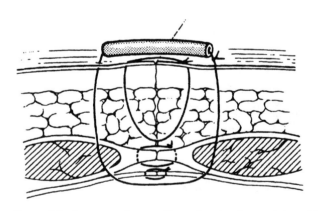

Figure 37.4   Retention Suture. (Reproduced with permission of WHO. *Surgical Care at the District Hospital*, WHO 2003.)

Chest tubes: Thoracostomy: When the chest wall is opened or a subpleural bleb ruptures, a pneumothorax occurs. Sucking chest wounds, open to the air, are closed emergently with petrolatum gauze, a moist pack, or a plastic bandage sealed with tape. If large, the wound should be closed in several layers in the operating room with positive pressure anesthesia. After closure, the air can be removed with a needle.

Closed thoracostomy is used for a large pneumothorax, a tension pneumothorax, or an empyema (see Figure 37.5, Chest Tube Drainage).

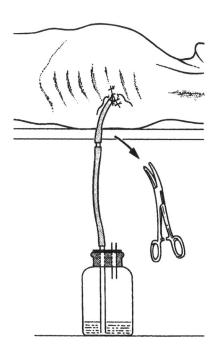

Figure 37.5 Chest Tube Drainage. (Reproduced with permission of WHO. *Surgical Care at the District Hospital*, WHO 2003.)

The third intercostal space in the midclavicular line is used for treating a pneumothorax, the ninth interspace in the posterior auxiliary line for an empyema. Confirm the presence of pus with an exploratory needle aspiration.

- Prep the skin and place local anesthetic in the skin, subcutaneous tissue, and intercostal muscle.
- Make an incision along the top of the rib to avoid the intercostal artery and nerve, wide enough for the trocar/chest tube.
- Plunge the trocar into the pleural space or use a large hemostat to open the tract.
- Guide the chest tube (1–2 cm diameter) over the trocar or grasp it firmly with the hemostat and introduce it into the pleural space. A fenestrated tube may help to drain an empyema.
- Introduce the tube 2–3 cm for a pneumothorax and far enough to encourage drainage from an empyema.
- Place a heavy stitch to securely anchor the tube.
- Set up a water seal drain as shown above. The bottle can be placed in a bucket to allow the patient to ambulate.
- Keep a clamp handy in case of a break in the continuity of the system.

Wait several days before removing the tube, when air leakage has stopped for 36 hr or until drainage ends, and the empyema is resolved (exam or CXR). Cut the stitch, have the patient take a deep breath, and remove the tube quickly. Cover the wound with a sterile watertight dressing.

Tendon Repairs

Tendon lacerations are common in regions where people carry bush knives for cutting firewood. The wound must be clean and less than 4 hr old. If these conditions are not met, clean the wound, close the skin leaving the disrupted tendon unsutured, and cover with antibiotics. A secondary repair can be carried out at another time in 4 to 6 wk. Flexor tendon repair is more difficult, and unless you have considerable experience, refer.

Repairs are best done in the operating room. Unless you are certain that only a single tendon is divided, review the anatomy (see Figure 37.6, Tendon Repair).

- Use a tourniquet; Bier's block provides adequate anesthesia. Maximum tourniquet time should be 1 hr.
- Keep the tendon moist with saline.
- Make the incision away from the tendon following skin creases if additional exposure is required.
- Irrigate the wound with saline and obtain hemostasis.
- Use nonabsorbable 5-0 suture (larger if needed for large tendons) and nontoothed forceps.
- Trim the proximal tendon end if necessary.
- Using a double-armed (2 straight needles), place the stitch shown in Figure 37.6.
- Release the tourniquet and ensure hemostasis.
- Close the skin; no drain is used.

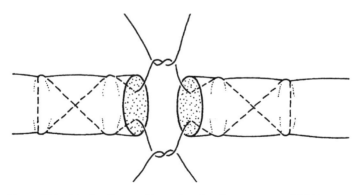

Figure 37.6 Tendon Repair. (Reproduced with permission of WHO. *Surgical Care at the District Hospital*, WHO 2003.)

Splint or cast the hand and wrist as indicated:

Lacerated wrist flexors: splint wrist in 45° flexion but leave the fingers free. Three wk splinting followed by another week of protected movement.

Lacerated wrist extensors: splint in 30° extension for 4 wk. Physical therapy should be arranged.

Abdominal Incisions

See Figure 37.7, Abdominal Incisions.

Only a few abdominal incisions will allow access for most surgeries. The object is to avoid cutting nerves, to provide adequate exposure, to ease closure, and to minimize pain, adhesions, and hernias.

Midline (A): The incision is straight forward; a lateral extension (a) may be used to increase exposure. The anterior and

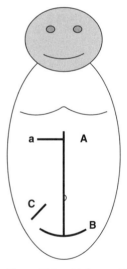

Figure 37.7 Abdominal Incisions.

posterior sheaths are cut and the intact muscle retracted laterally. Close the rectus sheaths first then the midline.

Pfannenstiel (B): An option to a lower midline incision. It takes longer and is more prone to bleeding and infection (Cochrane Database of Syst Rev 2007, Issue 1).

A transverse incision 10 cm long is made 4 cm above the pubis with a slight downward curve. The rectus sheaths are cut in the direction of the skin incision and dissected down to the pubis and about 8 cm upward. The rectus muscles are split, and the peritoneum is entered in the midline.

Transverse for appendectomy (C): Incise from the midline toward the iliac crest. Retract them medially or divide if necessary. Split the external, internal, oblique, and transversalis muscles laterally, parallel to their fibers. The peritoneum may be entered in any direction.

37.2 Fluids, Electrolytes

Monitoring electrolytes is usually impossible in most situations in developing nations. The practitioner is encouraged to prepare before their overseas posting by proactively managing IV fluids and electrolyte balance in their hospitalized patients. That is, carefully consider a patient's IV and electrolyte needs each day, aiming for a perfect balance the next day. Then, store this knowledge away for the time when you cannot obtain electrolytes.

Some general guidelines are given in Tables 37.1 and 37.2:

- Use normal saline if hypovolemic.
- Give crystalloid solution at a rate of 3 × equal to loss to restore intravascular volume.
- Hold potassium chloride (KCl) until renal function assured. D5 one-quarter NS with 10 mEq KCl or one-half strength Darrow's solution will usually keep the electrolytes unchanged with normal renal function (mmol = mEq).

Table 37.1   24-hour Basal Requirements

Age	Water	Sodium	Potassium
Adult	2500 ml	100 mEq	20 mEq
Child < 2 yr/kg	120 ml	2–3 mEq	1–2 mEq
Child > 2 yr/kg	80 ml	2–3 mEq	1–2 mEq

Table 37.2   Composition of Replacement Fluids

Fluid mEg/L	Na	K	Ca	Cl	Base	Colloid Osmotic Pressure
Normal saline	154	0	0	154	0	0
Ringer's/Hartmann's solution	130–140	4–5	2–3	109–110	28–30	0
Albumin 5%	130–160	< 1	variable			27
Normal plasma	140	4	2.5	105	40	27
Half strength Darrow's solution	60	17		52	25	2.5% dextrose

Electrolyte concentrations of body fluids:
Gastric: sodium Na 45 mEq/L, K 10 mEq/L
Pancreas: Na 110 to 150 mEq/L, K 2.5 to 7.5 mEq/L
Diarrhea: Na 100–140 mEq/L, K 5–35 mEq/L

Oral Rehydration Solutions

WHO ORS is usually available and contains mEq/L: Na 90, K 20, Cl 80, HCO_3 30, and glucose 20 gm (110 mmol).

Or, make your own: (1 teaspoon, tsp = 5 ml)

6 tsp sugar + one-half tsp salt + one-half tsp sodium bicarbonate and squeeze of citrus in 1 L clean water, or

Rice water (water left in rice after it is completely cooked) 1 L + one-half tsp salt + squeeze of citrus juice. Green coconut water adds K.

Replacement fluids can be given IV, intraosseous, via NG tube (do not use expensive prepared sterile IV fluids but do use old IV sets and bags), normal saline only subcutaneously via abdominal site (Am Fam Physician 2001;65:1575), or rectally as an enema as appropriate.

37.3 Transfusions

The Clinical Use of Blood, WHO Handbook 2001
Rules:

Whole blood is more commonly available in rural hospitals. In general it contains:

- Volume of blood ~450 ml per unit.
- Volume of anticoagulant + preservative 63 ml.
- No functioning platelets, factor V or VIII.
- H & H ~12 g/ml and 40%.
- May transmit HIV-1, HIV-2, HTLV, hepatitis A-E, syphilis, malaria, Chagas diseases, and occasionally others.
- Risk of volume overload.
- Type and cross ABO and RhD.
- Use a line with a blood filter.
- Never add medications, heat in hot water, leave unused outside of refrigerator over one-half hour. Only NS can be added/ mixed with blood for transfusion.
- Complete use by 4 hr.
- Change IV line every 4 units or 12 hr.
- Monitor patient (vital signs and I + O) during transfusion: when started, 15 min later, hourly, at end, 4 hr after completion.

Mild Reactions

Cause: Histamine release, mild reaction

Epidem: 1% to 2% of patients.

Sx/Si: Urticarial rash and pruritus.

Rx: Slow transfusion, administer antihistamine; if no improvement, stop transfusion and manage as moderately severe reaction.

Moderate-Severe Reactions

Cause: Possible mismatch, patient's preexisting antibodies, bacteria contamination (0.4%).

Epidem: Frequently transfused patients, lab, or ward error.

Sx/Si: Flushing, urticarial rash, fever with rigors, tachycardia, headache, mild dyspnea.

Rx: Stop transfusion, start NS, and give antihistamine and, if appropriate, antipyretic (not aspirin), steroids, and bronchodilators. Send transfusion set, urine, and 2 tubes of blood drawn from the other arm (one clotted and one in an anticoagulant tube) to lab. Collect urine for 24 hr and check for hemolysis. If not improved in 15 min, manage as life-threatening severe reaction below.

Life-Threatening Reaction

Cause: Probable mismatch with hemolysis, septic shock, anaphylaxis.

Epidem: Acute intravascular hemolysis usually occurs when 10 to 50 ml of transfused blood given.

Sx/Si: Anesthetized or unconscious patient may only show hypotension and bleeding; red urine; loin, back, chest, infusion site pain, dyspnea.

Rx: Give oxygen, assess for bleeding, pass urinary catheter, and look for hemoglobinuria. Give furosemide 1 mg/kg IV and consider broad spectrum antibiotics.

Delayed Hemolytic Transfusion Reactions

Cause: Rare antigen incompatibility

Epidem: Appears 5 to 10 d post transfusion.

Sx/Si: Fever, jaundice, anemia, occasionally hemoglobinuria.

Rx: Usually no treatment necessary except maintain hydration and urine output.

Indications for Transfusion

General guidelines for transfusion taken from *The Clinical Use of Blood Handbook* are listed below. A diuretic such as furosemide may be necessary to prevent volume overload. Packed RBCs are recommended. Hb in g/dL.

- β thalassemia major keep Hb at 10 to 12.
- Decompensated anemia.
- Malaria if Hb < 4 or very ill and < 6.
- Sickle cell crisis and Hb < 5 or > 2 below normal baseline. Goal is 7 to 8.
- Acute GI bleeding keep Hb > 9 until rebleeding unlikely.
- Pregnant < 36 wk and Hb < 5.
- Pregnant < 36 wk with CHF, malaria, severe infection, or heart disease and Hb < 7.
- Pregnant > 36 wk and Hb < 6.
- Pregnant > 36 wk and ill (as above) with Hb < 8.
- Infants and children Hb < 4.
- Infants and children with malaria and hyperparasitemia > 20% or hypoxia and Hb < 6.
- Surgery for minor procedures Hb < 7 to 8.
- Major surgery or decompensated patient may require a higher Hb.

Autologous Blood Transfusion

Useful when the blood supply is inadequate or suspect for infection. The patient's blood to be reinfused must be sterile and free of any contaminate. Ideal situations are blood in the abdomen from a ruptured spleen or ectopic pregnancy. Blood older than 6 hr should not be used.

Collect the blood with a small vessel and strain through a sterile sponge. Pour the blood into a transfusion bag containing anticoagulant whose top has been washed and cut off with a sterile blade. Transfuse through an IV blood filter.

Coagulopathy: Disseminated Intravascular Coagulation

The Clinical Use of Blood, WHO 2001

Cause: Infection, bacterial sepsis, malaria

Obstetrical, preeclampsia, abruption, amniotic fluid embolus, retained products of conception, retained dead fetus

Trauma

Malignancy, leukemia

Snake venom

Sx/Si: Bleeding, bruising, oozing at IV sites, organ dysfunction with respiratory, renal, hepatic, CNS failure. Palpable and petechial rash

Lab: Place 3 ml venous blood in clean test tube; keep it warm in your pocket. Time when a clot forms; 4 to 11 min is normal, longer with DIC, often > 20 min. Fragmented RBCs and decreased platelets on smear. ESR = 0.

If available, elevated prothrombin, partial thromboplastin, thrombin times. Decreased fibrin and increased fibrin split products (D-dimer).

Rx: Treat the underlying cause urgently. Give fresh whole blood if bleeding and give fresh frozen plasma 1 pack/15 kg body weight. Give cryoprecipitate and platelets if available and count < 20 000. Avoid heparin.

37.4   Burns

General Rules

- A serious burn is > 10% body area of child, > 15% in adult (see Table 37.3).
- These require IV fluid resuscitation.

Table 37.3   Estimating Surface Area of Burns %

	Adult	Infant-Child			
		Age < 1 yr	1–4 yr	5–9 yr	10–14 yr
Head + neck	9 (7 + 2)	21	19	15	13
Trunk + buttocks	31 (13 + 13 + 5)	31	31	31	31
Arm	9.5 each	9.5	9.5	9.5	9.5
Leg	20 each	14	15	17	18
Perineum	1	1	1	1	1

- Consider airway, breathing, circulation.
- Consider underlying conditions, seizure-causing fall into fire.
- First and second (partial thickness) burns have sensation and hurt.
- Third degree (full thickness) burns do not hurt as the nerves are killed.
- Hospitalize serious, circumferential, full thickness, head, face, hands, feet, and perineum burns. Also infants, elderly, trauma victims, otherwise ill, and those with inhalation injury.
- Give tetanus immunization.

Fluid Requirements in Burns

Adults: 3 × weight in kg × % burned (maximum 45%) plus:
    Maintenance: kg × 35 ml
    Increase if indicated
    Give 50% in first 8 hr and 50% over next 16 hr
    Next day give:
    1 × weight in kg × % burned plus
    Maintenance: kg × 35 ml
Give over 24 hr
Children: Same calculation for % burned (maximum 35%) plus
    Maintenance: first 10 kg = 100 ml/kg

second 10 kg = 75 ml/kg

subsequent > 20 kg = 50 ml/kg

Give 50% in first 8 hr and remainder over 16 hr

Next day give:

1 × weight in kg × % burned plus

Maintenance as children above

- Replacement fluid for burn NS or LR or Hartmann's solution.
- Maintenance fluid one-half strength Darrows or D5 ¼ NS.
- Monitor urine output; keep at 0.5 ml/kg/hr in adults, 1.0 ml/kg/hr in children.
- Elevate burned limbs and head.
- Cover partial thickness burns.
- Insert urinary catheter.
- Use NG tube for vomiting, abdominal distention, burns > 20% of body.
- Give antacids or gastric mucosa protectors.
- Feed when possible 90 cal/kg, protein 3 gm/kg.
- Protect from flies with a mosquito bed net.
- Give multivitamins and iron (if necessary).
- Consider escharotomy for circumferential burns of limbs or chest.
- Provide physiotherapy.
- Give antibiotics only for contaminated burns.
- Use aseptic techniques.
- Transfer severe burns if able or seek expert advice.
- Debridement and skin grafting: remove all necrotic tissue and bullae; gently wash with 0.25% chlorhexidine or other water-based antiseptic. Cover with topical antibiotic (0.5% aqueous $AgNO_3$ inexpensive), nonstick petroleum gauze, and then dry gauze. Change 1 to 2 × daily when seepage.
- Skin grafting sometimes necessary for second degree and always for third degree.

37.5 Abscesses

Infect Dis Clin North Am 2006:20
General Principles (see Figures 37.8 thru 37.13).

- Incision and drainage is necessary to remove the pus.
- Many abscesses are fluctuant, tender, warm, with shiny skin.
- Deep abscesses may have none of these signs; do an exploratory needle aspiration using a ≤ 18-gauge needle.

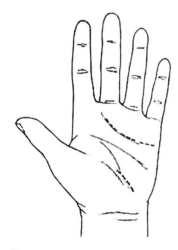 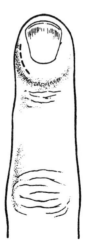

Figure 37.8 Incisions for Drainage of the Hand. (Reproduced with permission of WHO. *Surgical Care at the District Hospital*, WHO 2003.)

Figure 37.9 Drainage of Paronychia. (Reproduced with permission of WHO. *Surgical Care at the District Hospital*, WHO 2003.)

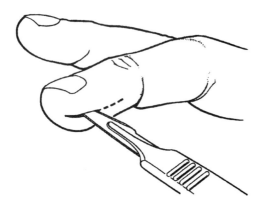

Figure 37.10 Drainage of Felon. (Reproduced with permission of WHO. *Surgical Care at the District Hospital*, WHO 2003.)

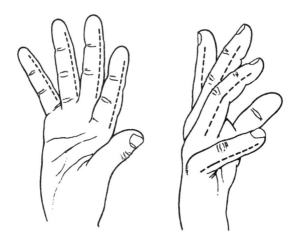

Figure 37.11 Drainage of Fingers. (Reproduced with permission of WHO. *Surgical Care at the District Hospital*, WHO 2003.)

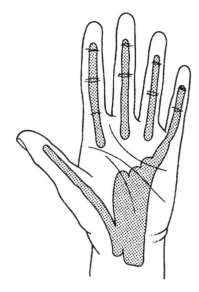

Figure 37.12 Palmar Fascial Spaces. (Reproduced with permission of WHO. *Surgical Care at the District Hospital*, WHO 2003.)

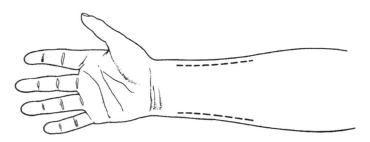

Figure 37.13 Drainage of Arm. (Reproduced with permission of WHO. *Surgical Care at the District Hospital*, WHO 2003.)

- Local anesthetics do not work in pus; do a field block or use ketamine or general anesthesia.
- Make a large enough incision at the midpoint of the abscess.
- Open the cavity with forceps; then use your finger to break down loculations.
- Culture and gram stain pus.
- Irrigate the cavity with saline.
- Pack the cavity with petroleum gauze or sew in a latex drain.
- Use gravity to facilitate drainage.
- Antibiotics are not usually necessary but give if fever, cellulitis, or abscess of hand, ear, or throat.
- Remember TT if needed.
- The mother may continue to breast feed from a treated breast abscess unless HIV+.

    In general:

- Use skin incisions as shown in figures.
- Follow palmar creases.
- Splint hand in position of function (as holding tennis ball).
- Remove drains in 1 to 2 d.

37.6   Pyomyositis

Usually caused by *Staphylococcus aureus*; *Streptococcus pneumonia*, and unusual pathogens in AIDs patients but occasionally associated with a preceding viral infection.

Common in tropical countries; etiology unclear.

Pus is found in the muscle. Most frequently the thigh, buttock, calf, shoulder, or abdominal muscles are involved. X-ray if appropriate to rule out underlying osteomyelitis.

Fever, pain, swelling, and restricted movement are present.

Treatment is wide I & D and debridement. Follow the abscess cavity with your fingers. If you touch bare bone, consider osteomyelitis and drain the bone (see chapter 39.4). Culture and gram stain pus. Keep the drain in until it stops draining, usually 2 to 3 d.

Cloxacillin (50 mg/kg/dose) 4×/d IV or IM until culture report.

37.7 Techniques

Burr Holes

Essential Surgical Care, WHO
When to do a craniotomy:

- unconscious with focal signs
- deteriorating consciousness with secure ABCs
- unconscious, lucid interval, now unconscious
- open skull fracture and deteriorating
- coma due to head injury with no improvement

Time is urgent; look for hemiparesis, seizures, pupillary dilatation, decreased pulse, and increasing BP.

- Use general anesthesia if possible or local anesthesia with epinephrine (never ketamine).
- Place a urinary catheter.
- Shave the entire scalp and prep for surgery.
- Give prophylactic antibiotic dose.
- Operate first on the side with the dilated pupil or contralateral to hemiparesis.
- Location of a temporal burr hole is 3 cm above the midpoint of the zygomatic arch.
- Incise the skin, separate the muscle, control bleeders as necessary. Insert a retractor.
- Incise and reflect the periosteum using an elevator or scalpel handle.
- Use a Hudson Brace or similar drill to penetrate the bone using the sharp perforator bit until the inner table is just perforated.

- Change to a burr bit and widen the cone-shaped hole into a cylinder; the dura is now visible.
- Wash out any epidural hematoma with a syringe.

    If blood is beneath the dura (it is blue or tense), open it by pulling it up with a dural hook or a bent needle.

- Make a cruciate incision.
- Remove the epidural or subdural blood with gentle suction.
- If a clot has formed and cannot be extracted, a craniectomy is necessary.
- Extend the skin incision vertically.
- Remove the bone following the clot or active bleeding. Use bone nibblers or rongeur to open the skull as necessary.
- Tie off any arterial bleeders or undersew them using silk sutures. Or use cautery. Venous bleeders will stop with application of crushed temporalis muscle or gelatin sponge. Use bone wax on the burr hole bone edges.
- Close the dura tightly to prevent leakage.
- Place a drain (IV tubing or similar) if the dura is not opened or has been closed tightly with no leakage.
- Elevate any depressed fractures.
- Close the scalp in 2 layers.
- Perform burr holes in the frontal (in line of pupil at hairline) and parietal areas if no blood is found. Six holes may be needed. If blood was found, remember epidural hematomas are bilateral in 2% of cases.
- Nurse with the head up.
- Avoid vomiting.

Chapter 38
Urology

38.1 Techniques

Paraphimosis-Dorsal Slit

- Obtain a dorsal nerve block or a ring block of the penis using plain lidocaine (see chapter 42).
- Attempt to reduce the foreskin with gentle pressure on the glands to reduce edema. Press the glands downward with both thumbs and use the fingers to pull up on the prepuce.
- A dorsal slit may be made and the cut edges of the wound oversewn with fine running absorbable suture if reduction is unsuccessful.

Suprapubic Cystostomy

See Figures 38.1 through 38.8.

Useful for removal of stones and bladder drainage with urethral or prostate obstruction. Local, regional, or general anesthesia may be used.

- Fill the bladder if necessary.
- Place the patient in Trendelenberg position.
- Make a median or transverse incision 2 cm above the pubis extending through the fascia.
- Separate the muscles and push the peritoneal reflection and perivesical fat upward.
- Place 2 stay sutures or Allis clamps at 3 o'clock and 9 o'clock on the bladder to mark the incision site.

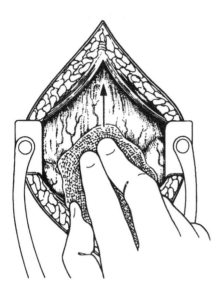

Figure 38.1 Suprapubic Cystostomy. (Reproduced with permission of WHO. *Surgical Care at the District Hospital*, WHO 2003.)

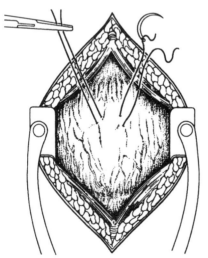

Figure 38.2 Suprapubic Cystostomy. (Reproduced with permission of WHO. *Surgical Care at the District Hospital*, WHO 2003.)

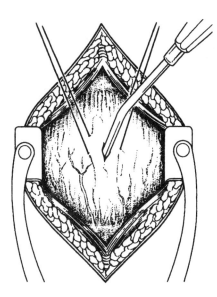

Figure 38.3 Suprapubic Cystostomy. (Reproduced with permission of WHO. *Surgical Care at the District Hospital*, WHO 2003.)

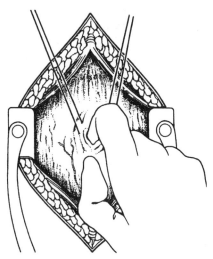

Figure 38.4 Suprapubic Cystostomy. (Reproduced with permission of WHO. *Surgical Care at the District Hospital*, WHO 2003.)

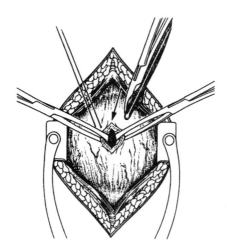

Figure 38.5 Suprapubic Cystostomy. (Reproduced with permission of WHO. *Surgical Care at the District Hospital*, WHO 2003.)

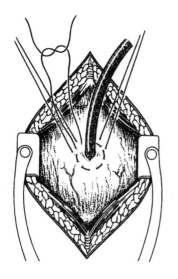

Figure 38.6 Suprapubic Cystostomy. (Reproduced with permission of WHO. *Surgical Care at the District Hospital*, WHO 2003.)

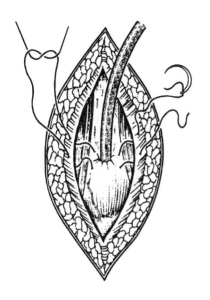

Figure 38.7 Suprapubic Cystostomy. (Reproduced with permission of WHO. *Surgical Care at the District Hospital*, WHO 2003.)

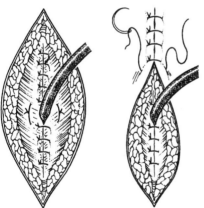

Figure 38.8 Suprapubic Cystostomy. (Reproduced with permission of WHO. *Surgical Care at the District Hospital*, WHO 2003.)

- Drain the bladder to prevent wound contamination.
- Make the incision and place a catheter, inflate the balloon, and close the wound with a purse string suture using absorbable sutures.
- Close with 2 layers of absorbable sutures if the bladder incision was larger than just enough room for a catheter and place the suprapubic catheter on the superior end of the incision away from the pubis.
- Sew the bladder to the rectus sheath if long-term placement is planned, as in Figures 38.6 and 38.7.
- A drain is placed in the perivesical space. The abdominal wound is closed.

Circumcision

Circumcision may be used as the definitive treatment for a prior dorsal slit after swelling has subsided, for religious purposes, and to prevent transmission of STIs.

Use a dorsal nerve block (see chapter 42).

The Gomco clamp can be used in infants, children, and adults. For children and adults, the crimped edges should be reinforced with interrupted absorbable sutures.

Free hand circumcision:

- Secure the preputial skin edges with straight clamps at 3 o'clock, 6 o'clock, and 9 o'clock.
- Break up adhesions with a straight clamp.
- Crush the skin at 12 o'clock from its edge to the corona.
- Cut the crushed skin creating a dorsal slit.
- Insert a stitch of fine plain catgut at the apex of the incision for traction.
- Cut the flap down to the frenulum with sharp scissors.
- Clamp and ligate any bleeders.
- Coapt the skin and mucous membrane with interrupted absorbable stitches.
- Apply petroleum gauze as dressing.

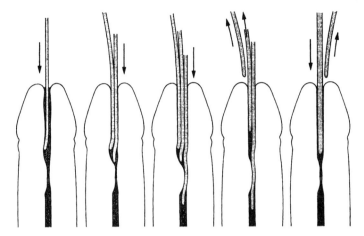

Figure 38.9 Urethral Dilatation. (Reproduced with permission of WHO. *Surgical Care at the District Hospital*, WHO 2003.)

Urethral Stricture

See Figure 38.9, Urethral Dilatation.

Common with untreated urethritis. If unable, proceed to suprapubic drainage.

- Sedate patient if necessary.
- Wash area with antiseptic.
- Start antibiotic to cover urinary pathogens.
- Instill 5 cc lidocaine gel into urethra and wait 5 min.
- Lubricate small filiform catheter and continue to add others until one passes, gradually working up in size.
- Perform dilatation with gradually increasing curved bougies once stricture passed.

UROLOGY

Chapter 39

Orthopedics

39.1 General Principles

(Review site: http://wheelessonline.com/ortho)

General overview: This chapter is written for a medical provider with some experience in orthopedics. If you do not feel competent treating a fracture, provide first aid, stabilize the patient and fracture, and refer.

- Cover any exposed bone with sterile saline soaked gauze.
- Give TT for open wounds.
- Check for circulation, nerve damage, tendon or muscle damage (movement). Correct circulatory insufficiency emergently.
- Try and treat fractures with closed reduction as open reductions are technically beyond most readers' skills and prone to infection.
- Liberally admit patients to the hospital.
- Apply a splint before a cast if swelling is a concern.
- Elevate the injured limb or skull.
- Splint or cast in a position of function whenever possible.
- Begin physical therapy early.
- Change casts when they become loose or damaged.
- Bones become "sticky" at 7 to 10 d and difficult to reduce. Check the alignment of your reduced fractures at this time to detect slippage.
- Keep the casted limb elevated higher than the heart with pillows or traction.

- Check a casted limb at 6 hr and 12 hr for too tight an application and circulatory compromise. If a cast is too tight, split it to relieve pressure and reapply using an elastic wrap.
- General anesthesia is necessary for muscle relaxation for treating many fractures and dislocations.

39.2   Fractures in Children

The greater the potential for growth, the more acceptable is an imperfect reduction. Attempt an accurate reduction but accept the following:

- up to 30° angulation in the direction of movement of a joint
- the younger the child the more correction by growth is possible
- up to 20° rotation
- up to 2 to 5 cm overriding, expect increased growth after a fracture
- a "bone block" of a supracondylar fracture of the elbow with limited flexion

   Do not accept the following:

- inaccurate reduction of the lateral condyle of the humerus, especially one with rotation
- medial condylar fracture of the humerus into the joint
- tibial spine fracture with limitation of knee motion
- nonanatomic reductions of Salter II through V fractures (see Figure 39.1)

Idiopathic Congenital Talipes Equinovarus (Club Foot)

Rule out meningomyelocele (refer) and start treatment at birth.

- Prepare padding and plaster on an examination table.
- Have the mother hold the infant on its back.
- Watch the infant's face for signs of pain.
- Correct the forefoot adduction as much as possible.
- Evert the heel; this will correct the forefoot inversion.

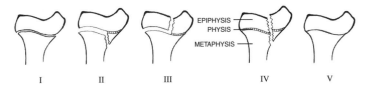

Figure 39.1 Salter II through IV Fractures. (From Diaz. LBB *Emergency Medicine* 2nd Ed 2006. Drawing by Michael Scholz.)

- Proceed if the lateral border of the foot is straight; if not, stop here and cast.
- Dorsiflex the foot as much as possible.
- Hold this position and prepare to apply the cast.
- Cover with 1 cm cotton padding, 1.5 cm on the medial heel and foot.
- Keep the knee flexed.
- Apply the plaster from medial to lateral over the dorsum of the foot.
- Mold the plaster as you go holding the foot in position.
- Reinforce the medial side of the cast with a slab of 4 to 6 layers of plaster.
- Cast from the tip of the great toe and the proximal interphalangeal joint (PIP) joints of the others.
- Apply plaster up to the hip (in fat newborns) or below the knee.
- Hold the plaster until it sets.
- Cut the plaster along the lateral side from toe to heel once set to allow for foot swelling.
- Recast about every 2 wk.
- Have the mother soak the cast off just prior to returning to the hospital to save time and a crying infant.
- Continue for 3 to 6 months.
- Refer if correction is unsuccessful.

- Continue casting until the child walks if correction succeeds, then night splints and club foot shoes.

39.3 Management of Dislocations and Fractures

Finger Fractures

Am Fam Physician 2006;73:827

Undisplaced phalangeal fractures can be "buddy taped" to an adjacent uninjured finger. Or, a small metal or plaster splint can be fashioned, secured at the wrist and along the finger. Watch for rotation of finger fractures, flexed finger tips should all point toward the thenar eminence.

Mallet Finger Fracture Evulsion

The insertion of the distal extensor tendon is torn off pulling a fragment of bone proximally. The finger cannot be fully extended.

Cast or splint the distal intraphalangeal joint (DIP) joint in hyperextension with the PIP joint flexed at 90°. Hold for 4 to 6 wk.

Metacarpal Fractures

Reduce angulation and hold with a short arm posterior splint that extends to the PIP joint, the wrist extended 30°, the metacarpal phalangeal (MP) joint flexed 30° in the position of function. Be sure to correct any rotation (the finger tips will overlap).

First carpal-metacarpal joint, Bennett's fracture: The base of the metacarpal is fractured, the distal fragment displaced laterally and pulled proximally.

- Use local, regional, or general anesthesia.
- Hang the thumb from an IV pole.
- Push on the distal fragment to obtain alignment

- Apply a "scaphoid cast" while still hanging, the thumb held at a 90° angle to the fingers.
- Recast at 2 to 3 wk and maintain for 6 wk.

Radial Fracture

Radial fracture with distal ulnar dislocation (Galeazzi) is difficult to reduce and may require surgery.

Distal Radius (Colles' Fracture)

Reduce if the distal fragment has > 15° angulation. A hematoma block usually is adequate.

- Prep the skin with Betadine.
- Approach through the dorsal wrist.
- Inject 5 to 10 ml 2% lidocaine without epinephrine into the fracture site.
- Have an assistant hold the upper arm for traction.
- Disimpact the fracture by pronating the arm, pulling on the hand while it is flexed.
- Push the displaced fragment down with your thumb.
- Apply a short arm cast when reduction is satisfactory, holding the wrist 15° flexed in ulnar deviation, the arm pronated.
- Watch carefully for vascular compromise from swelling.
- Cast 4 to 6 wk.

Ultrasound exam can be used in lieu of X-ray films (Acad Emerg Med 2006;13:966).

Reverse Colles' or Smith's Fracture

Reduce using the opposite maneuvers to that of the Colles' fracture. Maintain the wrist in dorsiflexion, the forearm supinated.

Fracture-dislocation Wrist, Barton's Fracture

The articular surface of the distal radius is sheared off with dislocation of the carpal bone(s). Hard to hold in reduction and best referred.

Scaphoid Fracture

Difficult to see on X-ray; compare with a film of the other wrist. If the scaphoid (snuff box) is tender, place a short-arm cast, which includes the thumb up to the DIP joint. The thumb and index finger should be able to touch as in the "OK" sign. Remove the cast in 2 wk and re–X-ray. The fracture may now be apparent. Recast for a total of 12 wk. Nonunion is of concern. Refer for bone grafting if it occurs.

Fracture of the Clavicle

Often caused by a direct blow or fall. An X-ray is often unnecessary. If a pneumothorax is suspected, an anterior-posterior (AP) CXR is adequate. A triangular sling is easy to apply and comfortable. Anatomical reduction usually is not crucial unless there is a proximal fracture pushed in past the sternum. Pull out with towel clips. Resume shoulder range of motion as soon as possible. Healing takes 3 to 6 wk.

Fracture of the Scapula

Caused by a direct blow to the chest. An X-ray is necessary and will identify associated rib fractures. Reduction is impossible. Treat as a clavicle fracture.

Fracture of the Proximal Humerus

Fractures of the greater or lesser trochanter and nondisplaced shaft fractures are treated with a triangular sling and early mobilization.

Displaced or fracture dislocations are aligned and reduced in the operating room under general anesthesia.

Place a bulky pad in the axilla and apply a triangular bandage and then another bandage holding the upper arm to the chest (sling and swathe). Start range of motion exercises when the pain decreases at about 2 wk. Healing takes 8 to 12 wk.

Midshaft Humerus Fracture

The radial nerve may be damaged; check for wrist dorsiflexion. If this is lost, you will need to keep the wrist in a functional position with a cock-up splint.

Reduce the fracture; usually general anesthesia is necessary in adults. Overlapping of the fragments is acceptable, but distractions will not heal. The bones must touch. Use a sling and swathe bandage or a U-shaped gutter splint, the bottom of the U at the elbow, the ends under the axilla and at the top of the shoulder.

Encourage the patient to begin range of motion exercises. Healing takes 8 wk.

Frozen Shoulder

A risk of any fracture or dislocation about the shoulder; a frozen shoulder occurs when the patient does not begin early mobilization. Explain to the patient that movement hurts, but it is necessary. Useful therapy includes the pendulum exercise:

- Lean over a table flexing the upper body to 90°. Hang the arm still in the sling (but not the swathe) over the table and swing the arm in a circle of ever increasing circumference.

- A second exercise is to "walk" the fingers up a wall to greater and greater heights sweeping forwards and backwards.

Elbow Fractures

The "sail sign" of a fat-fluid interface helps make the diagnosis in subtle cases; most are obvious intercondylar interarticular fractures.

Use general anesthesia in adults; usually an assistant is necessary to stabilize the arm. Closed reduction is followed by a posterior 90° splint.

Start supination and pronation in a few days and active flexion-extension at 2 to 3 wk. Keep the splint on for protection for 4 to 6 wk then use a sling for several more.

Olecranon Fractures

Nondisplaced fractures with intact triceps muscle insertion are treated as above. Displacement or tendon rupture require operative treatment with K wires and are best discussed with a specialist.

Radial Head and Neck Fractures

Caused by a fall on an outstretched arm. Try to reduce under anesthesia as necessary. Use a 90° posterior splint starting prona-tion-supination exercises in a few days and extension-flexion movements after.

Forearm Fractures-Dislocations

Try to reduce the displaced radial head and hold it in supination with the elbow flexed 90°. A long arm cast is needed for 6 to 8 wk. This Monteggia fracture is unstable and may require opera-tive repair in adults.

Single diaphysial fractures of radius or ulna are reduced by hanging the arm from an IV pole, the upper arm horizontal with a weight or counter traction on the upper arm. Reduce the fracture and apply a 90° long arm cast with the thumb up, the forearm in neutral (see Figure 39.2).

Radial and ulna fractures (both bones) are treated in a similar manner.

Elbow Dislocation

Caused by a fall on an outstretched hand and associated with ulnar nerve injury and medial epicondyle fracture, which occa-sionally is trapped in the joint.

- Use general anesthesia for reduction.
- Have an assistant stabilize the upper arm while you apply trac-tion, holding the arm at 30° flexion.
- Pull the olecranon toward you while guiding it laterally or medially depending on the direction of the dislocation.

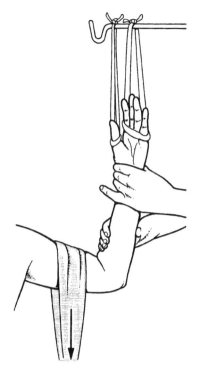

Figure 39.2 Forearm Fractures. (Reproduced with permission of WHO. *Surgical Care at the District Hospital*, WHO 2003.)

- Once corrected, the arm should have complete range of motion (ROM) and no valgus deformity—if not refer.
- Re–X-ray.
- Apply a posterior splint, the elbow at 90° and the forearm in neutral thumb up position.
- Start active ROM at 2 to 3 wk.
- Do not stretch or manipulate the elbow.
- Remove the splint at 4 wk (Clin Orthop 1987:165).

Radial Head Dislocation (Nursemaid's Elbow)

- Occurs in children.
- Place your thumb on the radial head.
- Extend the elbow.
- Supinate the forearm.
- Flex the elbow.
- Feel or hear a pop as the radius relocates.

Digit Dislocation

Am Fam Physician 2006;73:810

Dislocations of the MP and interphalangeal joints are usually posterior.

- Do a digital block.
- Pull the digit outward.
- Push at the base of the dislocated phalanx.
- Splint 2 to 3 wk.
- Refer if this fails.

Shoulder Dislocation

Most dislocations are anterior; the shoulder appears sunken and motion is impossible.

- Obtain AP and axillary (axial) X-rays.
- Avulsion of the great tuberosity or surgical neck of the humerus will probably reduce, but general anesthesia may be needed.
- Use IV diazepam and an analgesic for pain relief or general anesthesia.
- Place the patient prone on a table with the affected arm hanging down to the floor.
- Hang a bucket from the arm using a wide bandage around the wrist to the handle.
- Gradually add 10 to 15 lbs of weights (IV bags) to the bucket.
- Wait, watching for respiratory compromise.

- Use general anesthesia with traction on the moderately abducted arm while an assistant manipulates the humeral head through the axilla if this fails.
- Check circulation and axillary nerve.
- Apply a sling and swathe bandage.
- Mobilize early.
- Reduce recurrent dislocations simply by having the patient lie on their back, place your foot in their axilla for counter traction, and gently pull up 45° on the arm.

Pelvic Fractures

Single fractures of the pelvic ring are stable and require only symptomatic treatment and a cane or walker as pain subsides.

Most fractures occur at 2 spots; separation of the pubic symphysis counts as a fracture. These are unstable.

- Treat shock.
- Type and cross for 2 or more units of blood.
- Do an urethrogram (inject contrast up the urethra and X-ray) if there is blood about the urethra to prove there is an intact urethra.
- Pass a Foley or suprapubic catheter as indicated.
- Rig a strong sling in an orthopedic bed to elevate the pelvis and hold it together.
- Apply skeletal traction (see Placing a Tibial Pin below) with the hips in 30° abduction and 20° internal rotation, the knees at 10° flexion. A hip spica cast is an alternative.

Hip Dislocation

Often caused by an MVA, the posterior is the most common. The hip is flexed, adducted, with internal rotation, the knee overlying the opposite thigh.

- X-ray looking for fractures of the acetabulum, pelvis, and femur. Refer these.
- Examine for nerve palsy. Refer these.

- Use general or spinal anesthesia.
- Hang the dislocated leg over the table, the patient on their abdomen.
- Flex the hip to 90°.
- Apply traction downward.
- Push the femoral head into place by direct pressure and careful rotation of the leg. The hip should have normal ROM.
- Apply skin traction for 3 wk.
- Encourage gentle hip exercises and sitting up.
- Allow nonweight bearing at 6 wk, partial weight bearing at 12 wk, and off crutches at 4 months.

Femur Fractures

Fractures of the femur are best referred. Suspect with inability to bear weight. There is usually shortening and external rotation of the leg, but impacted fractures can be difficult to diagnose. Blood loss can be significant (1–3 L).

- Consider a femoral nerve block prior to transfer (Ann Emerg Med 2003;41:227)
- Transfer in a Thomas splint or use 2 pillows, 1 below the knee and 1 above, each between the legs. Bound with broad bandages.

Supracondylar femur fractures:
  The distal fragment is displaced posteriorly.

- Reduce the fracture if displaced while the patient is under general anesthesia.
- Hold the reduction with skeletal traction, the knee flexed 10° with pillows.
- Start quadriceps exercises and passive movement of the patella early.
- Begin to exercise the knee at 4 to 6 wk.

Femoral fractures in children:

- Often occurs when a carried infant is dropped but consider abuse.
- Children under 2 yr can be managed by applying skin traction to both legs and hanging them from ropes attached to an over-bed frame, their hips flexed at 90°. Have their buttocks resting on the bed for easy diaper changing.

Patellar Fracture

- Undisplaced fractures with the quadriceps mechanism intact are treated in a long leg cast or knee immobilizer for 3 to 4 wk.
- Any large hematoma is aspirated prior to cast application.
- At 4 wk, remove the cast and start ROM activities.
- Weight-bearing 8 to 12 wk starts later.
- Open fractures are best referred.

Lower Leg Fractures

Proximal Tibial Fractures:

- Simple fractures are reduced under anesthesia and immobilized by placing a tibial pin 3 to 4 inches distal to the fracture site.
- Quadriceps and knee bending exercises begin while still in traction.

Placing a tibial pin (see Figures 39.3 through 39.5):

- Prep the skin with antiseptic solution.
- Infiltrate the skin and subcutaneous tissue with local anesthetic on both sides of the tibia.
- Make a small vertical incision at a point 1 cm posterior to the tibial tubercle.
- Insert a Steinman pin until it touches the bone.
- Drill it through the bone perpendicular to the long axis of the bone.
- Make another nick with the scalpel as the pin approaches the skin to allow the pin to exit.

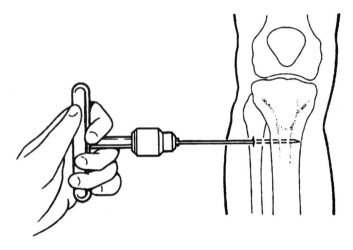

Figure 39.3 Placing Tibial Pin. (Reproduced with permission of WHO. *Surgical Care at the District Hospital*, WHO 2003.)

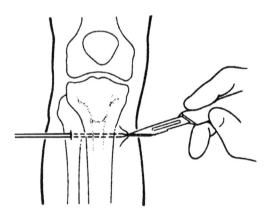

Figure 39.4 Placing Tibial Pin. (Reproduced with permission of WHO. *Surgical Care at the District Hospital*, WHO 2003.)

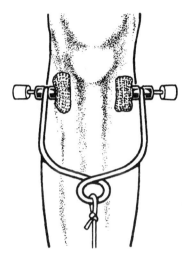

Figure 39.5 Placing Tibial Pin. (Reproduced with permission of WHO. *Surgical Care at the District Hospital*, WHO 2003.)

- Apply tincture of benzoin to the skin and then cover the pin with gauze.
- Cover the sharp ends of pin.
- Apply traction using ropes and pulleys.
- Use about 10% to 15% of body weight for the weights.

Midshift tibial fractures:

- Reduce while the patient is sitting, the leg hanging freely over a table.
- Apply a long leg cast to the groin, the knee flexed at 10°.
- Change to a short leg cast that covers the patella at 6 to 8 wk.
- Remember to pad the perineal nerve!

Proximal and midshaft fibular fractures:

- Managed without casting.

ORTHOPEDICS

Ankle fractures:

All are intra-articular and accurate reduction is essential.

- Reduce by traction and reversing the movement that caused the injury. Ligamentous injuries occur with the fracture. Closed reduction may be difficult and open reduction needed.
- Cast in a short-leg cast, the foot at 90° and neutral.
- Elevate the limb.
- Change the cast at 4 wk.
- Apply a new walking cast at 8 wk.
- Start crutches and careful weight bearing at 12 wk with the cast removed.

The Ottawa rules (JAMA 1993;269:1127) are used to determine when an ankle X-ray is necessary in patients > 16 yr old.

- pain near the malleolus, and
- inability to bear weight and walk 4 steps, or
- bone tenderness along the posterior or tip of a malleolus

Foot Fractures

Talus fracture:

Usually neck fracture with dislocation of subtalar joint as body of talus is pushed posterior and medially.

- Reduce if necessary with longitudinal traction pulling the heel forward while dorsiflexing the foot.
- Evert the foot and plantar flex.
- Apply a short leg nonweight bearing cast.
- Cast for 6 to 8 wk.
- Check for spine injuries.

Calcaneous fracture:

Either direct blow with force driving into subtalar joint and calcaneous body or avulsion Achilles tendon/tuberosity fracture.

- Apply compression dressing, short leg splint, and elevate.

- No weight bearing for 6 to 8 wk, then guarded weight bearing for another 6 to 8 wk.
- Check for spine, knee, and hip injuries.
- Refer Achilles tendon avulsions, which need to be fixed in place with screws.

Tarsometatarsal Joint Fractures (Lisfranc): Am Fam Physician 2007;76

X-ray should show medial borders of second metatarsal aligned with medial edge second cuneiform, fourth metatarsal aligned with cuboid.

- Suspect Lisfranc fracture-dislocation when widened space between first and second metatarsals, point tenderness at tarso-metatarsal joint, small fleck fracture at the base of the second metatarsal adjacent to the first, and loss of alignment between second metatarsal and cuboid (as above).
- Do a closed reduction if alignment abnormal.
- Elevate, apply a short leg splint.
- Refer for pinning if unable to reduce.
- Apply short leg nonweight bearing cast for 4 to 6 wk if successful.

Metatarsal fractures:

- Reduce fractures and dislocations if > 4 mm displacement or 10° angulation.
- Use a firm bottom shoe or short leg cast. Fracture of the fifth metatarsal tuberosity = firm shoe, distal fractures of diaphysis require casting for 6 to 8 weeks, then guarded weight bearing for another 8 to 12 wk.

39.4   Osteomyelitis

Cause: *Staphylococcus aureus* > 50%; *Salmonella sp.* (sickle cell); TB especially vertebral; other bacterial and fungal.

ORTHOPEDICS

Epidem: Common in children, compound fractures, leprosy.

Pathophys: Hematogenous spread of bacteria to metaphyseal side of epiphyseal place. Acute intramedullary infection if untreated becomes chronic with abscess formation. Pressure drives infection into cortical bone and under periosteum. Either drains through skin and/or dissects under periosteum cutting off blood supply to diaphysis resulting in dead bone (sequestrum). Periosteum lays down new bone (involucrum), which, if not damaged by infection or surgery, gives final support and function to bone.

Sx/Si: Acute stage fever and bone pain; chronic swollen limb, enlarged bone, draining sinus.

Crs: Chronic infection with pathological fracture, occasional dissemination.

Cmplc: Amyloidosis, altered limb growth.

Lab: Culture of draining pus not reliable. Bone biopsy positive in most.

Xray: Positive at 2 to 3 wk periosteal new bone and osteopenia. Ultrasound may show periosteal elevation

Rx:

- Obtain cultures of blood and bone if area identified.
- Appropriate IV antibiotics in acute disease covering *Staph* and *Salmonella* if needed.
- Give chloramphenicol 25 mg/kg IM or IV q 8 hr for children < 3 yr and with SS disease.
- Give cloxacillin IM or IV 50 mg/kg q 6 hr for children > 3 yr.
- Switch to oral medications once temperature down to normal for a total of 6 wk.
- X-ray at 3 and 6 wk.
- Operate and drain if abscess forms. Incise down to periosteum and drain; if no pus, drill multiple holes into medullary canal to drain. Culture and gram stain pus, irrigate, place drain on bone, and close wound loosely.

- Remove sequestrum when involucrum has formed sufficiently to support integrity of bone. This usually takes 6 to 12 months during which antibiotic therapy is not necessary.
- Protect involucrum when sequestrum removed, and cast limb to protect it after surgery.
- Refer for inadequate involucrum.
- Sequestrum is a nidus for recurrent infections.

Chapter 40

Ophthalmology

40.1 Conjunctivitis

Newborn

Cause: *Neisseria gonorrhea*

Epidem: Conjunctivitis in the newborn, ophthalmia neonatorum, occurs within the first 30 d of life.

Sx/Si: Acute, bilateral, purulent infection with swollen eyelids and profuse discharge of pus. The lids are hardened, and the red conjunctiva may protrude between them. Signs and symptoms always develop within 48 hr of birth.

Lab: Diagnosis is by gram stain of swabbing from the upper retrotarsal fold and culture.

Rx: Treatment must be started immediately. Hospitalize and irrigate the eyes hourly with normal saline or a 4% boric acid solution, then apply topical antibiotic ointment or drops (tetracycline, gentamicin, or chloramphenicol). Give ceftriaxone 50 mg/kg (up to 150 mg) IM once or kanamycin 25 mg/kg (up to 75 mg) IM once. Spectinomycin may also be used.

Prev: Treat the mother and father and report to public health officials. If only one eye is involved, cover the uninvolved eye to prevent spread.

Cause: *Chlamydia trachomatis*

Sx/Si: Infection usually appears several days after birth (range 1–60) with irritated red eyes without exudate.

Lab: Inclusion bodies are found in epithelial cells.

Rx: Treatment is with tetracycline or erythromycin eye ointment plus oral erythromycin for 14 d (Med Lett Drugs Ther 1995;35:117).

Cause: Other causes of conjunctivitis in the newborn include *Staphylococcus*, *Haemophilus*, *Streptococcus*, *E. coli*, *Pseudomonas*, *Moraxella*, and chemical conjunctivitis from silver nitrate.

Prev: Maternal screening when possible or eye prophylaxis of the neonatal at the time of birth.

Mechanically clean the eyes at birth with sterile saline then apply 1% tetracycline or erythromycin ophthalmic ointment or 1% to 2% silver nitrate solution. Irrigate the eyes 30 seconds after applying silver nitrate to avoid chemical conjunctivitis. Silver nitrate is inactivated by light and should be stored appropriately.

Child and Adult

Cause: Conjunctivitis may be due to chlamydia or gonorrhea (treat the same as neonate following local STI guidelines), but more likely it is viral (adenovirus), allergic, or bacterial (same agents as neonate). Suppurative keratitis may also follow agricultural injuries; those involving vegetable matter often result in *Aspergillus*, *Fusarium*, or *Candida* infections.

Lab: Diagnosis is by corneal swabbing and gram stain.

Rx: Treatment is topical antibiotic eye ointments or drops. If no response in 48 hr, consider adding a topical antifungal such as econazole 1%.

Topical NSAID or antihistamine eye drops/ointments may help allergic conjunctivitis. Cold 3% sodium bicarbonate eye drops are soothing as are artificial tears.

40.2   Glaucomas

Cause: Often but not always increased intraocular pressure.

Epidem: Glaucoma is classified into open and closed angle types, primary and secondary. Open angle glaucoma is prevalent in Black Africans, while acute closed angle is common in Asians. Strong genetic component so family history is important.

Sx/Si: Open angle glaucoma has an insidious onset. Only occasionally is there eye pain or headache. The intraocular pressure (IP) is usually elevated > 21 mmHg. The optic disc shows increased cupping, first on the temporal side, as it deepens. The cup:disk ratio approaches 1:2. The vessels may disappear at the cup's edge and reappear at its floor. Visual fields are decreased, initially in the nasal quadrants and later peripherally in all quadrants.

Diagnosis is by measurement of IP, visual fields, and funduscopic exam. A very rough guide of increased IP is to gently palpate the down-turned eye through the closed upper lid using your 2 index fingers to compare pressures in each eye. Tonometer is often available. It must be remembered that glaucoma can occur with a normal IP. A provocative test may be used if a tonometer is available. Have the patient NPO for 8 hours, measure the IP, then have patient drink a liter of fluid. Measure the IP every 15 min. An increase of 10 mmHg suggests glaucoma.

Rx: If glaucoma is diagnosed or suspected, referral is necessary. Surgery (trabeculectomy) is the preferred treatment in most situations as long-term compliance with eye drops is unlikely.

Sx/Si: Acute closure glaucoma usually presents as an emergency with acute, severe eye pain, headache, and sometimes vomiting. The eye is red and congested, the cornea often hazy, the pupil dilated and fixed. The iris is pressed flat against the cornea. The other eye is quiet, but its shallow anterior chamber can be viewed by shining a light across the eye from either side. Atropine-like drugs may precipitate the angle closure.

Rx: Acetazolamide 250 mg orally 4 × daily is the treatment. IV acetazolamide, mannitol, or oral glycerol may be used. Timolol maleate 0.5% 1 drop twice daily should be started. If referral for definitive surgery is delayed, continue acetazolamide with supplemental potassium, timolol drops, and add pilocarpine 1% to 4% 4 × daily.

Sx/Si: Secondary glaucomas may result from iridocyclitis complicating leprosy, TB, syphilis, and onchocerciasis. The fluid in the anterior chamber appears "dusty" when a light is shined through it like sunlight streaming through dust. The pupil may dilate irregularly. The iris is pushed toward the cornea. Hemorrhage into the anterior chamber (hyphema) is another cause. IP should be lowered with acetazolamide, and the patient referred for treatment of the underlying condition.

Congenital glaucoma results in a larger eye or eyes. Cupping of the disks may be seen. Refer is necessary.

40.3   Iridocyclitis

Cause: Inflammation of the iris and the ciliary body.

Epidem: An associated disease is often the cause: TB, sarcoidosis, syphilis, Reiter's syndrome, Behcet's syndrome, and ankylosing spondylitis. The type 2 hypersensitivity reaction in leprosy is another common cause of iridocyclitis. Many cases are idiopathic.

Sx/Si: (Iridocyclitis or anterior uveitis) may present in one or both eyes with a gradual onset of deep eye pain, photophobia, lacrimation, blurring of vision and visual loss, inflammation around the limbus rather than the entire conjunctiva, papillary constriction with sluggish response to light, and cloudiness of the anterior chamber. A slit lamp is needed to see the early aqueous flare; a more severe cloudiness can be seen with a hand lens and a light. Corneal precipitates appear as small yellow-white dots. The iris may be irregular from synechias. Initially the IP is normal, and the eye feels soft; later secondary glaucoma may occur. The eye may be anesthetic.

Crs: The differential is conjunctivitis and acute glaucoma. Blindness is a danger.

Rx: Pupillary dilatation, atropine or similar drug. Use hourly until the pupil dilates, then 1 drop 1 to 3 × daily. Ocular steroids, hydrocortisone 1%, drop every 4 hr. Treat the pain with anti-inflammatory drugs and warm compresses. Watch for and treat glaucoma with acetazolamide and drops.

40.4   Ocular Injuries

Corneal abrasions are managed with a mydriatic/cycloplegic drop (cyclopentolate 1%) once and ocular antibiotics for 3 to 5 d. A pressure patch is customarily applied for at least 24 hr.

Corneal foreign bodies can be removed under local anesthesia (amethocaine 1% or benoxinate 0.4%) using a cotton bud or a sterile hypodermic needle. A rust ring from a metallic object may be curetted with the needle but remember the central cornea is 0.5 mm thick. Apply 1 drop of a mydriatic/cycloplegic and antibiotic drops.

Blunt trauma is generally managed with bed rest, with the head elevated, and monitoring of the IP. Topical antibiotics are given with systemic antibiotics for bony fractures that involve the sinus or a break in the skin. Total or near total hyphema can be treated with a paracentesis.

Penetrating eye injuries are covered with a shield, given topical and parenteral antibiotics, and referred to a specialist. If referral is not available within 48 hr and the iris has prolapsed, it must be carefully excised, topical antibiotics applied, and the eye patched.

40.5   Retinal Detachment

The patient complains of a veil falling over an eye as the visual field defect arises. A large detachment can be seen with an ophthalmoscope. The detached retina is in focus with a higher plus diopter, the vessels are dark, and the retina gray colored. Ultimately, referral is needed to treat an underlying disease, occasionally a tumor.

40.6   Chalazion

Chalazion (meibomian cysts) may be removed after topical and local anesthetic injection and eversion of the eyelid with a chalazion clamp. Incise the cyst vertically (right angles to the lid margin) on the conjunctival surface and curette out the cyst. No stitches are necessary. Apply antibiotic drops or ointment. Injection of intralesional triamcinolone is a good alternative treatment.

40.7   Trachoma

Clin Infect Dis 2008;15:564; Am J Trop Med Hyg 2003;69:1 entire issue

Cause: *Chlamydia trachomatis* also causes the recurrent chronic eye infection of trachoma. Subtypes A through C are transmitted from eye to eye usually via eye-seeking flies and cause trachoma, while subtypes D through K largely cause genital STIs with occasional direct contact spread to the eye.

Epidem: Common throughout the world particularly where the 6 Ds are found: dry, dusty, dirty, dung (and flies), eye discharge, and high population density. The disease begins in infancy and over years may lead to eyelid scarring, eyelashes turning inward (entropion), and corneal inflammation (keratitis), scarring, and blindness. One hundred fifty million with disease, 6 million blind. It is the leading cause of preventable blindness in developing countries.

Sx/Si: Diagnosis is usually clinical and based on a grading system. A good light, a 2.5× magnification loop and a small rod or wooden applicator handle to evert the upper lid are used. Inspect the upper eyelid.

Grade 1. Inflammation-follicular (TF): 5 or more follicles > 0.5 mm in diameter. The follicles are round, elevated, and may be lighter in color than the conjunctiva. Contrast these follicles with the flattened angular cobblestones of allergic conjunctivitis.

Grade 2. Inflammation-intense (TI): Intense, red, edematous, inflammatory thickening with loss of > 50% of normal deep tarsal blood vessels.

Grade 3. Scarring (TS): White lines in tarsal conjunctiva, often featherlike.

Grade 4. Trichiasis (TT): At least one eyelash rubbing on the eyeball or evidence of eyelash removal.

Grade 5. Corneal opacity (CO): Visual impairment due to corneal scar covering at least part of the pupil.

Rx: Oral antibiotic treatment has supplanted topical ointments.

- azithromycin 20 mg/kg single dose
- doxycycline 100 mg daily for 21 d
- tetracycline 250 mg 4 × daily for 21 d

Epilation (lash removal) manually or cautery to the eyelash base treats trichiasis. Separating animal pens from humans and daily face washing are also effective.

Prev: Sanitation, face washing, and fly reduction.

Mass treatment with azithromycin reduced carriage in flies from 23% to 0.3% (Am J Trop Med Hyg 2007;36:129). *Musca sorbens* fly primary source of transmission; prefers to feed on human feces. So VIP (Ventilation Improved Performance) toilets are helpful.

Chapter 41

Dental

Where There Is No Dentist. Hesperian Foundation in print and online (www.hesperian.org/publications_download_dentist.php).

The teeth are numbered 1 to 32 as a backwards "⊃" as you look at the patient. Start at no 1, top right posterior, proceed anteriorly to the incisors then left to the third upper molar, then lower left posterior molar over to the right posterior, 3 molars, 2 premolars, canine, 4 incisors, canine, etc. Or, if you use the British system right upper quadrant, no 1 anterior incisor to no 8 posterior most molar, RUQ, RLQ, and LLQ.

The upper molars generally have 3 roots, the lower ones 2; the premolars 2 or 1 (upper) or 1 (lower). The upper teeth roots often touch the bottom of the maxillary sinus. Teeth have lingual and buccal surfaces.

41.1 Anesthesia

- Use a topical anesthetic applied to predried gums prior to injection.
- Apply local pressure with a cotton applicator, enough to blanch the mucosa, then quickly inject a drop or two of anesthetic in the blanched area (especially good for the palate) if topical anesthetic unavailable. Any local anesthetic will do (epinephrine will prolong the time the anesthetic works but is not necessary). Local anesthetics work poorly in abscess cavities.
- Inject slowly to minimize pain.

Anesthesia of the upper teeth is straightforward. Inject about the roots. Or, you can inject the maxillary nerve as it exits the bone. Start in sulcus over distal root of second molar, advance anteriorly over each tooth. Anesthetize the gum then advance the needle under the skin. Draw back in case you are in the artery, inject 0.5 to 1.0 ml. You also need to inject the palate side of the tooth, about 0.25 ml/tooth. Inject slowly; these hurt. One injection in the midline behind the upper incisors will cover the 6 front teeth.

For the lower teeth, you can use individual nerve blocks for each tooth or do nerve blocks on the inferior alveolar nerve, lingual, and long buccal nerve.

The inferior alveolar nerve block takes practice.

- Place your hand in the mouth, the thumb on the ramus of the mandible, the index finger outside the mouth on the other side of the ramus.
- Use a long needle, aim for a point midway between your fingers 1 cm above the top of the posterior molar. The needle will enter the mucosa at a 45° angle and should hit the bone about 2 cm past where you enter the mucosa.
- Be sure to inject a small amount of anesthetic when the needle enters the mucosa and to aspirate before injecting about 1½ ml at the nerve site.
- Wait 3 min if the lower lip is numb; proceed with other injections. If not, reinject.
- Do not do these nerve blocks on both sides at one time; the patient may aspirate their tongue. If you plan to work on the 3 posterior molars, a second block is necessary.
- Inject 0.5 ml anesthetic into the buccal side where the cheek meets the gum.

You can anesthetize all lower teeth in this manner; or, if only the anterior incisors require anesthesia, block the mandibular nerve where it exits the bone between the lower premolars. Inject 0.5 ml and massage the anesthetic into the area.

41.2 Extractions

When to pull teeth:

- Hurts all the time.
- It is fractured with an exposed root.
- It hurts when moved, and it is loose.
- Prior to oral radiation therapy for cancer.

Before you pull a tooth, check for the following:

- bleeding tendencies/anticoagulants: may need suturing
- valvular heart disease: will need endocarditis prophylaxis
- bisphosphamide use: may develop osteonecrosis bone
- allergies to drugs
- immune compromised: poor healing

You will need the correct instruments, usually a spoon or probe to separate the gum tissue from the tooth and an elevator to loosen the tooth and an upper universal forcep (150) and a universal lower forcep (151). Other specialized forceps cowhorn (87) for lower molars, right (17) and left (18) upper molar or hawk's bill (73) are available. Have suture equipment, cotton, silk, or absorbable 3-0 suture, gauze, and a good light source. Use an aspirating syringe for anesthesia if it is available. Treat an infected tooth with antibiotics for a week before attempting extraction.

How to pull a tooth:

- Obtain anesthesia.
- Reflect the gum tissue from the tooth to be removed (both sides).
- Loosen the tooth with the elevator by placing the sharp part of the elevator against the tooth.
- Slide it down under the gum as low on the tooth as possible.
- Rotate the elevator using the bone and adjacent tooth to loosen the bad tooth.

- Grasp the tooth with the forcep as low as you can toward the root. The object is to expand bone, like moving a fence post from the soil by rocking it back and forth.
- Apply a twisting motion for single-rooted teeth, attempting to rotate the tooth in larger and larger areas about its long axis.
- Tip back and forth or in a figure of 8 movement for 2 and 3-rooted teeth.
- Use your other hand to feel the bone expand around the tooth as it loosens. Anterior teeth come straight out. Molars usually come out buccally (toward the cheek).
- Feel that the tooth was extracted completely; root tips are smooth.
- Try not to leave roots. They may cause an infection.
- Remove upper root tips cautiously; it is possible to drive them into a sinus causing a fistula. Root tips ≤ 3 mm can be left in if removal is dangerous.
- Remember, when pulling deciduous teeth not to damage the permanent tooth below; never use a cowhorn forceps. If 2 or more teeth were removed, it may be necessary to suture the gums together.
- Control bleeding by squeezing the sides of the socket together; this will also compress any bone that loosened.
- Remove any bone chips, damaged or loose tissue.
- Have the patient bite down on cotton for ≥ 30 min to control bleeding.

   Antibiotics are not usually necessary.
   Extraction aftercare:
- Bite down on gauze to control bleeding.
- Bite down on a moistened tea bag if gauze is unsuccessful.
- Avoid smoking or sucking on straw for 3 d.
- Take first dose of pain medication before anesthetic wears off.
- Do not rinse mouth or drink hot fluids for several days.
- Eat soft foods.

- Rinse gently with warm salt water starting on day 2.

  Complications:

- Dry socket is a steady pain that begins a day or two after an extraction. It is caused by a disrupted clot. Apply oil of cloves (eugenol) on gel foam into the socket. If gel foam is not available, use cotton and change daily.
- Dislocated jaw.
- Nerve damage.

Dental (Periapical) Abscess

Cause: Anaerobic bacteria

Pathophys: Bacterial infection in tooth spreads to root and surrounding bone.

Sx: Pain, swelling, occasionally fever and lymphadenopathy.

Si: Tenderness when tooth moved, caries.

Crs: Will usually drain spontaneously with death of tooth.

Cmplc: Occasionally chronic osteomyelitis. Warm heat applied to painful tooth encourages drainage through skin and should be avoided.

Xray: Lucency about root of tooth.

Rx: Oral penicillin ± metronidazole or clindamycin; extraction of tooth after several days' wait.

Facial Fractures: Mandible

Cause: Due to trauma.

Sx/Si: May complain of paresthesia from nerve damage. Change in occlusion, ecchymosis, crepitus on palpation, limited opening. Left untreated high risk of malunion or osteomyelitis.

Xray: May show fracture; panorex is best.

Rx: Obtain reduction under local or general anesthesia with nasotracheal intubation if needed. Avoid any dental extractions.

Temporary immobilization can be obtained by applying wire loop ligatures around the mandibular and maxillary premolars and tying them together taking care to hide the sharp ends of the wire. Prestretch the wire before using.

For the 6 wk it will take to heal the fracture, arch bars should be wired to the teeth by a dentist or experienced provider and then connected to immobilize the jaw.

Chapter 42

Anesthesia

42.1   Ketamine Anesthesia

In many ways ketamine is an ideal anesthetic for use by an inexperienced provider in developing countries. But, it must be used with care as it induces a dissociative anesthesia. Patients have excellent analgesia and amnesia, have bronchodilatation with little respiratory depression, and the BP and heart rate rises. But limb movements, lack of muscle relaxation, and emergence delirium with hallucinations may be troublesome. Nystagmus, pupillary dilatation, and increased secretions are to be expected.

As it increases intracranial pressure, it should not be used for intracranial surgery or for those at risk of stroke. It should be avoided with penetrating eye injuries and in CAD.

Dissociative symptoms are less common in children. They can be decreased with concomitant administration of a benzodiazepine. Increased secretions are pretreated with atropine.

Administration is by IV, IM, or rectally. Induction doses are 0.5 to 2.0 mg/kg IV, 4 to 8 mg/kg IM, and 8 to 10 mg/kg rectally. The induction dose lasts 10 to 15 min. Maintenance doses are 25 to 100 μgm/kg/min. Refrigerate multidose vials after opening.

A typical 50 kg adult might be managed with induction using 50 mg ketamine, 0.5 mg atropine, and 10 mg diazepam IV followed by an infusion of 2.5 mg/min. Care must be taken that the patient not awaken during surgery in a dissociative state. The author has found the drug particularly useful in obstetrical emergencies requiring cesarean delivery in the face of massive bleeding. But, it is oxytocic and should not be used during pregnancy except as noted above or for forceps delivery.

General Anesthesia

General anesthesia is not covered in this book because anesthetic machines and drugs available vary greatly from hospital to hospital. The WHO has an excellent text, *Anesthesia in the District Hospital*, 2nd Ed, 2000.

Lidocaine

Lidocaine (Lignocaine) is one of the safest local anesthetics, which is often combined with epinephrine (1:50 000–1:200 000) to slow its absorption from tissue. Commonly used strengths are 0.5% to 2% for injection or infiltration and 2.5% to 5% for topical use. Preparations containing epinephrine should never be used IV or for injections around digits or the penis. Epinephrine prolongs lidocaine's action from around 1 to 2 hr. Metabolism occurs in the liver and becomes important when large doses are used. Toxicity causes CNS irritation ranging from sleepiness, confusion, to seizures. Circumoral and tongue numbness and eyebrow twitching are early warning signs. Tissue acidosis, as in abscess cavities, reduces potency. Lidocaine can be autoclaved. Approximate maximum dosage for infiltration is 4.5 mg/kg plain and 6 mg/kg with 1:100 000 epinephrine added. A 0.5% solution is adequate for infiltration, 1% for nerve blocks, and 2% for topical anesthesia. "Heavy" lidocaine (5% lidocaine in 7.5% glucose) is used for spinal anesthesia.

Tetracaine mixed with 6% glucose is used in spinal anesthesia. It is also used for corneal and conjunctival anesthesia. Instill a drop at a time and repeat as necessary.

42.2   Local Anesthesia Blocks

Field Block

Inject local anesthetic in a linear manner to block cutaneous nerves distal to the injection. Ideal on the limbs and scalp and for harvesting skin grafts.

Digital Block

Using 0.5% to 1% lidocaine without epinephrine, infiltrate about 1 ml on either side of the base of the proximal phalanx at the metacarpophalangeal joint (MCP) joint.

Dorsal Nerve Block of Penis

Use 0.5% to 1% lidocaine without epinephrine. Infiltrate 1 ml (newborn) to 10 ml (adult) about the base of the penis at 2 o'clock and 10 o'clock positions.

Intravenous Regional Anesthesia (Bier's Block)

Determine the systolic BP in the limb. Start a large bore IV line in the distal extremity. Elevate the limb for 5 min or apply an Esmarch or Ace bandage and drain the limb of blood. After 5 min, inflate the cuff to 30 mmHg higher than the systolic BP and inject 20 to 40 ml (arm) or 30 to 90 ml (leg) 0.5% lidocaine without epinephrine (4 mg/kg maximum in adults and 0.5 mg/kg in children). Keep the BP cuff pressure elevated and wait 5 min. Apply a second BP cuff distal to the first if the patient complains of pain and inflate this over the now paresthetic limb, then deflate the first proximal cuff. Keep the cuff pressure 30 mm over the systolic pressure at all times. Two hr is the usual maximum tourniquet time. At the end of the procedure, release the cuff slowly and allow the venous blood to intermittently return to the circulation over 15 to 30 min. Do not use this technique in patients with SS anemia. Be certain the cuff does not leak before you start!

Spinal Anesthesia

It is recommended that spinal anesthesia not be undertaken in the following:

- children
- shock or hypotension
- infection around the back
- any patient not generally fit such as those with cardiac disease
- unless adequate skilled assistants, suction, oxygen, and vasopressor drugs are available

Never give spinal anesthesia and operate alone!

Technique:

- Apply a sphygmometer and obtain a BP; start oxygen by nasal cannula.
- Adequately hydrate the patient with one or more liters of NS or LR (20 ml/kg children).
- Consider an injection of a vasopressor such as ephedrine 25 mg IM (Cochrane Database of Syst Rev 2006, Issue 4)
- Lay the patient on the table with a 5% tilt downward towards the head.
- Prep the back with an iodine solution.
- Have an assistant arch the patient's back to open the intervertebral spaces.
- Choose the widest space below L2. The iliac crest is at the level of the L3–L4 disc.
- Anesthetize the skin with a small wheal of local.
- Introduce the spinal needle carefully until the dura "pop" is felt, remove the stylet, and observe free flow of CSF. Repeat until successful or change to general anesthesia if unsuccessful.
- Inject the anesthetic such as tetracaine 0.2% in 6% dextrose solution or cinchocaine 0.25% in 6% dextrose. Three ml is usually adequate. Never use local anesthetic unless it is "heavy" with glucose solution.

- Remove the needle.
- Have the patient turn onto their back with the knees flexed for 10 min for middle abdominal surgery to allow the anesthetic to "fix" to the nerves. Keep the head tilted down at 5° for that time then level the table and position the patient for surgery. For one-sided operations such as hernia repair, leave the patient on their side for 5 to 10 min. For leg surgery, do the same, but the head need not be tilted down 5°.
- Be sure to ensure adequate venous return by propping a patient to one side with a wedge under the hip if she is pregnant or a large abdominal mass is present.
- Remain alert for hypotension and nausea and vomiting.
- Treat hypotension with IV fluid infusions, blood, ephedrine IM 5 to 10 mg at a time or an ephedrine IV infusion (30 mg in 500 ml).
- Keep the patient supine for at least 6 hr to avoid spinal headache.

Low Spinal or Perineal Anesthesia

The technique is the same as for spinal anesthesia except the needle may be inserted while the patient is sitting. Only 1 ml of anesthetic is used, and the patient should remain sitting for 5 min. This technique is ideal for instrumented vaginal deliveries and genitourinary (GU) surgery.

Pudendal Block

A useful block for complicated vaginal deliveries and third and fourth degree repairs. Use a pudendal nerve block kit with a needle guard (Iowa trumpet) or a spinal needle held between the second and third fingers.

- Hold a syringe containing 10 ml of 1% lidocaine in the left hand to block the right nerve.
- Identify the ischial spine with the index finger of your right hand.

- Advance the point of the needle 0.5 cm beyond the tip of the spine over the sacrospinalis ligament.
- Insert the needle 1 cm through the ligament; aspirate for blood, and if none, inject.
- Repeat the other side switching hands.

Because of the small volume of anesthetic, the blocks may be repeated if the nerve is missed.

Paracervical Block

Useful for surgical procedures on the cervix including dilatation of the os. No longer used during labor because of fetal bradycardia.

Technique:

- Identify the cervix-vaginal junction using a speculum or manually.
- Inject 10 ml 0.5% lidocaine at 3 o'clock and 9 o'clock 5 to 7 mm deep through the vaginal mucosa into the broad ligament using a special pudendal block set or a spinal needle.

Chapter 43

Geographical Distribution of Diseases

This listing of diseases by region is intended to assist the health-care provider in the diagnosis of conditions based on geographic areas. Knowing the distribution and prevalence of illness in their location of practice or in the area of origin of refugees or travelers is an important first step in formulating a differential diagnosis. This information is essential for advising a patient at a travel medicine clinic.

Conditions change and epidemics spread to new areas so this chapter is only a rough guide. Consideration must be given to local conditions, migrations, altitude and seasonal variations, population and individual practices, susceptibilities, and migrations.

For up-to-date information on epidemic and emerging diseases and outbreaks, consult the WHO and CDC Health Information for International Travel Web sites (http://www.cdc.gov).

See Table 43.1 from CDC, Health Information for International Travel 2008.

Table 43.1   Disease by Region

			Disease			
Region	Amebiasis	Endemic Mycoses[1]	Dengue	Filariasis	Hanta Viruses	Hepatitis A
North Africa	W	L	S	S		W
Central, E, W Africa	S	S,H	S,H	W	S	W
Southern Africa	S	S,H	S			S,H
North America	L	S,H	L		S,H	S,H
Mexico, Central America	W	S,H	S,H		L	W
Caribbean	S	S,H	S,H	S		S,H
Tropical South America	W	S,H	S,H	S	S,H	W
Temperate South America	S	S	L		S,H	S,H
East Asia	S	L	S,H	S	W,H	W,H
Southeast Asia	S	S	W,H	W	S	W,H
South Asia	W	L	S,H	W	S	W
Middle East	W	L	S,H	S		W
Western Europe	L	L			W,H	S,H
Eastern Europe & Northern Asia	S	L			W,H	W,H
Australia & South Pacific	L	L	S,H	S,H		S,H

Disease

Region	Hepatitis B	Polio	Diphtheria	HIV	Japanese Encephalitis	Viral Hemorrhagic Fevers
North Africa	S	S	S	S		
Central, E, W Africa	W,H	S,H	S,H	W,H		S,H
Southern Africa	W,H	L	S	W,H		
North America	S		L	S		
Mexico, Central America	S		L	S		
Caribbean	S		S	S		
Tropical South America	W		S,H	S		S,H
Temperate South America	S		L	S		S,H
East Asia	W		L	S	S,H	
Southeast Asia	W	S	S,H	S,H	W,H	
South Asia	W	S	S,H	S,H	W,H	
Middle East	W	S	S	S		L
Western Europe	S		L	S		
Eastern Europe & Northern Asia	W		S,H	S,H	L	
Australia & South Pacific	S,H		S,H	S	L	

GEOGRAPHICAL
DISTRIBUTION OF
DISEASES

Table 43.1 Continued

Region	Leptospirosis	Leishmaniasis	Malaria	Plague	Rabies	Rickettsiae
				Disease		
North Africa	S	W	S	S,H	W	W
Central, E, W Africa	W,H	W,H	W,H	W,H	W,H	W
Southern Africa	S	L	S,H	S,H	S	W,H
North America	S,H	L		S	S	S
Mexico, Central America	W,H	W	S	L	S	S
Caribbean	W,H	L	S		S	S
Tropical South America	W,H	W,H	S,H	S,H	W,H	S
Temperate South America	S	S	S	L	L	L
East Asia	W	S	S	S,H	W	W
Southeast Asia	W,H	S	W	S,H	W	W,H
South Asia	W,H	W,H	W,H	S,H	W,H	W,H
Middle East	S	W,H	S	L	W	S
Western Europe	S	S			S	S
Eastern Europe & Northern Asia	S	S	S	L	W	S
Australia & South Pacific	S		S,H			S

Disease

Region	Schistosomiasis	Tick-borne Encephalitis	Trypanosomiasis[2]	Tuberculosis	Typhoid & Paratyphoid Fever	Yellow Fever
North Africa	S,H			W,H	S,H	
Central, E, W Africa	W,H		S,H	W,H	S,H	S,H
Southern Africa	S,H		S	W,H	S	
North America				S	L	
Mexico, Central America			S	S	S,H	L
Caribbean	S			S,H	S	L
Tropical South America	S		S	S,H	S,H	S,H
Temperate South America	S		S	S	S	
East Asia	S			W	S	
Southeast Asia	W			W	W	
South Asia	L	S		W	W,H	
Middle East	S			W	S	
Western Europe		S,H		S	L	
Eastern Europe & Northern Asia		W,H		W,H	S,H	
Australia & South Pacific	S			S,H	S	

[1]Histoplasmosis, coccidioidomycosis, and paracoccidioidomycosis

[2]Including African trypanosomiasis (sleeping sickness) and American trypanosomiasis (Chagas' disease)

Key: L: local transmission documented but rare
       S: sporadic, focal, or seasonal transmission in region
       W: widespread transmission
       H: epidemic activity or high risk for infection in some areas
       Blank: No reported cases (does not necessarily mean that there is no risk)

Reproduced from Health Information for International Travel, CDC.

Index

for malaria, 137
reactions to, 451–453
for sickle cell disease, 336
for thalassemia, 332, 333, 334
whole, components of, 451–453, 454
blood type, 104
body fluids
electrolyte concentrations of, 450
HIV transmission through, 172–173,
200–201, 204
microfilariae analysis of, 101–102,
227–228
body language, in cross-cultural patient
interview, 20, 26
body mass index (BMI), in illness risk,
291, 303
body temperature, of neonates, 389,
391
bone marrow
biopsy, for lymphoma, 343
depression, in anemia, 330
bones
fracture management for, 474–487
fracture types in, 472–474
infection of, 487–489
sclerosis, with sequestrum, 107
X-rays for differential diagnosis,
106–108
Bordetella pertussis, 59, 250–251
boric acid solution, for conjunctivitis,
491
bradycardia
fever with, 117
in neonates, 388, 394
"brain drain," 1–2
breast cancer, 345
breast feeding, 202, 245, 389, 460
breast milk, expressed, 390
breech presentation, in labor and
delivery, 410–412, 427

bronchodilators, for transfusion
reactions, 452
brown recluse spiders, 369
brucellosis, 256–257
Brugia sp., 81, 82, 227
budgets, for health services, 53
bugs, vector control of, 80–88
BUN, 104
Burkholderia pseudomallei, 252
Burkitt's lymphoma, 343
burns, 454–456
burr holes, for craniotomy, 461–462
Buruli ulcer, 353–354
button spider antivenom, 369

C

calcaneous fractures, 486–487
calcifications
intracranial, 106
liver, 112–113
pericardium, 290
urinary bladder, 113
calcium channel blockers, 288
calcium gluconate
for bites and stings, 365, 369
for magnesium overdose, 408
calcium supplements, for rickets, 380
calicivirus, in diarrhea, 209
calories (kcal), for Kwashiorkor, 383
Campylobacter sp., 74
in diarrhea, 209, 210, 211
cancers, 339–345
bladder, 344
breast, 345
Burkitt's lymphoma as, 343
cervical, 43, 73, 339, 341–343
cultural considerations of, 20–21
epidemiology of, 339–340
gastrointestinal, 307, 308
hepatocellular, 312, 344–345

environment (*cont.*)
  in geographical distribution of
      diseases, 511
  in health promotion research, 41,
      44
enzyme immunoassays (EIA), for HIV
      diagnosis, 178–179
eosinophilia
  fever and, 118–119
  in urine, 96
eosinophilic meningitis, 239
ephedrine, with spinal anesthesia, 508,
      509
epidemiology, 75–80
  definitions for, 76–77
  practical applications of, 44, 79–80
  prevention programs in, 77
  screening programs in, 77–79
  surveillance in, 79
epiglottis, 358
epilation, for trachoma, 497
epinephrine
  in lidocaine anesthetic, 499, 506,
      507
  neonatal emergency dose, 394
episiotomy, repair of, 427–428
epithelial cells, in urine, 96
Epstein-Barr virus (EBV), 343
equipment
  for births, 387
  for dental extractions, 501
ergometrine (Methergine), 406, 408,
      413, 421, 425, 428, 429
erythromycin, 251, 298, 431, 492
escharotomy, for burns, 456
Escherichia coli, 74, 209, 210, 211, 247
esophageal varices, 121, 307–308, 314
esophagitis, in HIV/AIDS, 195, 196
estimated date of confinement (EDC),
      400

ethambutol, for tuberculosis, 154,
      155–158
ethics code, for medical translators, 24
euphemisms, cultural, of current illness,
      115
Europe
  disease distributions in, 512–515
  HIV epidemiology in, 173
Eutrombicula sp., 87
evaluation, outcome *vs.* process, of
      health promotion projects, 41, 44,
      46, 47–48
expiration date, for drugs, 91
Explanatory Model, of patient beliefs,
      22
external cephalic version, during labor,
      413, 420
extractions, dental, 501–503
extremity surgery, anesthesia for, 507,
      509
eye contact, during patient interview,
      20, 26
eye irrigation
  for conjunctivitis, 491
  for snake spit, 371
eyeworm, 85, 229–230

F

facial fractures, 503–504
family counseling, for mental disorders,
      362
family planning, 436
family role, in patient care, 20–21
Fannia sp., 83
Fasciola sp., 224–226
fecal smear, direct, 100
feedings, supplemental/therapeutic
  for Kwashiorkor, 383–385
  for marasmus, 385
  for neonates, 390, 391, 392